FAITH AND HEALTH

Faith and Health

Psychological Perspectives

Edited by

THOMAS G. PLANTE
ALLEN C. SHERMAN

THE GUILFORD PRESS
New York   London

© 2001 The Guilford Press
A Division of Guilford Publications, Inc.
72 Spring Street, New York, NY 10012
www.guilford.com

Printed in the United States of America

This book is printed on acid-free paper.

Last digit is print number: 9 8 7 6 5 4 3 2 1

Library of Congress Cataloging-in-Publication Data
available from the Publisher
ISBN 1-57230-682-3

ABOUT THE EDITORS

Thomas G. Plante, PhD, ABPP, is Associate Professor and Chair of the Psychology Department at Santa Clara University, Clinical Associate Professor of Psychiatry and Behavioral Sciences at Stanford University School of Medicine, and Consulting Associate Professor in the School of Education at Stanford University. He is also a licensed psychologist, Diplomate in clinical psychology, and Fellow of the American Psychological Association. Dr. Plante is the author of *Contemporary Clinical Psychology,* editor of *Bless Me Father for I Have Sinned: Perspectives on Sexual Abuse Committed by Roman Catholic Priests,* and coauthor of *Getting Together, Staying Together: The Stanford University Course on Intimate Relationships.* He conducts research and writes on faith and health, ethics, and the psychological benefits of exercise, and has published more than 80 professional journal articles.

Allen C. Sherman, PhD, is Clinical Director of Behavioral Medicine and Associate Professor in the Department of Otolaryngology at Arkansas Cancer Research Center, University of Arkansas for Medical Sciences. He is a licensed psychologist and marriage and family therapist. Dr. Sherman's research focuses on quality of life and psychosocial adjustment among cancer patients, positive and negative adjustment to illness, psychological interventions, and psychosocial predictors of disease outcome.

CONTRIBUTORS

Emilia Bagiella, PhD, Department of Biostatistics, Joseph Mailman School of Public Health, Columbia University, New York, NY

Jack W. Berry, PhD, Department of Psychology, Virginia Commonwealth University, Richmond, VA

John T. Chirban, PhD, ThD, Department of Psychiatry, Harvard Medical School and The Cambridge Health Alliance, Cambridge, MA

Michele Dillon, PhD, Departments of Sociology and Anthropology, Purdue University, West Lafayette, IN

Natalie J. Dong, PhD, Rancho Los Amigos National Rehabilitation Center, Downey, CA

Alex H. S. Harris, MA, School of Education, Stanford University, Stanford, CA

Kamau R. S. Johnson, PhD, American School of Professional Psychology, Arlington, VA

Harold G. Koenig, MD, Departments of Psychiatry and Medicine, Duke University School of Medicine, Durham, NC

Michael McCullough, PhD, Psychology Department, Dedman College, Southern Methodist University, Dallas, TX

Doug Oman, PhD, School of Public Health, University of California, Berkeley, Berkeley, CA

Les Parrott III, PhD, Center for Relationship Development, Seattle Pacific University, Seattle, WA

Thomas G. Plante, PhD, ABPP, Department of Psychology, Santa Clara University, Santa Clara, CA; School of Education, Stanford University, and Department of Psychiatry and Behavioral Sciences, Stanford University School of Medicine, Stanford, CA

Tia Powell, MD, Department of Psychiatry, College of Physicians and Surgeons, Columbia University, New York, NY

R. Corey Remle, BA, Department of Sociology, Duke University, Durham, NC

Edward P. Shafranske, PhD, Department of Psychology, Pepperdine University, Irvine, CA

Naveen K. Sharma, Santa Clara University, Santa Clara, CA

Allen C. Sherman, PhD, Departments of Behavioral Medicine and Otolaryngology, Arkansas Cancer Research Center, University of Arkansas for Medical Sciences, Little Rock, AR

Stephanie Simonton, PhD, Department of Behavioral Medicine, Arkansas Cancer Research Center, University of Arkansas for Medical Sciences, Little Rock, AR

Richard P. Sloan, PhD, Department of Psychiatry, College of Physicians and Surgeons, Columbia University, New York, NY

Timothy W. Smith, PhD, Department of Psychology, University of Utah, Salt Lake City, UT

Siang-Yang Tan, PhD, Graduate School of Psychology, Fuller Theological Seminary, Pasadena, CA

Carl E. Thoresen, PhD, Department of Counseling Psychology, School of Education, Stanford University, Stanford, CA

Kenneth A. Wallston, PhD, School of Nursing, Vanderbilt University, Nashville, TN

A. Sandra Willis, PhD, Department of Psychology, Samford College, Birmingham, AL

Paul Wink, PhD, Psychology Department, Wellesley College, Wellesley, MA

Everett L. Worthington, Jr., PhD, Department of Psychology, Virginia Commonwealth University, Richmond, VA

PREFACE

There has been strong interest in the relationship between religious faith and health for thousands of years. Many people, across diverse religious traditions, have sought spiritual guidance and religious support to help avoid, recover from, or cope with both physical and emotional problems. In recent years, the mass media have paid a great deal of attention to these issues, with feature television programs and cover stories in the news weeklies examining the role of faith and health. At the same time, scientists have begun to evaluate empirically the relationship between religious faith and health outcomes. A growing number of well-conceived and methodologically rigorous studies have been conducted to examine whether religious beliefs and behaviors might be tied to either health benefits or health risks. Specifically, findings are not uniform, but several investigations have suggested that religiousness is associated with better health practices, enhanced ability to cope with illness and adversity, and lower rates of mortality from all causes. Other studies have noted links with lower depression, anxiety, and alcohol and drug use and higher self-esteem, marital adjustment, life satisfaction, and well-being. Research has also begun to explore whether forgiveness, hope, or service to others are associated with positive health outcomes, such as lower cardiovascular risks.

What types of health outcomes have been linked with what dimensions of faith? How robust or meaningful are these connections? For which individuals, in which circumstances, are these ties most important? How do we explain these relationships?

Although there are a growing number of studies that have examined relationships between faith and health, few contemporary comprehensive books exist that provide state-of-the-art thinking and findings from experts in this area of research and practice. The purpose of this book is to provide the reader with an up-to-date assessment of what we know about the rela-

ix

tionships between religious faith and health outcomes. We also hope that this book will help both research and clinical professionals to better understand the issues relevant to the faith and health connection, as well as outline a research and clinical agenda for professionals interested in this topic.

In order to avoid some of the disadvantages of edited books, which sometimes feel fragmented, and to increase the flow between chapters, the contributors participated in a 2-day conference at Santa Clara University on May 5 and 6, 2000, to present their chapters and get feedback about their work. All contributors read each other's draft chapters and provided written feedback. In doing so, the group worked as a team to fine-tune their thinking and writing. We believe that this conference resulted in a much more cohesive and seamless book.

*   *   *

Numerous people and organizations other than the author(s) assist in the development and completion of a book. Some provide help in a direct and concrete manner, whereas others provide help in less direct and more supportive ways. We would like to acknowledge the assistance of the many people who have helped in both ways and who have contributed to the development of this project.

First, we would like to thank the many wonderful people at The Guilford Press who have enthusiastically worked to publish this book. We would especially like to thank editor Jim Nageotte for his strong interest in the project, outstanding and thoughtful feedback, participation in our 2-day Santa Clara conference, and high level of professionalism and vision. We would also like to thank Katherine Lieber, Kim Miller, and Jeannie Tang.

Second, we would like to thank the John Templeton Foundation, the California Wellness Foundation, the Santa Clara University Bannan Institute for Jesuit Education and Christian Values (William Spohn, Director), and the Santa Clara University Thomas Terry Grant Program for their support in funding the conference that brought all of the authors to campus for several days' worth of discussions about the topic and book.

Third, we would like to thank our administrative assistant, Patricia Brandt, for her assistance with the conference and other matters related to this book. Thanks are due as well to our tireless research assistant, Umaira Latif.

Finally, we would like to thank friends, colleagues, mentors, and family who have been supportive and instructive in a variety of diverse ways over the years. For Thomas Plante, these include mentors Peter Merenda, John Sousa, and Gary Schwartz; spiritual advisors Frs. Sonny Manuel and Steve Privett; and family members Lori and Zachary Plante, Eli and Marilyn

Goldfarb, Marcia Plante, Mary Beauchemin, Lee Sperduti, Henry and Anna McCormick, and Margaret Condon. For Allen Sherman, these include Stephanie Simonton, who provided invaluable support and encouragement for this project. Thanks are due as well to Daniel Brown, Jack Engler, and Deborah Hulihan for their mentorship and to Robert and Judith Sherman, David and Gina Sherman, Ora and Eric Gelb, and Mirjam Wheeler for offering incisive helpful feedback about the project and serving as role models of the quest to live spiritually.

CONTENTS

Part II
FAITH AND HEALTH IN SPECIAL POPULATIONS

Part III
FAITH AND HEALTH IN THE CLINIC

Part IV
COMMENTARIES ON RESEARCH CONCERNING FAITH AND HEALTH

1

-◀O▶-

RESEARCH ON FAITH
AND HEALTH

New Approaches to Old Questions

THOMAS G. PLANTE
ALLEN C. SHERMAN

In recent years there has been a surge of interest in relationships between religious faith and health. Domains that traditionally have been viewed as separate are coming together in new ways. This heightened interest is evident not only in academic conferences and journals but also in the popular press. Social and biomedical scientists have focused on religion for more than 100 years and have forged a rich research tradition within psychology, as well as in sociology, gerontology, epidemiology, and nursing (e.g., Durkheim, 1897/1951; James, 1902/1985; Osler, 1910; for reviews see Johnstone, 1997; Levin & Vanderpool, 1991; Wulff, 1991). Typically, however, this work was regarded with a measure of indifference or derision within mainstream psychology and medicine (Levin & Schiller, 1987; Wulff, 1991). Science and faith were viewed as separate worlds with little common ground. Thus the breadth and intensity of current interest, particularly with respect to health, represents a significant change. The landscape has shifted.

Does religious faith influence health? Are religious practices associated with altered risks for morbidity or mortality? Do religious or spiritual individuals tend to enjoy better well-being or mental health across the lifespan? Does spiritual or religious involvement change the way individuals adapt to the demands of chronic illness? This volume brings together some of the

1

leading investigators who have explored these intriguing questions. Though research is in its early phases, the chapters that follow review some of what we have learned and begin to trace the outlines of the many mysteries that remain.

FAITH AND HEALTH: IRRECONCILABLE DIFFERENCES?

Historically, religion and healing have been closely tied. In Western culture, according to Kuhn (1988), the first known medical license was issued by the church in the 12th century; the license was forfeited in the event of excommunication. These links were largely eroded as medicine became increasingly grounded in Enlightenment rationalist sensibilities and Cartesian philosophy of science, which viewed mind and body as fundamentally separate. The body and corporeal world were seen as the appropriate focus for science, whereas the mind and soul were the purview of the church. Over the past several decades, the dualistic, biomedical model that evolved from this perspective has been increasingly supplanted by a broader, biopsychosocial paradigm (Engel, 1977). Health and illness are viewed as a reflection of reciprocal interactions among biological, psychological, and social influences. This change has been driven in part by massive evidence that psychological and cultural factors have an important impact on health. Is it possible that religious faith is among the tapestry of psychosocial factors that influence health and morbidity?

Some individuals are uncomfortable with inquiry in this area. Methodological and ethical objections have been raised both by scientists (Sloan, Bagiella, & Powell, 1999) and by clergy (*Christian Century*, 1999). Interestingly, some of these reservations would sound familiar to social scientists who embarked on the study of religion a century ago. Some researchers have been hesitant to endorse this line of investigation because the methodological and conceptual challenges seem too daunting. How can one approach scientifically something so ineffable, intangible, and mysterious as religious experience? The arena seems inherently too "fuzzy" and obscure to be conducive to empirical investigation. As noted, however, there is a long history of research on religion in the social and health sciences; although the scientific rigor of these studies varies widely, a broad foundation is in place to support investigations concerning the health correlates and consequences of faith. Moreover, as in any complex field of study, one can expect the methodology to become more rigorous and the questions more refined as the field progresses.

Conversely, another objection is that scientific inquiry will obscure the vitality and richness of religious expression. Attempts to approach religion from a scientific vantage point are destined to be grossly reductionistic and oversimplified. Clearly, spirituality is, at its core, intensely personal and experiential, and cannot be distilled in a test tube or captured on a questionnaire. The question is whether there are modest traces of the experience that are conducive to scientific investigation, and that can be approached in a meaningful way. We believe the answer to that question is yes, that the question can be approached in much the same manner in which investigators have sought to explore other complex, dynamic experiences (e.g., emotions, family dynamics) without confusing the map with the territory.

Others have objected that focusing on the health correlates of religiousness conveys an implicit message that religion should be evaluated based on whether it is functional according to some arbitrary criterion: "Does it work?" Challenging a utilitarian approach to religion, VandeCreek (1999) argues that "such attempts are degrading to religious faith and practice whose driving force can never be intentional self-enhancement. . . . We need to remind ourselves regularly that true religiousness is a positive end in itself even if it contributes to poorer health" (pp. 200–201). Obviously, irrespective of whether some aspects of religious observance are associated with favorable or unfavorable health outcomes for some individuals, the value of a religious life rests on much broader concerns and commitments. Health researchers do not study religion per se; they do not "test" the veracity of doctrinal beliefs or pass judgment on the merits of different theological positions (Hood, Spilka, Hunsberger, & Gorsuch, 1996). Happily, their task is much more modest and prosaic—to study the psychosocial functioning and medical status of human beings engaged in religious pursuits.

TRACING THE CONNECTIONS BETWEEN FAITH AND HEALTH

In their attempts to understand the relationships between psychosocial factors and health, health psychologists have focused on several broad areas of inquiry. One area concerns health behaviors and beliefs, which influence risk of morbidity and mortality (e.g., diet, smoking, alcohol consumption, hygiene, contraceptive use, seeking medical care). A second area concerns adjustment to illness (e.g., coping, quality of life). Life may change in dramatic ways in response to a particular disease—how do patients and their families manage these burdens? A third area concerns physiological functioning and disease end points. How do psychosocial factors influence neuroendocrine activity, immune function, or disease onset and progression?

Religious or spiritual involvement may have relevance for each of these broad areas. It is widely recognized that some health behaviors, such as alcohol consumption or premarital sex, are strongly influenced by religious proscriptions among certain religious communities (Levin & Vanderpool, 1991; Vaux, 1976). As Van Ness (1999) wryly observes, "violent deaths among pacifist Quakers and automobile fatalities among the mostly pedestrian Amish are relatively infrequent" (p. 17). The health implications of religious guidelines are usually positive (e.g., lower rates of smoking-related cancer among Mormons; Troyer, 1988), but they may be negative as well. For example, teenagers from denominations with strict prohibitions against drinking are more likely than other adolescents to abstain from alcohol, but they may be at elevated risk for binge drinking when they decide to indulge (Kutter & McDermott, 1997). Aside from their impact on risky health behaviors, religious beliefs may also shape attitudes toward preventative health practices, such as contraceptive use, cancer screening, and vaccinations (Conyn-van Spaendonck, Oostgvogel, van Loon, van Wijngaarden, & Kromhout, 1996; Erwin, Spatz, Stotts, & Hollenberg, 1999, Studer & Thornton, 1987)

Once an illness is diagnosed, religiousness or spirituality may also be important in understanding how individuals adapt. A growing number of studies have focused on faith as a resource for coping with illness and its impact on adjustment and quality of life (Baider et al., 1999; Hughes, McCollum, Sheftel, & Sanchez, 1994; Keefe et al., 2000; Koenig, Pargament, & Nielsen, 1998; Saudia, Kinney, Brown, & Young-Ward, 1991; Tix & Frazier, 1998). In the wake of a debilitating disease, religion may offer a reassuring sense of comfort, a source of social support from other church members, a framework for deriving meaning in adversity, or guidelines for how to cope. Alternately, for a Christian Scientist who has recently discovered a breast lump, religious convictions may contribute to dangerous avoidance of conventional medical care. For a lesbian woman raised in a Fundamentalist Church, with HIV, religion may evoke depleting feelings of shame and guilt. How patients interpret symptoms, define the type of assistance that is needed, and communicate about their problems may all be colored by religion (Walsh, 1999).

More provocatively, religious or spiritual engagement may influence physiological functioning and host vulnerability to disease. A growing number of epidemiological studies point to connections between attendance at services and all-cause mortality among community residents (e.g., Hummer, Rogers, Nam, & Ellison, 1999; Oman & Reed, 1998; Strawbridge, Cohen, Shema, & Kaplan, 1997; McCullough, Hoyt, Larson, Koenig, & Thoresen, 2000; see McCullough, Chapter 3, this volume). Other studies have examined associations between religiousness and survival among individuals who are seriously ill (e.g., Kune, Kune, & Watson, 1992; Oxman, Freeman, & Manheimer, 1995; Ringdal, 1996). These findings are intriguing, though their interpretation is not without controversy (see Sloan, Bagiella, & Powell, 1999; Sloan, Bagiella, & Powell, Chapter 14, this volume). Relative to the large number of population-based studies on religion and health, there are fewer clinical studies that examine medical outcomes among patients with established disease (e.g., myocardial infarction among patients with coronary heart disease), and still fewer physiological investigations that focus on putative mechanisms of action (e.g., ischemic episodes). Moreover, most studies have examined only very narrow aspects of religion and spirituality, such as church attendance. Nevertheless, research in these areas is expanding rapidly, and our knowledge base is apt to become appreciably more sophisticated in the next few years.

Aside from the potential impact of religious faith on health, interesting questions are also being raised about the potential impact of health on faith (Andrykowski et al., 1996; Collins, Taylor, & Skokan, 1990; Feher & Maly, 1999; Moschella, Pressman, Pressman, & Weissman, 1997). How does a brush with serious illness or disability influence one's spiritual concerns? Under what circumstances does illness usher in stronger faith or painful doubts? How do these responses change over time, and how do they color other areas of life?

Thus there are compelling reasons for both health professionals and students of religion to focus on the interface between religion and health. For those interested in health, religious orientation carries with it a broad array of potential health influences, risk moderators, and coping responses, both positive and negative. For those interested in religion, major health changes are among the nodal transitions in life that may call forth the deepest spiritual needs and responses. There is ample room for collaboration.

DEFINING RELIGIOUSNESS AND SPIRITUALITY: BEYOND THE QUAGMIRE

Among the innumerable challenges of studying religion and health, one of the most fundamental problems concerns definitions. Religiousness and spirituality are both complex, multidimensional constructs—how are they best defined and distinguished? Like love, most of us "know it when we see it," but operationalizing these terms proves elusive. Unfortunately, research, theory building, and clinical coordination all require some reasonable consensus about how these terms are to be delineated.

Despite more than a century of research and theoretical work devoted to religion, there is no widely accepted definition. Research on spirituality is of a more recent vintage, and attempts to define it are even more challenging. Some writers have steadfastly refused to address issues of definition, whereas others have devoted endless pages to it (Hood et al., 1996). Most would probably agree with the conclusion reached by sociologist J. Milton Yinger more than 30 years ago: "any definition of religion is likely to be acceptable only to its author" (1967, cited by Hood et al., 1996, p. 4). For most health researchers, "religion" involves a social or institutional dimension. It includes the theological beliefs, practices, commitments, and congregational activities of an organized institution. "Spirituality" has increasingly come to mean a more personal experience, a focus on the transcendent that may or may not be rooted in an organized church or a formal creed (Burkhardt, 1989; Fetzer Institute/National Institute on Aging, 1999; King, Speck, & Thomas, 1994). Not everyone accepts these distinctions, however. Investigators in the field of psychology of religion often use the terms "personal religion" or "faith" to encompass some of what health researchers usually mean by "spirituality"—internalized beliefs and experiences, as opposed to the social and institutional aspects of organized religion (Hood et al., 1996; Wulff, 1991). "Religion" is seen as reflecting *both* personal and institutional qualities (Hill et al., 1998; Pargament, 1997). And, of course, the personal and social domains of religion are not always readily separated.

Just as definitions of religion differ in their emphasis on personal versus institutional dimensions, they also differ in their emphasis on substantive versus functional perspectives. Substantive approaches try to illuminate the central characteristics of religion, such as beliefs about God or the sacred, whereas functional approaches are concerned with how individuals make use of religion (e.g., as a means of managing the ultimate, existential challenges in life; Pargament, 1997; Zinnbauer et al., 1997). Pargament (1997) offers a useful definition that attempts to combine substantive and functional approaches. In his view, religion is a process, "*a search for significance in ways related to the sacred....* Religion has to do with building, changing, and holding on to the things that people care about in ways that are related to the sacred" (1997, p. 32, emphasis in original). He challenges the increasingly popular view that "spirituality" involves personal experience, whereas "religion" is primarily an institutional entity. Instead, spirituality is seen as the major function of religion—the search for the sacred.

Despite these divergent perspectives, most health researchers agree that investigations should encompass several broad dimensions of religious involvement. Which particular dimensions are included and how they are clustered together varies somewhat from one model to the next, but these generally include: religious values and beliefs, personal commitment, spiritual experiences, public or organizational religious practices, private or nonorganizational religious practices, fellowship, and religious or spiritual coping (Davidson, 1975; Fetzer Institute/National Institute on Aging, 1999; Glock, 1962; Hill et al., 1998; Hood et al., 1996). Thus there is some consensus about what elements should be studied even if particular definitions of religion remain a subject of debate.

Defining spirituality is more problematic. Traditionally, spirituality was viewed as part and parcel of religion, and it has been distinguished from religiousness only within the past few decades, as some segments of society became more secular and disenchanted with traditional religious institutions (Turner, Lukoff, Barnhouse, & Lu, 1995; Zinnbauer et al., 1997). Unfortunately, in the effort to separate highly personal experience from formalized theology and rituals, the literature sometimes implies that spirituality is "good," a mature developmental achievement, whereas religion is "bad," stymied by external trappings and social convention (Hill et al., 1998; Zinnbauer et al., 1997).

The nursing literature has been a particularly active forum for discussions about spirituality and health. A commitment to providing holistic care has been part of the impetus for work in this area and is reflected in attempts to avoid mechanistic or reductionistic explanations. Descriptions have focused on concepts such as life principle or unifying force, unfolding mystery, inner strength (e.g., joy, peace), and harmonious interconnectedness with self, others, a higher power, and the environment (Burkhardt, 1989; Dombeck & Karl, 1987; Emblen, 1992; Granstrom, 1985). From a research vantage point, some of these constructs are problematic because their referents are so broad and vague, and because they include some of the health outcomes that they purport to predict (e.g., hope, peacefulness, self-esteem, social affiliation). However, most writers seem to agree that spirituality involves a personal concern with meaning and transcendence—a belief that "what is 'seen' is not all there is" (Elkins, Hedstrom, Hughes, Leaf, & Saunders, 1988). These concerns may or may not be grounded in institutional beliefs and practices. Whether this concern for the transcendent, for something outside of oneself, necessarily involves the sacred is a matter of some debate (Hill et al., 1998). We would suggest that the sacred is an important element. Being captivated by a sunset, a sports team, or a political campaign is not intrinsically a spiritual experience simply because one feels connected to something larger than oneself. However, if these experiences are imbued with a sense of connection with the sacred, or ultimate reality, or things as they really are, then that would represent a spiritually significant experience. The ordinary activities of everyday life can thus become invested with spiritual meaning, as is the case for a Buddhist focusing mindfully on sweeping the steps or eating a raisin, a Jew reciting a prayer while washing her hands, or a Catholic who views preparing a meal as a sacrament (Emmons & Crumpler, 1999).

In sum, religion and spirituality are multifaceted, overlapping constructs whose specific definitions remain a subject of debate; however, there is some agreement about the general outlines and boundaries of these terms. The recent consensus report issued by the National Institute for Healthcare Research (Hill et al., 1998) is a good example of collaborative efforts to identify the basic characteristics of these constructs; both religiousness and spirituality were seen as reflecting "the feelings, thoughts, experiences, and behaviors that arise from a search for the sacred" (p. 21). In this volume, we use "spirituality" to refer to personal concerns with the transcendent—with something sacred, ultimate, or beyond superficial appearance. Spirituality may or may not be embedded in a formal, established religious tradition. We use the general terms "religiousness," "religious involvement," and "religious orientation" synonymously to refer to both the personal and social/institutional aspects of engagement with an established faith tradition. Relative to these broad terms, we use "religious or spiritual coping" more specifically, to designate particular efforts to manage the demands of a specific, challenging situation (e.g., diagnosis of heart disease, coronary artery bypass surgery). However, given the lack of consensus about specific definitions, in the following chapters the contributors have been invited to delineate what they mean by religiousness or spirituality in the context of their work.

OVERVIEW OF THE BOOK

The chapters that follow review recent findings concerning the intriguing connections between faith and health. They offer a broad survey of current scientific activity that examines physical and mental health outcomes among populations ranging from healthy adults to those with specific clinical disorders, spanning adolescence to old age. We explore emerging trends and highlight areas of controversy. Though most research has focused on white Christian participants, we include discussion of other ethnic and cultural groups. It is difficult for a single volume to do justice to such an expansive field. Of necessity, we have neglected relevant areas of inquiry, such as altruism; important disease entities, such as heart disease; and influential perspectives, such as pastoral care. Nevertheless, we hope this volume provides an engaging overview of a rapidly expanding field.

The first part of the book examines ties between faith and health in the general population. Thoresen, Harris, and Oman (Chapter 2) offer a broad review of the epidemiological and clinical literature. They summarize findings concerning medical and mental health outcomes and highlight important methodological and conceptual issues that need to be considered as the field moves forward. McCullough (Chapter 3) examines links between religious involvement and mortality—a topic that has sparked intense interest and debate. He sifts the evidence from large population-based studies, focusing on insights from a recent meta-analytic review. Wink and Dillon (Chapter 4) share results from a longitudinal study of older adults, currently in their late 60s to mid-70s, who have been followed with repeated assessments since adolescence. Their investigation offers unusually rich data about prospective relationships between religiousness and a broad range of physical and mental health outcomes. The chapter by Worthington, Berry, and Parrott (Chapter 5) shifts from research to theory. They offer an intriguing conceptual model of forgiveness, which is an area that has commanded growing attention in the past few years. Finally, Sherman and Simonton (Chapter 6) discuss assessment of religiousness and spirituality in health research. They review some of the measures that seem practical for use in health settings and that have established or promising psychometric properties.

The second part of the book moves the focus from the general population to groups of special interest. The first two chapters consider how religious and spiritual involvement shape responses to life-threatening illness. Sherman and Simonton (Chapter 7) examine connections between religious or spiritual variables and adjustment to cancer. Remle and Koenig (Chapter 8) explore faith and health among individuals with HIV. Willis, Wallston, and Johnson (Chapter 9) examine the impact of religious involvement on health behaviors among adolescents and young adults. They explore whether smoking and alcohol use are associated with religious faith, God locus of control, and religious coping. Plante and Sharma (Chapter 10) review ties between religiousness and mental health outcomes. In particular, they discuss depression, anxiety disorders, schizophrenia, substance abuse, and general psychological well-being.

The third part shifts the discussion from descriptive research to clinical practice. Chirban (Chapter 11) discusses clinical assessment of spiritual and religious concerns in the psychotherapy setting. He offers specific guidelines for conducting a clinical assessment that offer rich, qualitative information unavailable in brief research measures. In addition, he considers how assessment of religious concerns might be influenced by the clinician, as well as the client. Tan and Dong (Chapter 12) discuss the use of spiritual interventions in treatment. They examine a number of religiously based treatment strategies, some of which might be offered by an individual clinician and others by the broader religious community. Shafranske (Chapter 13) surveys personal and professional attitudes toward religion among rehabilitation psychologists and physicians. He examines the role of religion in their personal lives, the religious issues they encounter in treatment, and their use of religious interventions.

The final part of the book offers commentaries about the current status of the field. Sloan, Bagiella, and Powell (Chapter 14) provide a critical appraisal. They highlight methodological weaknesses in research concerning faith and health. They also discuss ethical reservations about clinical applications, questioning the appropriateness of physicians offering spiritual interventions. Smith (Chapter 15) reviews the field from the vantage point of health psychology. As a leading investigator in health research rather than in religious studies, he offers the perspective of an informed "outsider." In the conclusion (Chapter 16), we weave together some of the themes expressed in prior chapters and offer reflections and recommendations about future directions for the field.

REFERENCES

Andrykowski, M. A., Curran, S. L., Studts, J. L, Cunningham, L., Carpenter, J. S., McGrath, P. C., Sloan, D. A., & Kenady, D. E. (1996). Psychological adjustment and quality of life in women with breast cancer and benign breast problems: A controlled comparison. *Journal of Clinical Epidemiology, 49*, 827–834.

Baider, L., Russak, S. M., Perry, S., Kash, K., Gronert, M., Fox, B., Holland, J., & Kaplan-Denour, A. (1999). The role of religious and spiritual beliefs in coping with malignant melanoma: An Israeli sample. *Psycho-Oncology, 8*, 27–35.

Burkhardt, M. A. (1989). Spirituality: An analysis of the concept. *Holistic Nursing Practice, 3*, 69–77.

Christian Century. (1999, January 27). Faith's benefits, p. 77.

Collins, R. L., Taylor, S. E., & Skokan, L. A. (1990). A better world or a shattered vision? Changes in life perspectives following victimization. *Social Cognition, 8*, 263–285.

Conyn-van Spaendonck, M. A., Oostvogel, P. M., van Loon, A. M., van Wijngaarden, J. K., & Kromhout, D. (1996). Circulation of the poliovirus during the poliomyelitis outbreak in the Netherlands in 1992–1993. *American Journal of Epidemiology, 143*, 929–935.

Davidson, J. D. (1975). Glock's model of religious commitment: Assessing some different approaches and results. *Review of Religious Research, 16*, 83–93.

Dombeck, M., & Karl, J. (1987). Spiritual issues in mental health care. *Journal of Religion and Health, 26*, 183–197.

Durkheim, E. (1951). *Suicide: A study in sociology* (J. A. Spaulding & G. Simpson, Trans.). New York: Free Press. (Original work published 1897)

Elkins, D. N., Hedstrom, L. J., Hughes, L. L., Leaf, J. A., & Saunders, C. (1988). Toward a humanistic–phenomenological spirituality: Definition, description, and measurement. *Journal of Humanistic Psychology, 28*, 5–18.

Emblen, J. D. (1992). Religion and spirituality defined according to current use in nursing literature. *Journal of Professional Nursing, 8*, 41–47.

Emmons, R. A., & Crumpler, C. A. (1999). Religion and Spirituality? The roles of sanctification and the concept of God. *International Journal for the Psychology of Religion, 9*(1), 17–24.

Engel, G. L. (1977). The need for a new medical model: A challenge for biomedicine. *Science, 196*, 129–136.

Erwin, D. O., Spatz, T. S., Stotts, R. C., & Hollenberg, J. A. (1999). Increasing mammography practice by African American women. *Cancer Practice, 7*, 78–85.

Feher, S., & Maly, R. C. (1999). Coping with breast cancer in later life: The role of religious faith. *Psycho-Oncology, 8*, 408–416.

Fetzer Institute/National Institute on Aging. (1999). *Multidimensional measurement of religiousness/spirituality for use in health research.* Kalamazoo, MI: John E. Fetzer Institute.

Glock, C. Y. (1962). On the study of religious commitment. *Religious Education, 57*(Research Suppl.), S980–S110.

Granstrom, S. L. (1985). Spiritual nursing care for oncology patients. *Topics in Clinical Nursing, 7*, 39–45.

Hill, P. C., Pargament, K. I., Swyers, J. P., Gorsuch, R. L., McCullough, M. E., Hood,

R. W., & Baumeister, R. F. (1998). Definitions of religion and spirituality. In D. B. Larson, J. P. Swyers, & M. E. McCullough (Eds.), *Scientific research on spirituality and health: A consensus report* (pp. 14–30). Rockville, MD: National Institute for Healthcare Research.

Hood, R. W., Jr., Spilka, B., Hunsberger, B., & Gorsuch, R. (1996). *The psychology of religion: An empirical approach* (2nd ed.). New York: Guilford Press.

Hughes, M. A., McCollum, J., Sheftel, D., & Sanchez, G. (1994). How parents cope with the experience of neonatal intensive care. *Children's Health Care, 23,* 1–14.

Hummer, R. A., Rogers, R. G., Nam, C. B., & Ellison, C. G. (1999). Religious involvement and U. S. adult mortality. *Demography, 36,* 272–285.

James, W. (1985). *The varieties of religious experience.* Cambridge, MA: Harvard University Press. (Original work published 1902)

Johnstone, R. L. (1997). *Religion in society: A society of religion* (5th ed.). New York: Wiley.

Keefe, F. J., Affleck, G., Lefebvre, J., Underwood, L., Caldwell, D. S., Drew, J., Gibson, J., & Pargament, K. (2000, March). *Coping with arthritis pain: The role of daily spiritual experiences and religious and spiritual coping.* Paper presented at the annual meeting of the American Psychosomatic Society, Savannah, GA.

King, M., Speck, P., & Thomas, A. (1994). Spiritual and religious beliefs in acute illness: Is this a feasible area for study? *Social Science and Medicine, 38,* 631–636.

Koenig, H. G., Pargament, K. I., & Nielsen, J. (1998). Religious coping and health status in medically ill hospitalized older adults. *Journal of Nervous and Mental Disease, 186,* 513–521.

Kuhn, C. C. (1988). A spiritual inventory of the medically ill patient. *Psychiatric Medicine, 6,* 87–100.

Kune, G., Kune, S., & Watson, L. (1992). The effect of family history of cancer, religion, parity, and migrant status on survival in colorectal cancer. *European Journal of Cancer, 28A,* 1484–1487.

Kutter, C. J., & McDermott, D. S. (1997). The role of the church in adolescent drug education. *Journal of Drug Education, 27,* 293–305.

Levin, J. S., & Schiller, P. L. (1987). Is there a religious factor in health? *Journal of Religion and Health, 26,* 9–36.

Levin, J. S., & Vanderpool, H. Y. (1991). Religious factors in physical health and the prevention of illness. *Prevention in Human Services, 9,* 41–64.

McCullough, M. E., Hoyt, W. T., Larson, D. B., Koenig, H. G., & Thoresen, C. E. (2000). Religious involvement and mortality: A meta-analytic review. *Health Psychology, 19,* 211–222.

Moschella, V. D., Pressman, K. R., Pressman, P., & Weissman, D. E. (1997). The problem of theodicy and religious response to cancer. *Journal of Religion and Health, 36,* 17–20.

Oman, D., & Reed, D. (1998). Religion and mortality among the community-dwelling elderly. *American Journal of Public Health, 88*(10), 1469–1475.

Osler, W. (1910). The faith that heals. *British Journal of Medicine, 1,* 1470–1472.

Oxman, T. E., Freeman, D. H., & Manheimer, E. D. (1995). Lack of social participation or religious strength and comfort as risk factors for death after cardiac surgery in the elderly. *Psychosomatic Medicine, 57,* 5–15.

Pargament, K. I. (1997). *The psychology of religion and coping: Theory, research, practice.* New York: Guilford Press.

Ringdal, G. (1996). Religiosity, quality of life and survival in cancer patients. *Social Indicators Research, 38,* 193–211.

Saudia, T. L., Kinney, M. R., Brown, K. C., & Young-Ward, L. (1991). Health locus of control and helpfulness of prayer. *Heart and Lung, 20,* 60–65.

Sloan, R. P., Bagiella, E., & Powell, T. (1999). Religion, spirituality, and medicine. *Lancet, 353,* 664–667.

Strawbridge, W. J., Cohen, R. D., Shema, S. J., & Kaplan, G. A. (1997). Frequent attendance at religious services and mortality over 28 years. *American Journal of Public Health, 87,* 957–961.

Studer, M., & Thornton, A. (1987). Adolescent religiosity and contraceptive usage. *Journal of Marriage and the Family, 49,* 117–128.

Tix, A. P., & Frazier, P. A. (1998). The use of religious coping during stressful life events: Main effects, moderation, and mediation. *Journal of Consulting and Clinical Psychology, 66,* 411–422.

Troyer, H. (1988). Review of cancer among 4 religious sects: Evidence that life-styles are distinctive sets of risk factors. *Social Science and Medicine, 26,* 1007–1017.

Turner, R. P., Lukoff, D., Barnhouse, R. T., & Lu, F. G. (1995). Religious or spiritual problems: A culturally sensitive diagnostic category in the DSM-IV. *Journal of Nervous and Mental Disease, 183,* 435–444.

VandeCreek, L. (1999). Should physicians discuss spiritual concerns with patients? *Journal of Religion and Health, 38,* 193–201.

Van Ness, P. H. (1999). Religion and public health. *Journal of Religion and Health, 38,* 15–26.

Vaux, K. (1976). Religion and health. *Preventive Medicine, 5,* 522–536.

Walsh, F. (1999). Religion and spirituality: Wellsprings of healing and resilience. In F. Walsh (Ed.), *Spiritual resources in family therapy* (pp. 3–27). New York: Guilford Press.

Wulff, D. M. (1991). *Psychology of religion: Classic and contemporary views.* New York: Wiley.

Zinnbauer, B., Pargament, K. I., Cole, B., Rye, M. S., Butter, E. M., Belavich, T. G., Hipp, K. M., Scott, A. B., & Kadar, J. L. (1997). Religion and spirituality: Unfuzzying the fuzzy. *Journal for the Scientific Study of Religion, 36,* 549–564.

PART I

—◀◉▶—

FAITH AND HEALTH
IN THE GENERAL
POPULATION:
RESEARCH AND THEORY

2

◄◦►

SPIRITUALITY, RELIGION, AND HEALTH

Evidence, Issues, and Concerns

CARL E. THORESEN
ALEX H. S. HARRIS
DOUG OMAN

Interest in the role of religious and spiritual (RS)[1] factors in health has a long history. Cultures from ancient to modern times have often viewed health and disease as directly related to a variety of religious beliefs and practices, as evidenced by the religious prescriptions of certain diets, physical activities, and types of quiet reflection and prayer (Rosen, 1993). During the past decade, claims and questions regarding possible RS–health connections have become popular in a bestselling sense. Several spiritually focused books have gained a place on the *New York Times* Top 10 list (e.g., Moore's [1994] *Care of the Soul*, Albom's [1997] *Tuesday's with Morrie*, and Chopra's [1999] *How to Know God*). Major news magazines such as *Time* and *Newsweek* have featured special articles about spirituality and health, and special issues have been published or will be published in scholarly journals (e.g., *American Psychologist, Annals of Behavioral Medicine, Journal of Health Psychology, Health Education and Behavior*). Several scientific meetings have featured invited speakers or symposia to address RS–health issues (e.g., Society of Psychosomatic Medicine, European Society of Health Psychology, Society of Behavioral Medicine) or are planning them. The American Psychological Association recently began publishing textbooks on the topic, such as those by P. Richards and Bergin (1997), Shafranske (1996), and W. R. Miller (1999).

In 1997, The John Templeton Foundation, in collaboration with the National Institute of Healthcare Research (NIHR), sponsored a series of conferences with medical and behavioral scientists to review the scientific evidence relating RS variables with physical health, mental health, alcoholism and other addictive disorders, and neurobiological factors (Larson, Sawyers, & McCullough, 1998). That effort helped trigger the Office of Behavioral and Social Science Research (OBSSR) at the National Institutes of Health (NIH) to establish a panel of behavioral scientists to critically and dispassionately review existing evidence presumably linking RS with health. In this chapter we briefly summarize some of findings in the Templeton/NIHR Consensus Report and some of the issues and concerns currently emerging in the OBSSR/NIH Panel.

Reactions to the popularity of RS issues and to the notion that RS factors influence health outcomes and need to be considered in health care have been varied. They tend to range from cynical skepticism on the one hand (e.g., Dawkins, 1999) to supportive advocacy on the other (e.g., Koenig, 1997). Some question the quality and validity of existing evidence, warning against physicians, for example, bringing spiritual and religious matters into their practice (Sloan, Bagiella, & Powell, 1999; Sloan, Bagiella, VandeCreek, Hover, & Casalone, 2000; see also Sloan, Bagiella, & Powell, Chapter 14, this volume). Others offer a less critical perspective on the quality of existing evidence linking RS to health and on what health professionals can consider doing in this area that meets their ethical responsibilities (e.g., Post, Puchalski, & Larson, 2000; see also Tan & Dong, Chapter 12, and Shafranske, Chapter 13, this volume).

This chapter seeks to familiarize readers with some recent empirical evidence about possible associations between RS factors and health outcomes. In considering this evidence, we believe a healthy skepticism is in order, an attitude that remains open to the possibility that RS-related beliefs and behaviors may indeed be important to health processes (in promoting, as well as in endangering, health) yet that also demands rigorous empirical evidence based on well-controlled studies to support claims and conclusions. We hope to introduce the dismissing critic to suggestive data that may create tempered doubt. We also hope to introduce the uncritical advocate (some might say "cheerleader") to issues and concerns that will encourage greater modesty in making claims and drawing conclusions.

To facilitate more informed perspectives on both sides of the debate, we address the following questions: Do specific RS factors influence specific health outcomes? Is there empirical evidence of sufficient quality to justify an answer to this question? What possible mechanisms might explain or account for a relationship if one exists? Are there any implications for health professionals based on the evidence at this point in time?

We first discuss some possible explanations for the "spiritual surge" and growing interest in the RS–health connection. Then we offer a brief historical comment on the scientific study of the RS–health area, followed by a brief discussion of definitional and conceptual concerns. Our comments on the scientific evidence that RS factors influence physical and mental health include the following:

- Some tentative conclusions about physical health from *Scientific Research on Spirituality and Health: A Consensus Report* (Larson et al., 1998).
- A consideration of some of the most recent well-conducted epidemiological studies to provide the reader with a more concrete sense of the state of the science on RS and health.
- A review of the few experimental (intervention) studies that have been conducted. An overview of the evidence linking RS factors to mental health.
- A brief summary of some issues and concerns emerging from the OBSSR/NIH panel mentioned previously.

We finish by discussing a few research issues that deserve attention and offering some brief observations and conjectures, including considerations for health professionals (for additional discussion of practice issues, see Chirban, Chapter 11; Tan and Dong, Chapter 12; and Shafranske, Chapter 13, this volume). Some initial steps to improve knowledge in this intriguing area are offered as well.

WHY THE SPIRITUAL SURGE AND INTEREST IN RELIGION–SPIRITUALITY AND HEALTH?

Several possibilities exist to explain the somewhat sudden surge of popular and scientific interest in the role of RS factors in health and illness over the past decade or so. First of all, scientific inquiry into the relationship between RS factors and health, essentially under way since the 1960s, has been gradually producing more and higher quality empirical evidence. These data from longitudinal studies suggest that religious factors (e.g., different religious affiliations or frequency of attending religious services) are related to lower mortality rates or disease risk. However, these published findings remained virtually unknown to if not ignored by the broader scientific community until very recently. Several factors may account for this gap, including the commonly accepted belief that anything with an RS flavor was by definition incompatible with science and its methods (Larson et al., 1998). There was also the perceived stigma in scientific cultures attached to conducting studies focused on RS phenomena (Sherrill & Larson, 1994), as well as a general lack of understanding by professionals (researchers and practitioners) of RS issues. Professional training and supervision have seldom focused on the topic until very recently. Related curricula have begun to emerge in medical education but remain, with few exceptions, absent in most professional psychology training programs (W. R. Miller, 1999; P. Richards & Bergin, 1997).

Are there any cultural or social trends that might contribute to this surge? Several possibilities come to mind: the rapidly aging population in this country and other industrialized nations (with advancing age often comes more attention to spiritual and religious concerns), the rapidly accelerating pace of life and the related difficulty of taking time to develop and maintain close intimate connections (growing levels of depression, anxieties, and hostility), concern about the loss of civility and common courtesy toward others, the changing nature of careers and relative loss of job security, and a diminishing sense of any community responsibility, with a kind of "rugged individualism" that has become excessive (e.g., Frank & Cook, 1995; Bellah, Madsen, Sullivan, Swidler, & Tipton, 1985; Schor, 1991; Thoresen, 1999).

Myers (2000a) and others (e.g., Csikszentmihalyi, 1999) write of the American paradox, in which wealth and consumption have increased exponentially for many people yet violence, despair, and isolation have also sharply increased, and a sense of community and connectedness have diminished. It seems as if Americans, among others, are not getting happier as they get richer. In fact, the relationship commonly believed ("If I had more money, I would be more happy") appears not to be valid (Csikszentmihalyi, 1999). Indeed, the association turns out to be negative beyond a modest level of wealth. People may be questioning their faith in materialism and success defined as wealth, recognition, and status. They may also be seeking sources of meaning and purpose not available through material means.

Perhaps the public popularity of religion and spirituality is best evidenced by the often unknown fact that most Americans, despite their growing diversity, report the following: they believe in God (96%), are affiliated with a religion (92%), are members of a church or synagogue (67%), and view their religion as "important or very important" (60%). Many also attend some kind of religious service regularly (42%) (Gallup, 1995). Furthermore, Gallup data (cited in Myers, 2000a) recently revealed that Americans reported a sharp increase in their need to "experience spiritual growth," from 54% in 1994 to 82% in 1998. As discussed in more detail subsequently, just what these survey data actually mean in terms of what a person does, thinks, and feels in specific life situations remains very unclear. Many factors influence how a person responds to any questionnaire item, including issues of social desirability and those associated with matters beyond one's conscious awareness (e.g., Bargh & Chartraud, 1999; Kirsch & Lynn, 1999). Also note that these data represent national averages, involving considerable differences between communities, states, and regions of the United States.

HISTORICAL PERSPECTIVES

Interest in the role of RS factors and health dates back hundreds of years. In the 19th century, empirical studies of possible relationships between RS factors and health started to appear, often as observations of a relationship between an RS factor, such as religious denomination, and a disease, such as cancer (Billings, 1891; Travers, 1837). At the end of the 19th century, Emile Durkheim (1897/1951), a founder of modern sociology, noted that suicide rates differed by religious affiliation. William James (1902/1985), a pioneering psychologist, commented on how religiousness, broadly defined, played a role in overall health. Also at this time, Sir William Osler, the founder of modern cardiology and a distinguished scholar and clinician, wrote in the *British Medical Journal* (Osler, 1910) on the power of faith and belief in God in the medical care of patients. Osler advised physicians to utilize the patient's faith as a major healing factor in treatment. In many ways, James and Osler recognized the power of enhancing positive response expectancies in influencing patients to heal, what many have perhaps incorrectly called the placebo effect (e.g., Kirsch & Lynn, 1999).

At midcentury Gordon Allport, a noted Harvard psychologist concerned with the intensive study of individual personality factors, commented on the absence of any attention to RS factors in psychology: "Among modern intellectuals, especially in the universities, the subject of religion seems to have gone into hiding. . . . Even psychologists, to whom presumably nothing of human concern is alien, are likely to retire into themselves when the subject comes up" (1950, p. 1). Allport saw religious issues as a major source of human motivations and goals. He described two different motivational styles or orientations that people seemed to have about religious involvement: extrinsic or intrinsic. That is, some people appeared to view religious experiences and goals from a more outgoing, interpersonally active framework (extrinsic), such as serving on committees and making social connections. Others, however, seemed more intrinsically motivated, more deeply and personally focused, and more concerned with the quality of their faith and connectedness with God (in whatever form). Though the behaviors of two people may be similar, Allport emphasized that their motivations for performing the behaviors might differ greatly. Significantly, Allport was one of the first psychologists to operationalize his conception of religious orientation (intrinsic/extrinsic) by developing a questionnaire, thus setting the stage for the study of individual differences within religion (Gorsuch & Miller, 1999).

Early Modern Studies

With few exceptions, controlled empirical studies on RS variables and health in the 20th century really got started in the late 1960s and have sharply increased ever since. Here we mention very briefly a few of the initial studies in this period that help set the epidemiological stage for understanding current findings that may link RS factors to health.

In the 1960s and 1970s, studies generally reported relationships between health variables and religious affiliation (e.g., Christian, Jewish) or denomination (e.g., Protestant or Catholic). Occasionally attendance at religious services was compared with a health outcome, such as all-cause mortality or major disease morbidities (e.g., Scotch, 1963). For example, one study examined coronary heart disease and mortality among Seventh-Day Adventists (SDAs), a Protestant denomination with strict rules against smoking, caffeine, and alcohol use, strong recommendations about eating a vegetarian diet, and a major emphasis on family life (Phillips, Lemon, Beeson, & Kuzma, 1978). They studied more than 27,000 Californians for 6 years in terms of dietary habits and found that the death rates for SDA members were dramatically lower than for other Californians. For example, SDA men had 74% lower mortality rates and women had 66% lower mortality than similarly aged Californians (ages 35 to 64). For all ages, SDAs had 50% fewer deaths.

In a follow-up study, Phillips, Kuzma, Beeson, and Lotz (1980) also found denominationally related differences in cancer deaths. Contrary to an explanation that related smoking to more deaths, cancer mortality was 50% less among SDAs than among *non*smoking Californians. That is, differences in death rates did not seem accounted for by group differences in smoking. Enstrom (1975) reported one of many prospective (that is, longitudinal) studies on Mormons and overall mortality. Mormons in California, compared with other Californians, revealed a type of dose–response relationship (i.e., more medicine or religion, for example, related to less pain or disease): very religiously active Mormons had fewer deaths than less religiously active Mormons, who had fewer deaths than inactive Mormons. Death rates were also substantially lower (over 50%) for most types of cancer. Significantly, smoking or abusing alcohol did not explain differences in most cancer deaths.

Comstock and colleagues (Comstock & Partridge, 1972; Comstock & Tonascia, 1978) conducted an 8-year study that was noteworthy because they moved away from looking only at religious denomination as a predictor and examined the effects of a more specific RS behavior on physical and mental health: how often one attended religious services. With almost 50,000 adults, after controlling for race, gender, age, smoking, marital status, and having a bathroom in the house, they found reduced disease risk for those who more frequently attended religious services. For example, compared with female nonattenders, women who regularly attended (once weekly or more) had lower relative risks for several diseases, such as a 52% lower risk for cardiovascular disease. They also found less anxiety and fear of death or dying among regularly attending women. Comstock and colleagues controlled for (i.e., ruled out) several covariates or possible factors that could have explained these differences (often called confounding variables) and still saw differences based on frequency of attending services.

What do these earlier studies tell us? Mostly that there is something about being involved in a religious organization, activity, or group that relates to better health status, including reduced risk of mortality. Designs of more recent studies have been more sophisticated, attempting to equate people statistically on more potentially relevant confounding variables (i.e., possible predictors of mortality). These studies have essentially revealed what earlier studies suggested: being religiously involved is associated with better health. The reason for this, however, has remained elusive and deserves attention. As Comstock and Partridge (1972) noted, attending religious services does not seem to reduce death rates directly, but it may serve as a "nonspecific factor" in diminishing death and disease. Note that the term "nonspecific" was also used widely in psychotherapy research at that time (Kiesler, 1966), setting the scientific stage for seeking what might be more specific and clearly identifiable factors that could explain health outcomes.

Keep in mind that there may be a central, if not controversial, issue about such data. On the one hand, these earlier studies undoubtedly failed to control for several factors, such as specific behavioral and psychosocial characteristics, that could in some sense have "explained" or accounted for the observed association. Perhaps members of a particular religious group, such as Mormons or SDAs, followed the rules of their religion about not smoking, about dietary restrictions, and about respecting the body's need to remain active and fit. Perhaps they also spent more time with their immediate family and with other church members because of the many opportunities and expectations provided by their religious community. If more recent studies, in controlling for these more specific factors, now demonstrate that the relationship found earlier has been "accounted for" by members thinking and behaving in more health-promoting ways, does that disprove or nullify any contribution of religious involvement to health? One can argue that it is the specific healthful actions and attitudes that count, not any general religious or spiritual factors that are important. However, others can view this situation as one in which one's religion or overall spiritual orientation to life provides a general and indirect context (sometimes called a distal factor) in which the more specific (proximal) factors, such as particular health-enhancing behaviors, are more likely to happen. One can argue the issue persuasively either way, depending in part on the conceptual perspective or orientation that has been adopted (Oman & Thoresen, 2001). We return to this conceptual and analytic issue later in this chapter. But first we comment on how the terms "spirituality" and "religiousness" have been and are being

used. This issue looms as a major problem, because confusion about terms
has impeded progress in trying to clarify relationships between RS factors
and health.

RELIGION AND SPIRITUALITY: IDENTICAL OR DISTINCT CONCEPTS?

As discussed more fully by Plante and Sherman (Chapter 1, this volume), the
meaning of the terms "religion" and "spirituality" has been a matter of controversy (Pargament, 1997). The following basic questions seem to be at
issue: Are religion (or religiousness) and spirituality the same? If not, in what
ways do they differ? Need spirituality be subsumed within a religious framework, or is religion one potential manifestation or feature of spirituality?

Broadly speaking, the concept of religion is often viewed as a societal
phenomenon, involving social institutions with rules, rituals, covenants, and
formal procedures. By contrast, a typical view of spirituality refers to the
individual's personal experience, commonly seen as connected to some formal religion but increasingly viewed as not necessarily associated with any
organized religion (W. R. Miller & Thoresen, 1999). However, the term
"religiousness" is often used to convey the individual's personal experience
as part of an organized religion (James, 1902/1985, used the term in this
way). In certain contexts, the term "religiousness" can be synonymous with
"spirituality." For example, in several Northern European countries, one
commonly speaks of religiousness in ways in which the term "spirituality" is
increasingly used by many in the United States (Stifoss-Hanssen, 1999).

The *Oxford English Dictionary* offers 10 pages of reference material on
the concept of spirituality (Simpson & Weiner, 1989). Two related themes
seem to dominate in this material: first, the notion of spirituality being concerned with life's most animating or vital qualities (the term *spiritus* in Latin
means "the breath," that which is most vital to life). Second, spirituality
involves the more immaterial features of life, as distinct from the body or
other more tangible and material things, including our senses, such as sight
and hearing.

Some contend that religion is the more inclusive concept, with spirituality as its major focus: "Religion is a search for significance in ways related to
the sacred" (Pargament, 1999, p. 11). Others contend that spirituality is the
more inclusive term, of which religion and religiousness may or may not be
a part. We opt for the view that these constructs may be viewed as two overlapping circles (Venn diagrams), with spirituality being the larger circle,
sharing with religion many overlapping areas, although each has some distinct, nonoverlapping areas (W. R. Miller & Thoresen, 1999; Thoresen,
1999).

We suspect that spirituality, if it is to mean something more than any idiosyncratic personal belief, involves seeking a sense of being or becoming connected to something much greater than just oneself (e.g., "beyond the ego"; Walsh & Vaughn, 1995), something that provides meaning and purpose to one's life, if not something sacred or holy (Thoresen, 1999). A more extended discussion of the many cultural, psychological, and theological issues is well beyond the scope of this chapter (see Emmons & Crumpler, 1999; Pargament, 1999; Stifoss-Hanssen, 1999).

In considering different conceptual approaches, we are mindful of those who may find it insensitive and improper, if not impossible, to approach matters of God, religion, and spirituality from a scientific orientation (e.g., Dawkins, 1999; Thomson, 1996). Many features or dimensions of religiousness and spirituality may remain well beyond the realm of what science can study. Yet we believe that at their best, scientists "love a mystery" and can work collaboratively with nonscientists to create ways to better understand RS phenomena and potential linkages to health. The perspective we suggest seems to fit the following assumptions about spirituality and religiousness.

- Religiousness and spirituality as concepts represent primarily functional or process-oriented phenomena (e.g., coping, social integration), not fixed structural characteristics (e.g., religious denomination). That is, RS factors are concerned with the changing nature of what the person does, thinks, feels, and subjectively experiences within particular social and cultural contexts. They commonly are not fixed traits or unchanging characteristics.

- Both religion and spirituality are multidimensional in nature. Some dimensions can be easily observed (e.g., attending services), and some dimensions have latent (underlying or unseen) qualities that are not readily observed (e.g., feeling closeness to God). In this way they are much like the concepts of personality, health, and love. Just as personality is more than behavior, health more than blood pressure, and love more than sexual arousal, spirituality is more than feeling connected to life, and religiousness is more than attending church services.

- Religiousness and spirituality are not adequately assessed by questionnaires with one or a few items, nor are they comprehensively measured using just one mode of assessment (e.g., only questionnaires or only personal accounts or narratives). Unlike fixed traits, most spiritual and religious factors change with time and circumstances; therefore, multiple assessments appear more desirable than single assessments in representing these constructs.

W. R. Miller and Thoresen (1999) have recommended one way to conceptualize religiousness and spirituality that seems to fit existing methodological and assessment approaches in the behavioral sciences. Their approach includes four major dimensions that are probably related to each other but still are distinct enough to be assessed separately. These include (1) *overt behaviors* (e.g., practices that are viewed by the individual as religious or spiritual, such as attendance at services, reading spiritual material, meditation, forgiveness, or serving others); (2) *beliefs* (e.g., perceptions of God as loving or punishing, self-efficacy concerning spiritual practices, sense of responsibility to and for others); (3) *motivations, values, and goals* (e.g., daily strivings, reasons for participating in spiritual practices); and (4) *subjective experiences* (e.g., feeling a sense of inner peace, mystical experiences). In reflecting on these dimensions, keep in mind that one of the major shortcomings in current research has been the failure to disaggregate the multiple dimensions of spirituality and religiousness. That is, studies until very recently essentially employed very simple assessments (e.g., a few items on denomination, frequency of service attendance, or frequency of prayer) with large samples (often in the thousands). Examining religiousness at a more micro or specific level (e.g., specific beliefs and behaviors related to attending services) has been rare (Hill & Hood, 1999). Assessment is discussed more extensively by Sherman and Simonton in Chapter 6 and Chirban in Chapter 11 of this volume.

WHAT IS KNOWN REGARDING THE RS FACTOR–HEALTH CONNECTION?

Interesting if not surprising associations between religious involvement, broadly defined, and health have been reported. The vast majority of the research examining potential relationships between religious factors and physical health status, including mortality, has been epidemiological and/or correlational in nature. Note that almost all of the research conducted to date has focused on religion or religiousness, not on spirituality seen as relatively or completely independent from religion. Furthermore, as noted previously, religious involvement usually has been limited to a person's reported affiliation with any organized religion (or the person's particular denomination within a religion) or to frequency of attendance at religious services. In addition, questions about religion often have been limited to a few questionnaire items administered on one occasion.

Scientific Research on Spirituality and Health: A Consensus Report: Physical Health (1998)

In the NIHR Consensus report, Matthews, Koenig, Thoresen, and R. Friedman (1998) cited studies providing evidence that seemed to link religious involvement, usually frequency of religious service attendance, with physical health factors. Here are some examples:

- Lower rates of coronary disease, emphysema, cirrhosis, and suicide (Comstock & Partridge, 1972).
- Lower blood pressure (Larson, Koenig, & Kaplan, 1989).
- Lower rates of myocardial infarction in an Israeli sample (Madalie, Kahn, & Neufeld, 1973).
- Improved physical functioning, medical regime compliance, self-esteem, and lower anxiety and health-related worries 1 year after surgery in heart transplant patients (R. C. Harris et al., 1995).
- Reduced levels of pain in cancer patients (Yates, Chalmer, St. James, Follansbee, & McKegney, 1981).
- Better perceived health and less medical service utilization (Frankel & Hewitt, 1994).
- Decreased functional disability in the nursing-home-dwelling for the elderly (Idler & Kasl, 1992, 1997).

Some Recent Well-Controlled Epidemiological Studies: Religious Attendance and Mortality

Some of the work in this area has not adequately taken into account other factors that could explain the reported relationships linking lower disease rates with higher religious involvement. For example, cigarette smoking is clearly related to morbidity and mortality. Failure to adequately control for smoking in any health-related study involving RS factors raises questions about what can be concluded about the role played by RS factors in reducing disease risk, including death, in the study. Recently the focus has been on using state-of-the-art epidemiological designs, often with fairly large samples, to see if RS factors predict health status, especially mortality, when many other factors related to health outcomes are included in the analysis. Table 2.1 describes four such studies recently completed (see McCullough, Chapter 3, this volume, for a detailed discussion of empirical studies linking RS factors to reduced mortality).

Several things are noteworthy about these four studies, such as the effort to include many covariates that could compete, so to speak, with the RS factors in predicting health outcomes. One can see from these studies that even with 12 or more control variables used in the analysis, the frequency of attending services still predicted all-cause mortality. In addition, the studies compared different statistical models containing various combinations of factors in an attempt to learn which specific factors, such as attending religious services, still remain significant predictors and which failed to remain significant when others are added to each model.

Keep in mind that these studies do not demonstrate that statistically significant RS factors, found in multivariate analyses to be independently predictive, cause or produce lower mortality or better health. Prediction is not the same as explanation. These data remain correlational, indicating that a

TABLE 2.1. Recent Controlled Studies of RS–Physical Health Relationships

Study/focus	Sample characteristics	Predictor variable(s)	Control variables	Outcome variables	Results and conclusions
Hummer, Rogers, Nam, & Ellison (1999) Epidemiological study of religious involvement and U.S. adult mortality, with an 8-year follow-up.	A national sample of 21,204 participants in the Cancer Risk Factor Supplement of the 1987 National Health Interview Survey	Religious service attendance (never, less than once per week, weekly, more than once per week)	Age Sex Family income Education Marital status Geographic region Race/ethnicity Health status Health behaviors Social support	Mortality analyzed by cause of death	In the full model (all covariates included) across all cause-of-death categories, those never attending services have a hazard ratio of 1.50 (i.e., 50% greater, $p < .01$), less than once a week 1.24 ($p < .05$), and the weekly group 1.21 ($p < .5$) compared to more-than-once-a-week reference group (RG). In full model those never attending services were at greater risk for death from respiratory disease (hazard ratio = 2.11, $p < .05$) and residual causes (hazard ratio = 2.42, $p < .05$) than RG and at marginally greater risk ($p < .10$) for circulatory and infectious diseases, cancer, diabetes, and external causes.
Musick, House, & Williams (in press) Epidemiological study of religious involvement and U.S. adult mortality with 7.5 year follow-up	A national sample of 3,617 from the Americans' Changing Lives study. Participants had a mean age = 47.1, were 53% female. African Americans and people over 60 were sampled at twice the rate of other groups.	Religious service attendance (never or less than once per month, one to three times a month, weekly, more than once weekly)	Age Sex Family income Education Marital status Race/ethnicity Health status Health behavior variables Social support Mental health Employment status Other religious factors Theodicy/beliefs	Mortality	In the full model, compared with the less-than-once-a-month reference group, those who attended services one to three times a month had a relative risk (RR) = .75 (25% less), those attending weekly RR = .65 (35% less), those attending more than once per week RR = .61 (39% less). This relationship was unexpectedly stronger among persons under 60 years old. Other religious behaviors and beliefs did not explain, and sometimes suppressed, the inverse association between service attendance and mortality. For example, private religiousness suppressed the effects of public religiousness (attending services) on mortality. Need for more specific religious/spiritual factors demonstrated.

Study	Sample	Religious service attendance	Covariates	Outcome	Findings
Oman & Reed (1998) A prospective study of religious service attendance and all-cause mortality over 5 years	A sample of 1,931 older residents of Marin County, California. Participants were 55 or older at baseline, 95% non-Hispanic whites, 44% male.	Religious service attendance (never, less than once per week, at least once per week)	Age Sex Family income Education Marital status Geographic region Race/ethnicity Health status Health behavior variables Social support Mental health Employment status Years of residence in county	Mortality	In the full model, weekly attendees of religious services had lower mortality than non-attendees, relative hazard (RH) = .72 (28% less, 95% CI = .55–.93). Contrary to hypothesis, religious attendance tended to be slightly more protective for those with high social support. It is concluded that lower mortality rates for those who attend religious services are only partly explained by demographic variables, health status, physical functioning, health habits, social functioning and support, and mental health.
Strawbridge, Cohen, Shema, & Kaplan (1997) Epidemiological study of religious involvement and mortality in a regional sample over 28 years	A sample of 5,286 Alameda, California residents, mean age 65.3 in 1994, 12.7% African American, 52.8% female. Assessed 1965, 1974, 1983, and 1994.	Religious service attendance (infrequent attendees, never to once to three times a month, and frequent attendees, once a week or more)	Age Sex Education Race/ethnicity Health status variables Health behavior variables Social support variables Mental health variables Religious affiliation	Mortality, improved health practices, increased social contacts, and stable marriages	Frequent attendees of religious services had lower mortality than infrequent attendees, R= .64 (95% CI: .53–.77] and the effect was significant for women, not for men. In the full model, females RR = 0.77 (23% less, 95% CI: .64–.94), males RR = .90 (23% less, 95% CI: .78–1.15). At follow-up, frequent attendees were more likely to stop smoking (RR = 1.90), increase exercise (RR = 1.38), increase social contacts (RR = 1.58), and have stable marriages (RR = 1.50).

nontrivial and nonrandom association was found between a particular RS factor, such as religious service attendance, and mortality. Furthermore, the presence of a significant statistical relationship between greater attendance and reduced all-cause mortality, even if found within a prospective, well-controlled design, does not mean that religious attendance benefits everyone or even benefits most people (Ellison & Levin, 1998). What it does tell us is that, on average, religious service attendance is associated with lower mortality from all causes. It is not a chance or random relationship. However, finding such a relationship in itself seldom sheds light on *which* persons may benefit more or less, nor does it clarify the mechanisms explaining the benefit.

To be fair, however, a relationship consistently demonstrated across various studies conducted by different researchers in various settings, especially if done using an experimental design, does provide very valuable information. Such relationships have often led to important clinical procedures that improve health and prevent disease without fully understanding all or even many of the mechanisms that explain just why one factor does lead to change in another factor. Some common examples include the relationship between taking aspirin and reduced pain and the relationship between eating limes (and other citrus fruits) and preventing scurvy. Both were used very productively for many decades without an understanding of the actual mechanisms involved. The ability to predict does not imply a causal relationship, and the establishment of a causal relationship (through experimentation) does not necessarily imply that one understands the causal mechanisms.

The study by Musick, House, and Williams (in press) illustrates an attempt to unpack or disaggregate broad, complex dimensions, such as "religious involvement." Perhaps the researchers revealed the "tip of the iceberg" in this study by using various combinations of factors to best clarify the relationship between RS and mortality. They found that once health behaviors (e.g., smoking, exercise) were entered in the analysis, religious involvement (a combination of attending services, prayer, listening to religious TV programs, and reading Scripture from the Bible) no longer independently predicted mortality. However, when they decided to separate religious involvement into two categories—private and public religiousness—they found that attending religious services predicted lower death rates but that private activities, such as watching religious TV and reading Scripture, were not predictive. Instead, these private activities seemed to take away the power of overall religious involvement to predict lower mortality. Stated differently, private religiousness "suppressed" the benefits of public religiousness (essentially, of attending services) in predicting mortality. How this might be explained raises fascinating questions.

Such findings revealed the urgent need to assess more specific factors within the broader RS concepts now being used (Thoresen & Harris, in press). One can readily conjecture, given the way constructs have been measured, that some of the RS and health relationships may actually turn out to be much stronger or much weaker than current evidence suggests. Examining more specific features of RS factors may also help clarify possible negative or harmful relationships—a topic that has received little attention in the empirical literature (Gartner, Larson, & Allen, 1991). Incorporating additional psychological factors within these studies would also be important, because it would permit examination of possible interaction effects of certain person factors with certain religious factors (e.g., how narcissistic personality characteristics interact with religious attendance or with a person's beliefs about God) in predicting positive and negative health outcomes.

Beyond Baseline Prediction

A clear need exists for studies that probe how specific psychological and contextual factors influence specific RS and health relationships. Given results of recent studies in which religious attendance independently predicted all-cause mortality (see McCullough, Chapter 3, this volume; McCullough, Hoyt, Larson, Koenig, & Thoresen, 2000, for a meta-analytic review), how can these findings be explained? Few argue that the relationship is direct or straightforward. Longitudinal studies often use a "unique variance" approach, in which one tries to identify factors that are unrelated enough to others in the model that each will predict health outcomes independently from other predictors. One of the problems with this analytic strategy is that in reality factors are often related to each other (e.g., religious attendance may be significantly and positively related to perceived social/emotional support, nonsmoking, religious coping style, healthy diet, and active physical activities). The problem essentially is this: There is only so much independent variance to go around. Most predictors of health outcomes are related to each other, limiting the available variance to predict a health outcome.

By analogy, many studies in this area may suffer from a "first come, first serve" situation. Consider, for example, that there are only so many seats on the overbooked 10:14 AM flight to Chicago. Those arriving early at the airport (predictor variables first entered in the regression analysis because of high univariate correlation with the outcome variable) are guaranteed seats in tourist class, whereas those with equally valid tickets who arrive just before flight time may not be allowed to board because their assigned seats have been given to those who came early. There is simply no more room in tourist class. However, those holding tickets in business or first class are not affected because those tickets are different (i.e., those predictor variables not related). Thus some factors that do influence other factors directly or indirectly (or more distally rather than proximally) and that do influence health outcomes indirectly will not be considered. Why? Because they failed to demonstrate their ability to contribute unique variance in predicting health. Their seats were already occupied. What is lost in this perspective of honoring only independent contributors is that potentially important factors in religiousness and spirituality may not receive the attention they deserve. This is not a problem if we are interested only in predicting a health outcome, but it is problematic if we hope to explain the functional relationship between variables, such as religious service attendance and mortality.

W. R. Miller and Thoresen (1999) have observed that when predictor or control variables are related to each other, too often they fail to be considered for further study because they are found to be statistically insignificant in epidemiological studies. They suggest that experimental and repeated-measures designs can answer many of the questions raised by epidemiological studies that are limited to assessing RS factors on a single occasion. Little progress can be made by using only broad measures on one occasion and assuming that what was assessed is permanent and unchanging, much like a fixed trait or characteristic (e.g., eye color or gender). Chatters (2000) makes this point in discussing the very modest literature on contextual factors in RS and health. Typically, most measures of context are used with the assumption that they will not change over time and that broad concepts, such as "being religious," black American, or elderly, validly capture all persons assigned that label. Clearly, for example, not all elderly or religious persons are the same.

Which Comes First?: The Temporal Sequence Issue

Related to the state-of-the-art studies cited in Table 2.1 is the problem of temporality. In what order do variables influence or relate to the health outcome? Do they function sequentially or concurrently? Often it is the sequence of events that ultimately may influence health that remains unclear. For example, might one variable (e.g., attending weekly services) occur initially before another (e.g., daily meditation or volunteering in the community) but then take place concurrently with other factors? Clarifying what the sequence is can greatly improve our understanding of possible multiple causes and how they may function over time.

T. Miller (1997) offers a useful example of ways to reduce this confusion and a caveat about relying upon popular cross-lag panel and structural equation models (SEMs). Many predictor and outcome variables are themselves variable, as the name implies, rather than constant or highly stable factors. If there is fluctuation in an RS predictor, such as a specific RS behavior, cognition, or experience, then correlational research designs assessing RS factors on only one occasion can create invalid or misleading evidence. T. Miller (1997) demonstrated the problem of unstable temporal order of predictors in a study of what leads to marijuana use in teenagers. He found that cross-lag panel analysis and SEMs provided results indicating that participants' own use preceded friends' use of marijuana. However, use of either log-linear or discrete time-series analysis revealed a more complicated sequence. First-time use of marijuana was found to occur before friends' use, but what followed was participant and friend use occurring concurrently in terms of predicting continued marijuana use. Because the notion of reciprocal determinism is now often accepted in understanding human behavior (Bandura, 1997), studies are needed that examine how variables interact with each other, often concurrently, not just how they predict or relate in a unidirectional manner.

Cross-lag correlation, path analysis, and SEMs have been shown to be suspect in trying to tease out temporal or causal relationships even from longitudinal data, to say nothing of cross-sectional studies (Rogosa, 1987, 1988). Rogosa and others (e.g., Rogosa & Willett, 1985) have described the advantages and use of a growth-curve approach to modeling change over time, especially for understanding individual differences in change over time. These methods could greatly improve understanding of the influence of specific RS variables on health outcomes.

Experimental Studies

Unfortunately, relatively few experimental studies of RS factors and health exist. Worthington, Kurusu, McCullough, and Sandage (1996) reviewed almost 150 studies that focused on RS, counseling, and mental health. Roughly, only 7% involved experimental (as opposed to correlational or descriptive) designs. Experimental studies have been conducted primarily in the areas of meditation and prayer, mostly intercessory prayer, in which one or more persons pray for the recovery of someone suffering from a serious chronic disease. However, such studies, especially meditation studies, often have been conducted within a secular rather than a religious framework (e.g., Kabat-Zinn et al., 1998; see also W. R. Miller, 1999).

For example, Alexander, Langer, Newman, and Chandler (1989) conducted one of the few studies to date that compared transcendental mediation (TM), mindfulness meditation (MF), and relaxation training. In addition, an assessment control condition was used. All groups were assessed in terms of their impact on short-term mortality rates and the reversal of age-related declines in physical health for 73 residents of eight nursing homes (mean age = 81 years). After 36 months, the TM group was found most improved on measures of mental health (18-month follow-up, $p < .01$), and systolic blood pressure (3-month follow-up, $p < .01$), followed by the mindfulness training group, the relaxation group, and the assessment control group, respectively. After 3 years, the survival rate for the TM group was 100%, compared with 87.5% for the MF group, 65% for the relaxation group, and 62.5% for the assessment control group ($p < .00025$). Other controlled studies using an RS factor as an intervention or adjunct to therapy have been conducted. Propst, Ostrom, Watkins, Dean, and Mashburn (1992) found cognitive-behavioral therapy using religious imagery to be somewhat more effective with religious clients than a nonreligious version, although the benefit was not maintained at follow-up.

Intercessory Prayer/Distant Healing

In recent years the effects of praying for others, often people unknown personally to those praying for them and living at a distance, have been studied using experimental designs. (As noted, meditation and intercessory prayer stand almost alone among RS factors as the objects of experimental research.) The results of these studies are intriguing and worthy of careful consideration. Here we can only touch the surface (see Dossey, in press; Targ, 1997).

Byrd (1988) and Sicher, Targ, Moore, and Smith (1998) have reported double-blind studies on the effect of intercessory prayer on mortality and other health outcomes. For example, among patients recovering from acute myocardial infarction, Byrd found that patients in the prayer condition did substantially better than control patients on a number of health-related outcome categories, such as 7% fewer antibiotics required at discharge ($p < .005$) and 6% less need for intubation ($p < .002$). In addition, they had 6% less pulmonary edema ($p < .03$), 6% less congestive heart failure ($p < .03$), and 5% less cardiopulmonary arrest ($p < .02$), although these differences were less significant when adjusted at the experiment-wide $p < .05$ level.

In a well-conducted replication of the Byrd study published in *Archives of Internal Medicine*, W. S. Harris et al. (1999) found that a prayed-for group of coronary intensive care unit (CCU) patients had better overall CCU course scores (an index of several major in-hospital procedures and outcomes, ranging from need for medications to bypass surgery, reinfarction, and death), than the usual-care group. However, the length and number of hospital stays did not differ significantly. Importantly, researchers in this study controlled for response expectancy effects (Kirsch & Lynn, 1999), which are often very powerful, by obtaining permission from their institutional review board not to inform anyone, including patients, about the prayer intervention. Thus the attending physicians, nurses, and patients themselves remained uninformed about the study.

Results such as these deserve serious attention. Although they do not shed light on how intercessory prayer works, they clearly provide evidence that the effects of prayer can be studied using empirical methods and can include objectively measurable and clinically important health outcomes. Not all intercessory studies, however, have demonstrated significant effects when experimental designs are used with participants randomly assigned to conditions. Needed at this point is replication of such effects by other researchers using very similar procedures. For a review of other religiously oriented health interventions, the reader is referred to A. Harris, Thoresen, McCullough, and Larson (1999).

RS Factors and Mental Health

As discussed by Plante and Sharma in Chapter 10 (this volume), certain types of religious and spiritual involvement appear to be associated with a variety of desirable and undesirable mental health outcomes (e.g., Bergin, 1983; Exline, Yali, & Sanderson, in press; Gartner, Larson, & Allen, 1991; Levin, Markides, & Ray, 1996; McCullough, Larson, & Worthington, 1998; Pargament, Smith, Koenig, & Perez, 1998; Worthington et al., 1996). Certain indicators or forms of RS involvement, such as greater frequency of church attendance, have been related to greater subjective well-being and life and marital satisfaction, as well as decreased depressive symptoms, suicide, delinquency, and substance abuse (McCullough et al., 1998). Other researchers have found certain RS factors, such as the presence of religious strain (Exline et al., in press), difficulty forgiving God (Exline, Yali, & Lobel, 1999), and "negative" religious coping styles (Pargament et al., 1998; see Sherman & Simonton, Chapter 7, this volume), to be related to undesirable mental health outcomes, such as greater stress, depression, and suicidality.

Worthington et al. (1996) noted that the relationships observed between RS variables and health outcomes depend greatly on which features of these multidimensional constructs are measured and made central to operational definitions. Consistent with this view, Gartner et al. (1991) observed that most studies linking religious commitment to psychopathology employed paper-and-pencil personality tests, whereas research linking religion to positive mental health has focused on behavioral events that could be reliably observed and measured. Of the 30 studies reviewed by Worthington et al. (1996), some found RS involvement to be associated with desirable mental health variables (e.g., Ellison, 1991), some found RS involvement unrelated to poor health (e.g., Masters, Bergin, Reynolds, & Sullivan, 1991), and two studies found certain forms of religious involvement or experience to be positively associated with undesirable mental health, such as shame (P. Richards, Smith, & Davis, 1991) or negatively associated with desirable variables such as well-being (Galanter, 1986). In a review of 139 research studies published in the *American Journal of Psychiatry* and *Archives of General Psychiatry* from 1978 through 1989, Larson et al. (1992) generally found a positive relationship between religious commitment and mental health. However, it is possible that studies failing to find any relationship or finding negative effects may not have been submitted for publication or published.

The current state of empirical research in the mental health area is very suggestive but still modest. As already mentioned, studies using single measures of RS variables, such as church attendance, have provided correlational results promising enough to warrant more study. However, specific interpretations or insights into possible underlying mechanisms, as noted, will not be gleaned with such measures or research designs. Although many studies of RS factors and mental health have suffered from sampling, measurement, and analytic limitations, some recent studies have addressed these issues by employing better sampling strategies, controlling for relevant covariates, and using multiwave prospective, instead of cross-sectional, designs (e.g., Levin et al., 1996). Some studies have begun to look more seriously at the role played by specific contextual factors, such as the extent to which community residents adhere to a single religion or a small number of faiths (i.e., homogeneity of religious beliefs within a community; see Ellison, Burr, & McCall, 1997). These studies have found a generally favorable association between religious involvement and well-being for specific populations, while controlling for relevant covariates. More of this type of study is needed to further clarify what type of religious involvement is associated with what mental health variables under what conditions and for whom. Table 2.2 is intended to familiarize the reader with these and a small selection of other studies that examined the religious involvement–mental health relationship.

Besides being directly associated with mental health and illness in some studies, RS factors may be important factors in the treatment process or therapeutic relationship (see Chirban, Chapter 11; Tan & Dong, Chapter 12; and Shafranske, Chapter 13, this volume). Substantial differences have been found in religious values between clients and treatment providers; these differences may affect treatment, especially for highly religious clients (Worthington et al., 1996). There is scant evidence to date that religiously or spiritually modified secular interventions, such as cognitive-behavioral therapy (CBT), may be more effective under certain conditions than standard cognitive-behavioral treatment for some religious clients (e.g., Propst et al., 1992).

The fairly extensive RS factor–mental health literature, which is primarily cross-sectional in design, leads us to think that RS involvement may be positively, negatively, or negligibly influential for mental health status, depending on the extent and form of the RS involvement and a host of person and context factors. As mentioned, the current wave of theoretical and empirical attention devoted to establishing the salutary effects of RS involvement may have been an understandable reaction to the previous pathologizing of religious involvement and spiritual experience by scientists generally and psychologists in particular (e.g., Ellis, 1971; Freud, 1961). A more balanced view and research agenda will allow a more rigorous and open-minded approach to the health implications of various forms of RS involvement and the possible moderating or mediating roles that various person and context factors may play. In particular, evidence of possible negative or deleterious relationships should be pursued, if a balanced and, to some, a believable perspective on this topic is to be achieved.

STATE OF THE SCIENTIFIC EVIDENCE: THE OBSSR/NIH PANEL

In 1999 the Office of Behavioral and Social Sciences Research in the National Institutes of Health (OBSSR/NIH) created an expert panel of social and behavioral scientists under the leadership of Norman Anderson and William R. Miller to report on the state of the science concerning RS factors and health. One of us (Thoresen) has been serving on that panel in preparing two chapters on physical health and on basic constructs and methods. In this chapter we can review only briefly some of the current issues and concerns and offer a glimpse of some initial findings from the panel's work. (Publication of the panel's full report, composed of several papers, will appear as a special issue of the *American Psychologist*, the major overview journal of the American Psychological Association).

The panel is organized into several working groups, called Constructs and Methods, Physical Health, Measurement, Possible Psychosocial Mediators, Neurobiological Pathways, and Contextual Factors. Each group is reviewing the quality of the scientific evidence linking RS factors with various health-related processes or outcomes. To evaluate the quality of studies, a system is used to rate studies from A for excellent to C for having serious methodological problems. In addition, the panel is evaluating the strength of evidence (rated from "persuasive" to "insufficient" or "no evidence") in different RS dimensions (e.g., public religiousness, depth of religiousness, or private religiousness) concerning specific health outcomes (e.g., all-cause mortality, cardiovascular morbidity, physical disability). Each study is judged on the adequacy of how RS had been conceptualized and assessed and the quality of the research design (e.g., how many and what kind of control variables or covariates were included, use of cross-sectional or prospective designs, appropriateness of statistical methods).

Of the many issues discussed, a primary concern remains the limited quality of many studies in terms of research designs and types of measures used. Some of these issues have already been voiced in this chapter and by several others (e.g., Larson et al., 1998; Thoresen, 1999; see also

TABLE 2.2. Selected Studies Examining the RS Factor–Mental Health Connection

Study/focus	Sample characteristics	Predictor variable(s)	Control variables	Outcome variables	Results and conclusions
Ellison & Gay (1990) A cross-sectional study examining religion, religious commitment, and life satisfaction in black Americans	A nationally representative sample of 2,107 black adults interviewed for the National Survey of Black Americans.	1. Religious affiliation (denominational preference) 2. Religious service attendance (1–4 scale) 3. Self-described religiosity (1–4 scale) 4. Frequency of personal prayer (1–4 scale)	Age Sex Family income Education Marital status Geographic region Urban/rural residence Personal stress Measures of friendships and perceived family closeness	"In general, how satisfied are you with your life as a whole these days? Would you say you are very satisfied, somewhat satisfied, somewhat dissatisfied, or very dissatisfied?"	In the full model, religious service attendance, but not subjective religiosity or frequency of personal prayer, was positively associated with perceived assessment of overall life quality ($r^a = .065$, $p < .05$). This association was stronger among nonsouthern blacks, for whom differences in denominational preference, age, and private religiosity related to differences in life satisfaction.
Idler (1987) A cross-sectional study examining patterns of religious involvement, health status, functional disability, and depression	A sample of 2,756 elderly adults (1,139 male, 1,617 female) from the Yale Health and Aging Project.	1. A two-item index of public religiousness (attendance at religious services and number of congregation members known to respondent) 2. A two-item index of private religiousness (self-reported religiosity and "How much is religion a source of strength and comfort to you?")	Age Family income Education Marital status Race/ethnicity Health status variables Health behavior variables Social support variables Housing stratum Optimism Fatalism	Functional disability (Activities of Daily Living) Depression Psychological Distress (Center for Epidemiologic Studies Depression Scale, CES-D)	In the full model, inverse associations of public religiousness with depression were found for women ($r = -.079$, $p < .01$) and with functional disability for men ($r = -.075$, $p < .05$) and women ($t = -.169$, $p < .001$). For men, increased private religious involvement weakened the association of health status with disability and the association of disability with depression.

36

Study	Sample	Measures	Covariates	Outcome	Results
Koenig, George, & Peterson (1998) A prospective study of religiosity and remission of depression in medically ill older patients. Patients were assessed in four follow-up interviews 12 weeks apart.	94 patients diagnosed with depressive disorder (major depression or subsyndromal depression) by a psychiatrist using a structured interview, Hamilton Depression Rating Scale (HDRS; >11), and the Epidemiological Studies Depression Rating Scale (>16)	1. A 10-item intrinsic religiosity scale 2. "How often do you spend time in private religious activities such as prayer, meditation, or Bible study?" (1–6 scale) 3. How often do you attend church or other religious meetings?" (1–6 scale)	Four of 17 variables were identified as important covariates: Quality of life, change in functional status during follow-up, family psychiatric history, admitting status (general medicine vs. other)	Number of weeks to remission from depression, "as defined as 2 weeks or more of fewer than three of the nine traditional DSM-III criterion symptoms"	Higher intrinsic religiosity was independently related to less time to remission, but church attendance and private religious activities were not. In the model with four covariates, intrinsic religiosity hazard ratio = 1.70, 95% CI: 1.05–2.75.
Propst et al. (1992) A controlled intervention study examining the comparative efficacy of religious and nonreligious cognitive-behavioral therapy (CBT) administered by religious and nonreligious therapists for clinical depression in religious individuals. Pre-, post-, and two follow-up assessments used.	Fifty-nine religious, depressed patients (10 male, 49 female) with a mean age of 40 years	Patients were assigned to one of three treatment conditions or a wait-list control condition (WLC). The treatment conditions were 18 50-minute sessions of religiously modified CBT (RCT), traditional CBT (NRCT), or pastoral counseling (PCT). The RCT presented Christian religious rationales for the procedures, used religious arguments to counter irrational thoughts, and used religious imagery procedures.	Patient and therapist religiosity Patient and therapist evaluation of treatment	Beck Depression Inventory, Modified Hamilton, Global Severity Index, Social Adjustment Scale, Symptom Checklist—Revised	The RCT but not the NRCT patients reported lower posttreatment depression and better adjustment scores than the WLC. No differences in improvement between the three treatment conditions were found at 3-month and 2-year follow-up. At 3 months, there was a therapist belief by treatment interaction effect, with nonreligious therapists in the RCT condition outperforming their religious therapist counterparts.

[a]Standardized regression coefficient in the full model.

McCullough, chapter 3; Sherman & Simonton, Chapter 7; and Sloan, Bagiella, & Powell, Chapter 14, this volume). For example, although cross-sectional studies can provide useful data in some areas, especially in the early stages, prospective or longitudinal studies are essential to understand what changes occur over time. Cross-sectional snapshots are no substitute for "real time" films. Yet sometimes prospective designs also are not "real" enough in the pictures they provide; often, for example, RS and other social and psychological factors are assessed on only one occasion, as if they were all fixed characteristics that never change. One's religious affiliation, such as Christian or Jew, may remain stable, but many specific factors associated with spirituality and religiousness, such as beliefs and practices, may vary with circumstances and contexts over time.

A related issue cited by the panel is essentially the absence, with rare exception (i.e., intercessionary prayer and meditation), of experimental research in this area. Understanding how RS factors might lead over time to changes in health status will require expanding the type of research studies that have been conducted to date, especially in terms of performing more experimental studies that probe what factors alter or influence (mediate and moderate) RS and health factors.

What conclusions will the panel likely reach? Although the answer remains to be determined, we can offer a glimpse forward. The evidence to date probably supports the view that the association between RS factors and health is not trivial, nor is it a random artifact. A relationship indeed exists that is not readily explained by several other known health-related factors, such as health behaviors (e.g., smoking), perceived social support and social networks, or various demographic factors. Furthermore, the areas of contextual and psychological factors, along with neurobiological research and the use of experimental designs, will be recognized as the least well developed yet in many ways the most promising areas in clarifying and advancing understanding. That said, a host of questions exist, with a fair amount of confusion and controversy about just what this nontrivial RS and health relationship is all about and what are, if any, the implications for health care training and practice. Further, the fact that some RS factors may indeed be hazardous to health will emerge as an area of study deserving much more attention than it has received thus far.

RESEARCH ISSUES AND RECOMMENDATIONS

Several conceptual, methodological, and analytic issues are relevant to the improvement of RS-factor research. Here we build on what has been presented in this chapter and elsewhere, briefly discussing some important issues and "next steps" in clarifying RS factor–health relationships, including possible mechanisms underlying these relationships.

The Value of the Behavior/Belief/Motivation/ Experience Framework

Why does attending religious services weekly predict lower overall mortality in well-controlled studies (McCullough, Hoyt, Larson, Koenig, & Thoresen, 2000)? How do we explain, for example, how serving others ("selfless service" or volunteering in the community) predicts lower mortality even when conventional risk factors, including social support, are controlled (Oman, Thoresen, & McMahon, 1999)? Answers to such questions based on empirical data require more detailed information about just what those persons involved in such studies are doing, thinking, and feeling.

Here are three examples that illustrate recent efforts to move away from large macro-level concepts (e.g., religious affiliation or denomination) toward the kind of specificity needed to unravel these relationships. The first study asked if certain kinds of religious coping would lead to stronger positive relationships with mental health outcomes. Pargament et al. (1999) found that, among family members waiting for a relative to undergo major surgery, those who used a "collaborating with God" style of religious coping, compared with a more self-directing or pleading-with-God style, had better coping outcomes and better religious outcomes. They also found that this collaborative coping style mediated the effect of depression and anxiety on psychological and religious outcomes, whereas other religious and secular kinds of coping (e.g., planning, instrumental social support) failed to do so.

In another study, Tix and Frazier (1998) looked at religious coping, as well as other psychosocial factors, as possible mediating variables in patients' adjustment to kidney transplant surgery and in how well their significant others coped with the operation. Religious coping was a significant predictor of overall life satisfaction at 3 and 12 months after surgery, particularly for Protestant, as opposed to Catholic, patients. Religious coping remained a significant predictor of satisfaction even when cognitive restructuring, locus of control, and demographic factors were considered.

A third study (Keefe et al., in press) examined RS factors among patients with arthritis and explored how RS factors were related to daily positive and negative emotions (moods), as well as to experienced pain. They used a unique research design in which each participant completed daily ratings of RS factors, mood and emotional states, social and emotional support, pain self-efficacy, and pain level over 30 consecutive days. RS factors were studied in considerable detail in terms of daily spiritual experiences (e.g., "Feeling deep inner peace or harmony"; "Desired to be closer to, or in union with God"), religious and spiritual coping (e.g., "Looked to God for strength, support, and guidance"; "Thought about how my life is part of a larger spiritual force"), religious and spiritual efficacy (e.g., "extent my religious or spiritual coping allowed me to control my pain today") and perceived salience of religion each day in relation to pain. Although higher levels of religious and spiritual efficacy predicted greater reduction in pain, the combination of daily spiritual experiences with perceived social support predicted the greatest increases in positive mood and the largest reductions in negative mood. Significantly, this study demonstrated that RS factors are clearly related to daily mood (positive and negative) and to religious or spiritual efficacy factors. When viewed independently of each other, these factors may be misrepresented in the actual experiences of people. By using a research design that reveals not only between-person differences but also within-person variability (in this case change from day to day over 30 days), a more complete and informative picture is produced. Interestingly, pain was at its lowest on those days when religious coping efficacy and daily spiritual experiences were higher, even though daily spiritual experiences by themselves were not related to pain.

These three studies illustrate the value of working with more specific concepts than have been assessed in the past, in ways that can yield more valid and reliable data. These studies further illustrate the need to look at possible interaction effects, such as type of coping (including daily coping), with certain person and contextual characteristics. In this way, progress can be made in identifying what variables increase or reduce the relationship between RS factors and health (Baron & Kenny, 1986).

How Might It Work?

Different models have tried to explain the relation between RS and health outcomes. Figure 2.1 presents a working model derived from a more detailed model that was developed for the OBSSR panel mentioned previously. The model tries to capture several factors that may be involved in the pathways connecting RS factors with health. Four points deserve comment. First, the model tries to show how RS factors might play a role in improving health. Second, any particular study would likely focus on only a slice of this RS–health conceptual pie (e.g., relationship of a spiritual factor with certain health behaviors and immune functioning). Third, some RS factors, under certain conditions, could diminish or endanger health. It is unlikely that all RS factors would benefit health under all conditions. Fourth, any model at this point is highly likely to be flawed in several ways, given limitations in our current knowledge. Any conceptual model is a work in progress, subject to continual revision. As such it can only attempt to capture the complex flow of events possibly linking RS to health. For example, the directionality suggested (linear from left to right) is undoubtedly oversimplified, as processes are almost always multidirectional and reciprocal.

Unfortunately, almost all empirical studies in this area to date have been designed not to test conceptual models or theory but to examine empirically

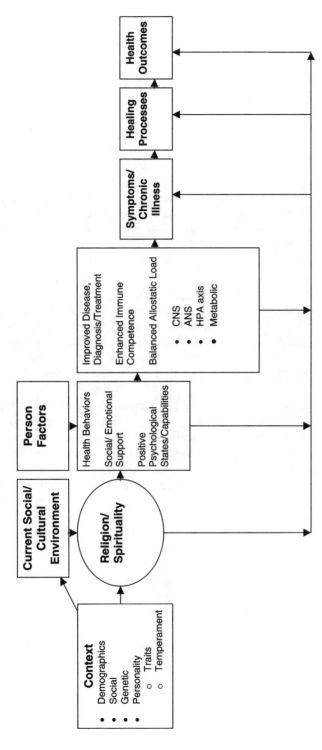

FIGURE 2.1. Religion/spirituality and better health. *Note:* Religion and spirituality may overlap but may also have distinct, nonoverlapping areas (e.g., spiritual beliefs or practices may or may not be related to any recognized religion). Also, although the above mode is presented with unidirectional arrows, clearly some factors may interact in bidirectional or multidirectional relationships. For example, although increased religious involvement may increase social support and in turn improve health outcomes, the direction of influence may be reversed for some people. In addition, more than one path to healing and health is proposed, some more direct than others.

41

whether relationships exist between an RS factor and some health outcome, often morbidity or mortality. An important next step is for researchers to describe more specific models and possible mechanisms and to design studies capable of providing supportive or disconfirmatory evidence.

For example, in a much publicized study, Oxman, Freeman, and Manheimer (1995) found both the lack of participation in social or community groups and the absence of strength and comfort from religion to predict mortality in patients who underwent elective heart surgery. For those interested in establishing a positive link between religious involvement and health, the tempting conclusion is that the strength and comfort that religion provides is what reduces mortality. Although this conclusion may be valid and seemed supported by the data, it is probably premature. While the data appeared to support the proposition, other possible explanations still exist. For example, it is possible that persons who report high levels of strength and comfort from their religion are people who also experience comfort from multiple sources, such as friendships, community, and marriage. It is possible that the capacity to experience much of life as comforting and strengthening predicts mortality independent of the source (such as one's religion). The question about strength and comfort from religion may also have been a proxy for optimism or another personality factor that was revealed in its religious manifestation but that is not tied to religion in an integral fashion.

As another example, in a prospective study examining the relationship between volunteering and mortality in a sample of elderly people, Oman, Thoresen, and McMahon (1999) statistically accounted for social functioning and social and emotional support through a number of measures. These included more than 10 variables, such as marital status, number of days out of the house per week, and religious service attendance. The purpose of including these other factors as covariates or controls was to estimate the independent effect of volunteering above and beyond the possible health benefits from several kinds of social contact and involvement. Although volunteering predicted over 40% lower mortality compared with those who did not volunteer in the community, even after accounting for social support variables, we cannot entirely dismiss the possibility that volunteering reduced mortality risk through increasing social support. This is so because of the limitations of the measures of social support that were used (e.g., marital status is a very narrow indicator of spousal or social support). Although this study explored and controlled for several competing explanations, results remain suggestive until more targeted studies are conducted. Again, failure to disconfirm a model (such as that volunteering reduces mortality), although important, is not the same as confirming it. Such confirmation in general requires evidence from experimentally designed studies (W. R. Miller & Thoresen, 1999).

The Importance of Linking Conceptualization and Measurement

Religion and spirituality are complex, multidimensional constructs. In designing studies and using relevant measurement tools, it is important to specify which features of the constructs are being measured, as well as a theoretical rationale for doing so. Ellison and Levin (1998) make a useful theoretical distinction between the functional and behavioral (or structural) aspects of religious involvement. They argue that identification and measurement of the possible functional roles of religion, such as providing an existential framework of meaning and purpose, specific coping strategies, or support for specific health behaviors, will pay dividends in terms of understanding the mechanisms through which health is influenced. Most but not all empirical studies have focused on behavioral or structural aspects of religious involvement, such as church attendance or rituals, and have not examined the functions that religious involvement may serve in people's lives.

An example of research that has focused on the functional aspects of religion is provided by Pargament and his colleagues (e.g., Pargament, 1997; Pargament et al., 1998). They have focused on religious coping as distinct from other religious or spiritual behaviors. They have identified different types of religious coping and have begun to examine the desirable and undesirable health correlates of each. This approach is grounded in the idea that one of the functions of religion is to help people cope more effectively with life's inevitable stressors. These researchers constructed definitions that distinguish between religious and nonreligious coping. In this way, the theoretical proposition that religion serves a coping function can be tested. Once different forms of religious coping have been characterized, then more precise and useful statements can be made. These statements would specify the health consequences of particular religious coping behaviors in particular situations by people with certain characteristics. Note that this is quite different from trying to answer a very general question such as, Does religion cause better health or does spirituality prevent disease? (See Oman & Thoresen, 2001, for extended discussion of these questions.)

Other Research Design Issues

Research questions should dictate, as much as possible, research designs. As questions become more sophisticated and precise, the need has developed to employ a greater variety of study designs. So far, the field has been dominated by cross-sectional–correlational research and prospective longitudinal research that examines the role of RS factors as independent predictors and, to a much lesser extent, as moderators or mediators of health status (e.g., Tix & Frazier, 1998). These designs will continue to be useful, particularly if they employ more precise, multidimensional, and well-validated measures of RS factors.

Other designs and methods, such as single-participant ($N = 1$) experiments (Hilliard, 1993), a variety of interview designs (see T. Richards & Folkman, 1997), daily monitoring methods (see Keefe et al., in press), and controlled intervention studies have been largely missing. Intervention studies in particular, such as those by Alexander et al. (1989) and W. S. Harris et al. (1999), illustrate the feasibility and explanatory power of experimental designs in RS factor research. Particularly for health professionals interested in applying culturally sensitive, empirically validated treatments, intervention research offers the double benefit of simultaneously developing efficacious treatment strategies as well as providing opportunities to test theoretical propositions concerning underlying mechanisms.

SOME TENTATIVE CONJECTURES AND CONCERNS

Conclusions about the emerging area of RS and health need to be highly tentative and stated more in the spirit of reasoned conjectures based on mostly suggestive evidence. The following conjectures and concerns seem justified at this point in time. In offering them we recognize the possibility that some readers may find them overly conservative and cautious, whereas others may see them as excessively optimistic. Hopefully, these conjectures will appear reasonable and justified enough to encourage colleagues to take the question of RS and health seriously and to elect to study facets of the topic.

• With the large number of Americans who currently profess a belief in God (96%), attend religious services regularly(42%), consider their religious and spiritual beliefs as very important in their lives (60%), associate frequent religious involvement with greater happiness (47%), and express the need for greater spiritual growth (82%), RS factors deserve careful and critical consideration by health care professionals in research and training and in conventional and alternative/complementary health care practice (Gallup, 1995; Myers, 2000b).

• RS factors appear to be associated with physical, mental, and overall health, but the lack of adequate controls and designs in many studies has seriously limited our understanding of these relationships.

• Evidence linking RS, assessed as frequent attendance at religious services, to reduced all-cause mortality has been impressive, but the nature of and explanation for this relationship remains quite unclear. In general, evidence from well-controlled prospective studies linking religious attendance and other RS factors to specific major diseases, such as various cancers (as opposed to all-cause mortality), remains insufficient and unclear.

• Missing in almost all major studies has been a more careful study of person and psychological factors (distinct from social support or social ties), such as self-evaluative processes and persistent socially situated cognitions, specific contextual or environmental factors, and various physiological processes that could clarify pathways linking RS to health outcomes.

• The need to use a much greater variety of research designs and assessment strategies, combining more qualitative with quantitative methods, seems imperative. Relevant problems and questions need to dictate the selection of particular designs and methods. Sometimes new or adapted methods are needed. Too often, conventional research methods and designs determine what is studied and how (Cook, 1985; Thoresen, 1999).

• Evidence that RS-related factors, such as providing help to others (selfless service or altruistic behavior), forgiveness, and meditation provide health benefits is generally lacking but seems very promising and deserving of careful study (e.g., McCullough, Pargament, & Thoresen, 2000).

• Conceptually, the notion that some RS factors could lead in time to greater subjective well-being, overall life satisfaction, quality of life, even joy and happiness, along with less disease and distress, seems theoretically plausible and worthy of study. A broad perspective that spans the social, behavioral, and medical sciences is needed, with the collaboration of those in the humanities, including theologians and spiritual practitioners (e.g., clergy).

Perhaps the new millennium represents a fitting occasion for scholars and practicing professionals concerned with health to reconsider their perspectives on the role of RS factors in health and well-being, as well as in disease and disability. Very few of us have received any professional training on this topic (see Shafranske, Chapter 13, this volume; Thoresen, 1998). Yet it remains a major concern for many of those we serve, as well as those we study. As with some issues of church and state, reproductive health, and morality and character, matters of the spirit often elicit involuntary, "knee jerk" reactions charged with lots of emotional energy. We believe, however, that the time has come to address this topic with solid rigor and with sensitive respect. There is much to be humble about.

Advocacy has its place, as does skepticism. But extremes of either seldom help clarify the complexities. Too often topics involving faith and health have fallen prey to reductionistic concepts, dichotomous thinking, and stereotyped images. The issues are highly complex and truly challenging. But they are not insurmountable. We face the prospect, at least potentially, of reaping significant improvements in health care effectiveness, quality of life, and well-being if we proceed with the sensitivity, patience, and perseverance required. Einstein (1993) was right back in the last century when he observed that science without religion is lame, and religion without science is blind. Perhaps the same is true of spirituality and health as well.

ACKNOWLEDGMENTS

Preparation of this chapter was supported, in part, by grants to Carl E. Thoresen from the Fetzer Institute and the John Templeton Foundation and from participation on the Spirituality, Religiousness and Health: State of the Science Panel, Office of Behavioral and Social Sciences Research (OBSSR) in the National Institutes of Health (NIH). Work by Alex H. S. Harris was partially supported by a Stanford Presidential Graduate Fellowship, and Doug Oman was partially supported by Training Grant No. T32 HL07365-21 from the National Heart, Lung, and Blood Institute (NIH). The support and encouragement of Tom Plante and Allen Sherman in preparing this chapter is gratefully acknowledged, as is the seminal work of several colleagues, especially William R. Miller, Michael M McCullough, and Ken I. Pargament, who are conducting empirical research in the area of spirituality, religion, and health. The views expressed in this chapter are, however, solely our own and not those of agencies and organizations who assisted us in the preparation of this chapter.

NOTE

1. We use the abbreviation "RS" throughout the chapter to signify "religious and/or spiritual" and "religion and spirituality" to save space. Spirituality and religion are often used interchangeably yet actually represent, at least for some persons, overlapping concepts, each with some distinct features. We discuss the topic more fully in this chapter.

REFERENCES

Albom, M. (1997). *Tuesdays with Morrie*. New York: Doubleday.

Alexander, C. N., Langer, E. J., Newman, R. I., & Chandler, H. M. (1989). Transcendental meditation, mindfulness and longevity: An experimental study with the elderly. *Journal of Personality and Social Psychology, 57,* 950–964.

Allport, G. (1950). *The individual and his religion*. New York: Macmillan.

Bandura, A. (1997). Health promotion from the perspective of social cognitive theory. *Psychology and Health, 19,* 1–27.

Bargh, J. A., & Chartraud, T. L. (1999). The unbearable automaticity of being. *American Psychologist, 54,* 1173–1182.

Baron, R. M., & Kenney, D. A. (1986). The moderator-mediator variable distinction in social psychological research: Conceptual, strategic, and statistical considerations. *Journal of Personality and Social Psychology, 51,* 1173–1182.

Bellah, R. N., Madsen, R., Sullivan, W., Swidler, A., & Tipton, S. (1985). *Habits of the heart: Individualism and commitment in American life*. Berkeley: University of California Press.

Bergin, A. E. (1983). Religiosity and mental health: A critical reevaluation and meta-analysis. *Professional Psychology: Research and Practice, 14,* 170–184.

Billings, J. S. (1891). Vital statistics of the Jews. *North American Review, 153,* 70–84.

Byrd, R. B. (1988). Positive therapeutic effects of intercessory prayer in a coronary care unit population. *Southern Medical Journal, 81,* 826–829.

Chatters, L. M. (2000). Religion and health: Public health research and practice. *Annual Review of Public Health, 21,* 335–367.

Chopra, D. (2000). *How to know God: The soul's journey into the mystery of mysteries.* New York: Random House.

Comstock, G. W., & Partridge, K. B. (1972). Church attendance and health. *Journal of Chronic Diseases, 25,* 665–672.

Comstock, G. W., & Tonascia, J. A. (1977). Education and mortality in Washington County, Maryland. *Journal of Health and Social Behavior, 18,* 54–61.

Cook, T. D. (1985). Postpositivist critical multiplism. In R. L. Shotland & M. M. Marks (Eds.), *Social science and social policy* (pp. 21–62). Beverly Hills, CA: Sage.

Csikszentmihalyi, M. (1999). If we are so rich, why aren't we happy? *American Psychologist, 54,* 821–827.

Dawkins, R. (1999). You can't have it both ways: Irreconcilable differences. *Skeptical Inquirer, 23,* 62–64.

Dossey, L. (in press). Prayer and medical science. *Archives of Internal Medicine.*

Durkheim, E. (1951). *Suicide: A study in sociology* (J. A. Spaulding & G. Simpson, Trans.). Glencoe, IL: Free Press. (Original work published 1897)

Einstein, A. (1993). *Einstein on humanism.* New York: Citadel Press.

Ellis, A. (1971). *The case against religion: A psychotherapist's view.* New York: Institute for Rational Living.

Ellison, C. G. (1991). Religious involvement and subjective well being. *Journal of Health and Social Behavior, 32,* 80–99.

Ellison, C. G., Burr, J. A., & McCall, P. L. (1997). Religious homogeneity and metropolitan suicide rates. *Social Forces, 76,* 273–299.

Ellison, C. G., & Gay, D. A. (1990). Region, religious commitment, and life satisfaction among Black Americans. *Sociological Quarterly, 31*(1), 123–147.

Ellison, C. G., & Levin, J. S. (1998). The religion–health connection: Evidence, theory and future directions. *Health Education and Behavior, 25,* 700–720.

Emmons, R. A., & Crumpler, C. A. (1999). Religion *and* spirituality? The roles of sanctification and the concept of God. *International Journal for the Psychology of Religion, 9,* 17–24.

Enstrom, J. E. (1975). Cancer mortality among Mormons. *Cancer, 36*(3), 825–841.

Exline, J. J., Yali, A. M., & Lobel, M. (1999). When God disappoints: Difficulty forgiving God and its role in negative emotion. *Journal of Health Psychology, 4,* 365–379.

Exline, J. J., Yali, A. M., & Sanderson, W. C. (in press). Guilt, discord, and alienation: The role of religious strain in depression and suicidality. *Journal of Clinical Psychology.*

Frank, R. H., & Cook, P. J. (1995). *The winner-take-all society.* New York: Free Press.

Frankel, B. G., & Hewitt, W. E. (1994). Religion and well being among Canadian university students: The role of faith groups on campus. *Journal for the Scientific Study of Religion, 33,* 62–73.

Freud, S. (1961). The future of an illusion. In J. Strachey (Ed. and Trans.), *The standard edition of the complete psychological works of Sigmund Freud* (Vol. 21, pp. 1–56). London: Hogarth Press and the Institute of Psycho-Analysis. (Original work published 1927)

Galanter, M. (1986). "Moonies" get married: A psychiatric follow-up study of a charismatic religious sect. *American Journal of Psychiatry, 143,* 1245–1249.

Gallup, G. (1995) *The Gallup Poll: Public opinion 1995.* Wilmington, DE: Scholarly Resources.

Gartner, J., Larson, D. B., & Allen, G. D. (1991). Religious commitment and mental health: A review of the empirical literature. *Journal of Psychology and Theology, 19,* 6–25.

Gorsuch, R. L., & Miller, W. R. (1999). Measuring spirituality. In W. R. Miller (Ed.), *Integrating spirituality into practice: Resources for practitioners* (pp. 47–64). Washington, DC: American Psychological Association.

Harris, A. H. S., Thoresen, C. E., McCullough, M. E., & Larson, D. B. (1999). Spiritually and religiously oriented health interventions. *Journal of Health Psychology, 4,* 413–433.

Harris, R. C., Dew, M. A., Lee, A., Amaya, M., Buches, L. D. R., & Coleman, G. (1995). The role of religion in heart-transplant recipients' long-term health and well-being. *Journal of Religion and Health, 34,* 17–32.

Harris, W. S., Gowda, M., Kolb, J. W., Strychacz, C. P., Vacek, J. L., Jones, P. G., Forker, A., O'Keefe, J. H., & McCallister, B. D. (1999). A randomized, controlled trial of the effects of remote, intercessory prayer on outcomes in patients admitted to the coronary care unit. *Archives of Internal Medicine, 159,* 2273–2278.

Hill, P. C., & Hood, R. W. (1999). *Measures of religious behavior.* Birmingham, AL: Religious Education Press.

Hilliard, R. B. (1993). Single case methodology in psychotherapy process and outcome research. *Journal of Consulting and Clinical Psychology, 61,* 373–380.

Hummer, R. A., Rogers, R. G., Nam, C. B., & Ellison, C. G. (1999). Religious involvement and U. S. adult mortality. *Demography, 36,* 272–285.

Idler, E. L. (1987). Religious involvement and the health of the elderly: Some hypotheses and an initial test. *Social Forces, 66,* 226–238.

Idler, E. L., & Kasl, S. V. (1992). Religion, disability, depression, and the timing of death. *American Journal of Sociology, 97,* 1052–1079.

Idler, E. L., & Kasl, S. V. (1997). Religion among disabled and non-disabled persons: II. Attendance at religious services as a predictor of the course of disability. *Journals of Gerontology Series B—Psychological Sciences and Social Sciences, 52B,* S306–S316.

James, W. (1985). *Varieties of religious experience.* New York: Random House. (Original work published 1902)

Kabat-Zinn, J., Wheeler, E., Light, T., Skillings, A., Scharf, M. J., Cropley, T. G., Hosmer, D., & Bernhard, J. D. (1998). Influence of a mindfulness meditation-based stress reduction intervention on rates of skin clearing in patients with moderate to severe psoriasis undergoing phototherapy (UVB) and photochemotherapy (PUVA). *Psychosomatic Medicine, 60,* 625–632.

Keefe, F. J., Affleck, G., Lefebvre, J., Underwood, L., Caldwell, D. S., Drew, J., Egert, J., Gibson, J., & Pargament, K. I. (in press). Living with rheumatoid arthritis: The role of daily spirituality and daily religious and spiritual coping. *Journal of Pain*

Kiesler, D. J. (1966). Some myths of psychotherapy research and the search for a paradigm. *Psychological Bulletin, 65*, 110–130.

Kirsch, I., & Lynn, S. J. (1999). Automaticity in clinical psychology. *American Psychologist, 54*, 504–515.

Koenig, H. G. (1997). *Is religion good for your health?: Effects of religion on mental and physical health*. Binghamton, NY: Haworth Pastoral Press.

Koenig, H. G., George, L. K., & Peterson, B. L. (1998). Religiosity and remission of depression in medically ill older patients. *American Journal of Psychiatry, 155*, 536–542.

Larson, D. B., Koenig, H. G., & Kaplan, B. H. (1989). The impact of religion on men's blood pressure. *Journal of Religion and Health, 28*, 265–278.

Larson, D. B., Swyers, J. P., & McCullough, M. E. (Eds.). (1998). *Scientific research on spirituality and health: A consensus report*. Rockville, MD: National Institute for Healthcare Research.

Larson, D. B., Sherrill, K. A., Lyons, J. S., Craigie, F. C., Thielman, S. B., Greenwood, M. A., & Larson, S. S. (1992). Associations between dimensions of religious commitment and mental health reported in the *American Journal of Psychiatry* and *Archives of General Psychiatry*: *1978–1989*. *American Journal of Psychiatry, 149*, 557–559.

Levin, J. S., Markides, K. S., & Ray, L. A. (1996). Religious attendance and psychological well being in Mexican Americans: A panel analysis of three-generation data. *Gerontologist, 36*, 454–463.

Madalie, J. H., Kahn, H. A., & Neufeld, H. N. (1973). Five-year myocardial infarction incidence: II. Association of single variables to age and birthplace. *Journal of Chronic Disease, 26*, 329–349.

Masters, K. S., Bergin, A. E., Reynolds, E. M., & Sullivan, C. E. (1991). Religious life-styles and mental health: A follow-up study. *Counseling and Values, 35*, 211–224.

Matthews, D. A., Koenig, H. G., Thoresen, C. E., & Friedman, R. (1998). Physical health. In D. B. Larson, J. P. Swyers, & M. E. McCullough (Eds.), *Scientific research on spirituality and health: A consensus report* (pp. 31–54). Rockville, MD: National Institute for Healthcare Research.

McCullough, M. E., Hoyt, W. T., Larson, D. B., Koenig, H. G., & Thoresen, C. E. (2000). Religious involvement and mortality: A meta-analytic review. *Health Psychology, 19*, 211–222.

McCullough, M. E., Larson, D. B., & Worthington, E. L. (1998). Mental health. In D. B. Larson, J. P. Swyers, & M. E. McCullough (Eds.), *Scientific research on spirituality and health: A consensus report* (pp. 55–67). Rockville, MD: National Institute for Healthcare Research.

McCullough, M. E., Pargament, K. I., & Thoresen, C. E. (Eds.). (2000). *Forgiveness: Theory, research, and practice*. New York: Guilford Press.

Miller, T. Q. (1997). Statistical methods describing temporal order in longitudinal research. *Journal of Clinical Epidemiology, 50*, 1155–1168.

Miller, W. R. (Ed.). (1999). *Integrating spirituality into treatment: Resources for practitioners.* Washington, DC: American Psychological Association.

Miller, W. R., & Thoresen, C. E. (1999). Spirituality and health. In W. R. Miller (Ed.), *Integrating spirituality into treatment* (pp. 3–18). Washington, DC: American Psychological Association.

Moore, T. (1994). *Care of the soul: A guide for cultivating depth and sacredness in everyday life.* New York: Harper.

Musick, M. A., House, J. S., & Williams, D. R. (in press). Attendance at religious services and mortality in a national sample. *Journal of Health and Social Behavior.*

Myers, D. (2000a). *The American paradox: Spiritual hunger in a land of plenty.* New Haven, CT: Yale University Press.

Myers, D. (2000b). The funds, the friends, and the faith of happy people. *American Psychologist, 55,* 56–67.

Oman, D., & Reed, D. (1998). Religion and mortality among the community-dwelling elderly. *American Journal of Public Health, 88,* 1469–1475.

Oman, D., & Thoresen, C. E. (2001). *Does religion cause health? Differing interpretations and diverse meanings.* Manuscript submitted for publication.

Oman, D., Thoresen, C. E., & McMahon, K. (1999). Volunteerism and mortality. *Journal of Health Psychology, 4,* 301–316.

Osler, W. (1910). The faith that heals. *British Medical Journal, 18,* 1470–1472.

Oxman, T. E., Freeman, D. H., & Manheimer, E. D. (1995). Lack of social participation or religious strength and comfort as risk factors for death after cardiac surgery in the elderly. *Psychosomatic Medicine, 57,* 5–15.

Pargament, K. I. (1997). *The psychology of religion and coping: Theory, research, practice.* New York: Guilford Press.

Pargament, K. I. (1999). Psychology of religion and spirituality. *International Journal for the Psychology of Religion, 9,* 3–16.

Pargament, K. I., Smith, B. W., Koenig, H. G., & Perez, L. (1998). Patterns of positive and negative religious coping with major life stressors. *Journal for the Scientific Study of Religion, 37,* 710–724.

Pargament, K. I., Cole, B., VandeCreek, L., Balavich, T., Brant, C., & Perez, L. (1999). The vigil: Religion and the search for control in the hospital waiting room. *Journal of Health Psychology, 4,* 327–341.

Phillips, R. L., Kuzma, J. W., Beeson, W. L., & Lotz, T. (1980). Influence of selection versus lifestyle on risk of fatal cancer and cardiovascular disease among Seventh-Day Adventists. *American Journal of Epidemiology, 112,* 296–314.

Phillips, R. L., Lemon, F. R., Beeson, W. L., & Kuzma, J. W. (1978). Coronary heart disease mortality among Seventh-Day Adventists with differing dietary habits: A preliminary report. *American Journal of Clinical Nutrition, 31,* S191–S198.

Post, S. G., Puchalski, C., & Larson, D. B. (2000). Physicians and patient spirituality: Professional boundaries, competency, and ethics. *Annals of Internal Medicine, 132,* 578–583.

Propst, L. R., Ostrom, R., Watkins, P., Dean, T., & Mashburn, D. (1992). Comparative efficacy of religious and non-religious cognitive–behavioral therapy for the treatment of clinical depression in religious individuals. *Journal of Consulting and Clinical Psychology, 60,* 94–103.

Richards, P. S., & Bergin, A. E. (1997). *A spiritual strategy for counseling and psychotherapy.* Washington, DC: American Psychological Association.

Richards, P. S., Smith, S. A., & Davis, L. F. (1991). Healthy and unhealthy forms of religiousness manifested by psychotherapy clients: An empirical investigation. *Journal of Research in Personality, 23,* 506–524.

Richards, T. A., & Folkman, S. (1997). Spiritual aspects of loss at the time of a partner's death from AIDS. *Death Studies, 21,* 527–552.

Rogosa, D. (1987). Casual models do not support scientific conclusions: A comment in support of Freedman. *Journal of Educational Statistics, 12,* 185–195.

Rogosa, D. R. (1988). Myths about longitudinal research. In K. W. Schaie, R. T. Campbell, W. M. Meredith, & S. C. Rawlings (Eds.), *Methodological issues in aging research* (pp. 171–209). New York: Springer.

Rogosa, D. R., & Willett, J. B. (1985). Understanding correlates of change by modeling individual differences in growth. *Psychometrika, 50,* 203–228.

Rosen, G. (1993). *A history of public health.* Baltimore: Johns Hopkins University Press.

Schor, J. B. (1991). *The overworked American.* New York: Basic Books.

Scotch, N. A. (1963). Sociocultural factors in the epidemiology of Zulu hypertension. *American Journal of Public Health, 53,* 1205–1213.

Shafranske, E. P. (Ed.). (1996). *Religion and the clinical practice of psychology.* Washington, DC: American Psychological Association.

Sherrill, K. A., & Larson, D. B. (1994). The anti-tenure factor in religious research in clinical epidemiology and aging. In J. S. Levin (Ed.), *Religion in aging and health: Theoretical foundations and methodological frontiers* (pp. 149–177). Thousand Oaks, CA: Sage.

Sicher, F., Targ, E., Moore, D., & Smith, H. (1998). A randomized double-blind study of the effect of distant healing in an advanced AIDS population. *Western Journal of Medicine, 169,* 356–363.

Simpson, J., & Weiner, E. (Eds.). (1989). *Oxford English Dictionary* (2nd ed.). New York: Oxford University Press.

Sloan, R. P., Bagiella, E., & Powell, T. (1999). Religion, spirituality, and medicine. *Lancet, 353,* 664–667.

Sloan, R. P., Bagiella, E., VandeCreek, L., Hover, M., & Casalone, C. (2000). Should physicians prescribe religious activities? *New England Journal of Medicine, 342,* 1913–1916.

Stifoss-Hanssen, H. (1999). Religion *and* spirituality: What a European ear hears. *International Journal for the Psychology of Religion, 9,* 25–33.

Strawbridge, W. J., Cohen, R. D., Shema, S. J., & Kaplan, G. A. (1997). Frequent attendance at religious services and mortality over 28 years. *American Journal of Public Health, 87,* 957–961.

Targ, E. (1997). Evaluating distant healing: A research review. *Alternative Therapies in Health and Medicine, 3,* 74–78.

Thomson, K. S. (1996). The revival of experiments on prayer. *American Scientist, 84,* 532–534.

Thoresen, C. E. (1998). Spirituality, health, and science: The coming revival? In S. Roth-Roemer, S. K. Robinson, & C. Carmin (Eds.), *The emerging role of counseling psychology in health care* (pp. 409–431). New York: Norton.

Thoresen, C. E. (1999). Spirituality and health: Is there a relationship? *Journal of Health Psychology, 4,* 291–300.

Thoresen, C. E., & Harris, A. H. (in press). Spirituality and health: What's the evidence and what's needed? *Annals of Behavioral Medicine.*

Tix, A. P., & Frazier, P. A. (1998). The use of religious scoping during stressful life events: Main effects, moderation, and mediation. *Journal of Consulting and Clinical Psychology, 66,* 411–422.

Travers, B. (1837). Observations on the local diseases termed malignant. *Medico-Chirurgical Transactions, 17,* 337.

Walsh, R., & Vaughn, F. (1995). *Paths beyond ego: The transpersonal vision.* New York: Plenum.

Worthington, E. L., Jr., Kurusu, T. A., McCullough, M. E., & Sandage, S. J. (1996). Empirical research on religion and psychotherapeutic processes and outcomes: A 10-year review and research prospectus. *Psychological Bulletin, 119,* 448–487.

Yates, J. W., Chalmer, B. J., St. James, P., Follansbee, M., & McKegney, F. P. (1981). Religion in patients with advanced cancer. *Medical and Pediatric Oncology, 9,* 121–128.

3

-◄(O)►-

RELIGIOUS INVOLVEMENT AND MORTALITY

Answers and More Questions

MICHAEL McCULLOUGH

The scientific study of the relationship between religion and mortality reaches back further than many might imagine. Indeed, scientists have been interested in the influence of religion on mortality and longevity for nearly 130 years. In 1872, Francis Galton (1822–1911), who was already well known for his groundbreaking research on scientific genius, reported the results of a study that sought to examine scientifically whether prayer had any objective influence on human mortality.

Galton began by assuming that certain groups of people—namely, ministers and missionaries—prayed more than did others. He reasoned that if prayer were efficacious, then "prayerful" people such as ministers and missionaries would most likely live longer than less prayerful people. So, when Galton (1872) found that ministers did not live substantially longer than did attorneys or physicians, he felt confident that he had adduced definitive evidence that prayer was not efficacious.

Galton also reasoned that the members of royal families were frequently the subject of people's prayers (e.g., "God save the queen!") and reckoned that if prayer were efficacious in deterring death, then sovereigns would typically live longer lives than other people as a result of the many prayers said on their behalf. Using actuarial tables, Galton demonstrated that members of royal houses actually had lower life expectancies than did people from other affluent sectors of English society (including lawyers, gentry, and military officers). Based on the unremarkable longevity of clergy and sovereigns, Galton (1872) concluded that no statistical evidence existed for the efficacy of prayer in promoting or preserving physical health.

Humble beginnings indeed to the scientific study of religion and mortality.

Another important figure in the history of social science who was interested in the links between religion and mortality was Émile Durkheim (1858–1917), the father of French sociology. Durkheim's lifelong intellectual project was to demonstrate how human phenomena can be explained at the sociological level, and in his book *Suicide*, Durkheim (1897/1951) argued that suicide was largely a sociological phenomenon rather than a psychological one. From this basic premise he reasoned that religions that encourage strong social ties and adherence to social norms should deter suicide, leading to low suicide rates among their practitioners, whereas religions that do not encourage strong social cohesion would be unable to generate the normative force necessary to deter suicide. To support this hypothesis, Durkheim adduced evidence that largely Roman Catholic European countries (e.g., Spain, Portugal, and Italy), which were presumed to foster stronger social ties and lifestyle prescriptions, had lower suicide rates than did largely Protestant European countries (e.g., Prussia, Saxony, and Denmark).

Galton's and Durkheim's thinking about possible links between religion and mortality has been influential. In the century after their initial work, scores of researchers have examined the links between religion and mortality (for reviews see Koenig, McCullough, & Larson, 2000; McCullough, Hoyt, Larson, Koenig, & Thoresen, 2000; McCullough, Larson, Koenig, & Lerner, 1999). In this chapter I review one dimension of the relationship between religion and mortality: the role of ordinal and interval levels of religious involvement (such as frequency of church attendance, belief in God, or frequency of prayer) as predictors of mortality.

ORGANIZATION OF THIS CHAPTER

This chapter is divided into three major sections. First, I briefly review the major findings from studies in which researchers have examined the associations between religious involvement and mortality. Second, I describe the results of a meta-analysis in which my colleagues and I summarized quantitatively the results from this area of research. Third, I outline what I believe to be the major questions still to be addressed in understanding the links between religious involvement and mortality.

IS RELIGIOUS INVOLVEMENT LINKED TO LONGER LIFE?

The studies that address the link between religious involvement and mortality can be divided roughly into two groups: (1) studies that have examined samples of basically healthy, community-dwelling adults; and (2) studies that have examined samples of medically ill adults.

Religious Involvement and Mortality in Community Samples

One of the first investigations of religious involvement and mortality in community-dwelling adults was conducted by Comstock and colleagues (Comstock & Partridge, 1972; Comstock & Tonascia, 1977) using data from an 8-year longitudinal study of residents of Washington County, Maryland. The primary measure of religiousness was a single-item measure of frequency of church attendance. Across the 8-year follow-up period, Comstock and colleagues found that frequent church attenders were significantly less likely to die than were infrequent church attenders, even after controlling for race, sex, age, marital status, education, the presence of a complete bathroom in the house, and cigarette smoking (Comstock & Tonascia, 1977). Earlier analyses had suggested that the religious involvement was related to reduced mortality resulting particularly from heart disease, emphysema, cirrhosis of the liver, and suicide (Comstock & Partridge, 1972).

Researchers (including Comstock and his colleagues) have criticized Comstock's results for failure to control for baseline health status. However, the study and its findings captured the interest of other researchers. After Comstock and Tonascia's (1977) groundbreaking study, a variety of researchers (e.g., Berkman & Syme, 1979; House, Robbins, & Metzner, 1982; Zuckerman, Kasl, & Ostfield, 1984) also conducted early investigations of the religiousness–mortality link.

Similar studies followed throughout the 1990s, with researchers from the United States (e.g., Hummer, Rogers, Nam, & Ellison, 1999; Koenig et al., 1999; Strawbridge, Cohen, Shema, & Kaplan, 1997) and Israel (e.g., Goldbourt, Yaari, & Medalie, 1993; Kark et al., 1996) conducting intensive examinations of the association of religious involvement and length of life in samples of community-dwelling adults.

Goldbourt, Yaari, and Medalie (1993), for instance, followed a sample of 10,059 male Israeli government workers for 23 years to examine the predictors of mortality. They assessed religious orthodoxy using a three-item measure consisting of (1) whether the respondent received a religious or secular education; (2) whether the respondent defined himself as "orthodox," "traditional," or "secular"; and (3) frequency of attending synagogue. Unadjusted data indicated that each standard unit increase in orthodoxy was associated with a 16% increase in odds of survival through the 23-year follow-up period (these data were adjusted for age but were not adjusted for other demographic, biomedical, and psychosocial variables).

More recently, Strawbridge et al. (1997) used 28-year data from the Alameda County study to examine the relationship between religious attendance and all-cause mortality. They found an association of mortality and religious attendance across the 28-year follow-up. Although adjustments for baseline health status accounted for some of the variance in the religious attendance–mortality relationship, the adjusted relationship was still significant, with a relative hazard = .67 (i.e., the probability of dying for highly religious people in any given year, given the number of respondents alive during the previous year, was only 67% as large as was the probability of dying during any given year for people who were less religious). Strawbridge et al. (1997) also found that people who frequently attended church at the beginning of the study were less likely to smoke or drink heavily than were people who attended church less frequently. They also had more social connections than did infrequent church attenders.

As important, Strawbridge et al. (1997) found that frequent church attenders were more likely to change their health behaviors for the better during the 28 years of the study. Even after adjusting for initial differences in health behaviors, frequent attenders were more likely to (1) quit smoking, (2) reduce their drinking, (3) increase the frequency with which they exercised, (4) stay married to the same person, and (5) increase their number of social contacts than were infrequent attenders. Thus initial differences in the health practices of frequent and infrequent church attenders did not tell the whole story: Religious attendance was related to *positive changes* in the study population's health behaviors, which might have been, in part, responsible for the relationship of religious attendance and mortality. Interestingly, religious people were significantly *more* likely to become obese during the 28 years of the study.

Hummer, Rogers, Nam, and Ellison (1999) reported the same basic finding. Using a nationally representative sample of more than 21,000 adults followed from 1987 to 1995, they examined the association of religious service attendance with survival. In 1987, respondents completed a single-item measure of frequency of attendance at religious services, along with a variety of other measures to assess demographics, socioeconomic status, health, social ties, and health behaviors. Hummer et al. (1999) found that frequency of religious attendance was positively related to length of life. For example, people of both sexes who attended religious services more than once per week were estimated to live for 62.9 years beyond age 20. For those who attended once per week, life expectancy beyond age 20 was 61.9 years. For those who attended less than once per week, life expectancy beyond age 20 was 59.7 years. Finally, for those who reported never attending religious services, the life expectancy beyond age 20 was 55.3 years. This represents a 7.6-year survival differential between the frequent attenders and the non-attenders.

After controlling for a variety of potential confounds and mediators that could explain the association of religious involvement and longevity (including age, gender, health, social status, social support, cigarette smoking, alcohol use, and body mass index), people who frequently attended religious services survived considerably longer than did people with lower levels of public religious activity. Indeed, people who reported never attending religious services had an 87% higher risk of dying during the follow-up period than did people who attended religious services more than once per week. People at intermediate levels of religious service attendance also experienced lower risks of death than did nonattenders.

Because of the large number of observations, Hummer and colleagues (1999) were able to examine the association of religious involvement and mortality from specific causes (including circulatory diseases, cancer, respiratory diseases, diabetes, infectious diseases, external causes, and all other causes). Religious attendance was associated with lower hazard of death from most causes, including circulatory diseases, respiratory diseases, diabetes, infectious diseases, and external causes. There was little evidence that religious involvement was related to reduced mortality from cancer. When demographics, health, socioeconomic status, social ties, and health behaviors were controlled, most of these survival differences became statistically nonsignificant, although the direction of the associations still indicated that frequent attenders were living slightly longer lives than were nonattenders. The fact that religious involvement was related to reduced mortality from so many causes led Hummer and colleagues (1999) to propose that religious involvement might actually be one of the "fundamental causes" of longevity (i.e., it works through such a multitude of pathways and mechanisms that controlling any single mechanism or cause of death does not cause the association to disappear).

Religious Involvement and Mortality in Clinical Samples

Along with the evidence derived from examinations of community-dwelling samples, researchers have also examined whether religious people have greater survival in the face of serious illness or medical procedures (e.g., Kune, Kune, & Watson, 1992; Oxman, Freeman, & Manheimer, 1995; Ringdal, 1996). Oxman et al. (1995), for instance, examined the 6-month survival of 232 older adults who had undergone elective open heart surgery.

Prior to surgery, patients were assessed on a variety of demographic, biomedical, and psychosocial variables, including depression, presence of mental disorder, social support, and impairment in basic activities of daily living. Oxman et al. (1995) found that people who reported not receiving strength and comfort from religion were considerably more likely to die during the 6 months following surgery than were people who reported receiving a great deal of strength and comfort from religion. This association persisted even after controlling for other biomedical and psychosocial variables (odds ratio [OR] = 3.25, $p < .05$). When four indicators of religious involvement (attendance at religious services, amount of strength and comfort derived from religion, number of people known in one's congregation, and self-rated religiousness) were combined into a single measure of religiousness, the relationship between religious involvement and odds of 6-month mortality fell to nonsignificance (OR = 0.82, $p < .05$), suggesting that perhaps some aspects of religiousness, but not others, are associated with mortality.

Of course, not all investigations of the association of religious involvement and mortality have revealed favorable associations (e.g., Idler & Kasl, 1992; Janoff-Bulman & Marshall, 1982; LoPrinzi et al., 1994; Reynolds & Nelson, 1981). For example, Koenig et al. (1998) examined whether the use of religion as a source of coping was a predictor of all-cause mortality in a sample of 1,010 older adult males who were hospitalized for medical illness. These 1,010 patients were followed for an average of 9 years. At the beginning of their involvement in the study, patients completed a three-item measure of the extent to which they used their religion to cope with stress. In both bivariate analyses and analyses that adjusted for demographic, social, and medical differences among the patients, those who relied heavily on religion for coping did not live any longer than did patients who did not rely heavily on religion for coping. Idler and Kasl (1992) reported similar results from analyses of a sample of basically healthy, community-dwelling adults.

Sifting the Evidence: A Meta-Analytic Review of the Research

As can be seen from this brief review, some studies on religious involvement and mortality have revealed positive associations, whereas others have not. Given this apparent inconsistency, the literature on religious involvement and mortality has the potential to generate a substantial amount of scientific controversy. To address this potential for controversy empirically, my colleagues and I (McCullough et al., 2000) conducted a meta-analytic review. Meta-analysis is a family of analytic tools for aggregating and making sense of the results of many different empirical studies (see Cooper & Hedges, 1994). After conducting an extensive search (using electronic data bases, searches through the reference sections of relevant studies, and leads from other investigators) for published and unpublished studies relevant to the topic, we retrieved 42 independent estimates of the association, or *effect sizes*, for religious involvement and mortality. These 42 estimates, or effect sizes, incorporated data from 125,826 people.

We coded these 42 effect sizes on a variety of variables, including (1) how religious involvement was measured; (2) percentage of males and females in the sample; (3) number of statistical adjustments made to the association; and (4) whether the sample was composed of basically healthy community-dwellers or medical patients. We also made a series of codings to represent whether each of 15 potential confounds and mediators of the religious involvement–mortality association were controlled (race, income, education, employment status, functional health, global health appraisals, clinical or biomedical measures of physical health, social support, social activities, marital status, smoking, alcohol use, obesity/body mass index, mental health or affective distress, exercise).

Using all 42 effect sizes (which were adjusted for a variety of covariates of religion and mortality in the studies from which we derived them), we found an association of religious involvement and mortality of OR = 1.29, indicating that religious people had, on average, 29% higher odds of survival during any follow-up period than did less religious people. Another way of saying the same thing is that religious people had, on average, only 1/ 1.29 (77.5%) odds of dying during any specified follow-up period compared with less religious people, adjusting for at least some covariates.

How robust is this finding? We calculated a fail-safe N for the omnibus analysis (k = 42 effects), which is a function of the z values associated with each of the effect sizes included in the meta-analysis. This revealed that 1,418 effect sizes with a mean OR of 1.0 (i.e., literally no relationship of religious involvement and mortality) would be needed to overturn the significant overall association of religious involvement and mortality (i.e., to render the resulting mean effect size non-significant, $p < .05$, one-tailed) that we found in our omnibus analyses. The large number of nonsignificant results that would be needed to overturn these findings makes it extremely unlikely that the association of religiousness and mortality that our meta-analysis revealed was due exclusively to having found an uncharacteristically favorable set of studies for inclusion.

These 42 effect sizes were not homogeneous, however. There was a considerable amount of variability among them, suggesting that the effect sizes might better be considered as estimates of more than one single population parameter. Because they were more variable than we could expect would be due to sampling error alone, we assumed that characteristics of the samples or the procedures used to collect and analyze the data could help to explain the inconsistency. Through a series of regression analyses, we found several variables that helped to explain these variations in effect size.

First, studies that used measures of public religious involvement (e.g., frequency of attendance at religious services, membership in religious social groups, membership in religious kibbutzim vs. secular kibbutzim) yielded consistently larger effect sizes than did studies that used private measures (e.g., frequency of private prayer, use of religious coping, etc.), measures that combined indicators of public and private religious involvement, and measures that could not be identified due to insufficient information in the study reports. Indeed, studies that used measures of public religious involvement yielded an omnibus effect size of OR = 1.43 (i.e., after controlling for covariates, people high in public religious involvement had 43% higher odds of being alive at follow-up). In contrast, the association of religious involvement and mortality for effect sizes that used nonpublic measures of religious involvement was nearly zero (OR = 1.04). This finding suggests that mortality is linked to involvement in public religious activity to a much greater extent than to measures of other dimensions of religiousness.

Another important predictor of effect size was the percentage of males in the study sample. The relationship between religious involvement and mortality was considerably stronger for women than for men. Indeed, we estimated that a sample with 100% males would yield an effect size of OR = 1.33, whereas a sample of 100% females would yield an effect size of OR = 1.59.

Finally, the degree of statistical control exerted over the religion–mortality association was negatively related to effect size. Better controlled studies (i.e., those including more covariates) yielded smaller associations. This result is quite intuitive: Adjusted effect sizes (after controlling for mediators or confounds) *should* be smaller than unadjusted effect sizes.

In a final set of analyses, we estimated how strong the relationship between public religious involvement and mortality would be if researchers were to conduct a study that controlled for all 15 of the potential covariates, mediators, and confounds that we identified. In such a study, one would expect an OR of 1.23, which indicates that people highly involved in public religious activities would be expected to have 23% higher odds of survival than would people who are less involved in religious activities, *even after controlling for a large array of potential covariates, mediators, and confounds*. In this final set of analyses, the OR of 1.23 was not statistically significant. The nonsignificance of this estimate was due to the fact that we were, in a sense, abusing the tools of multiple regression by estimating parameters for a relatively large number of highly correlated predictor variables with a relatively small number of effect sizes (24 in all). Indeed, the 15 predictor variables were so highly intercorrelated (a condition called multicollinearity) that it was mathematically impossible to arrive at a solution without throwing 3 of them out of the prediction equation altogether! The effects of such abuses of multiple regression on the certainty of one's parameter estimates are well known (e.g., Cohen, 1990), and so it is important to focus on the size and direction of the OR and not on whether it is *significantly different* from 1.0.

Magnitude of the Adjusted Association of Religiousness and Mortality

Our meta-analysis revealed that, on average, people who are highly religious have 29% higher odds of being alive at a given follow-up than do people who are less religious (after adjusting for some covariates). An OR of 1.29 corresponds to a tetrachoric correlation coefficient of $r_{tet} = .10$ (Davidoff & Goheen, 1953)—a "small" effect by Cohen's (1988) rules of thumb. The adjusted association is small, but does that mean that it is unimportant? One helpful way to portray the association of religious involvement and mortality is with Rosenthal's (1990) binomial effect size display (BESD; Rosenthal, 1990, 1991), which can be used to portray effect sizes in terms of the difference between two groups (100 people high in religiousness, 100 people low in religiousness) in the odds of dying, when the base mortality rate is 50%. If the OR of 1.29 derived from our meta-analysis is portrayed using Rosenthal's BESD, one sees that approximately 47 of the 100 people in the "highly religious" group would be dead at follow-up (53:47 odds in favor of surviving), whereas approximately 53 of the 100 people in the "less religious" group would be dead at follow-up (47:53 odds against surviving). Thus, among a group of 100 "religious" people and a group of 100 "less religious" people, we would expect six more of the religious people to be alive at the point in time when 50% of the sample had died.

The BESD obtained for the association of religious involvement and mortality can be compared with the BESDs obtained from examining how other psychosocial variables or medical interventions are related to all-cause mortality. Table 3.1 shows what the BESDs would look like for several other variables whose relations to all-cause mortality have been examined in recent meta-analyses. The BESD for participation in an exercise-based rehabilitation program following coronary heart disease (Jolliffe et al., 2000) is similar (see Table 3.1) to the BESD obtained for the association of religious involvement and mortality. Based on Jolliffe et al.'s (2000) effect size estimates, 54 people receiving only conventional cardiac care would be dead, whereas 54 people in an exercise-based rehabilitation program would still be living.

The BESDs obtained for the association of "hazardous" alcohol use (two to four drinks per day for women, four to six drinks per day for men) and mortality (Holman, English, Milne, & Winter, 1996) and for "harmful" alcohol use (more than four drinks per day for women, more than six drinks per day for men) and mortality (Holman et al., 1996) are of similar magni-

TABLE 3.1. Binomial Effect Size Displays for Several Variables Related to All-Cause Mortality

Religious involvement

Vital status at follow-up	Highly religious	Less religious	Total
Dead	47	53	100
Alive	53	47	100
Total	100	100	200

Exercise-based rehabilitation following coronary heart disease (Jolliffe et al., 2000)

Vital status at follow-up	Exercise rehabilitation	Conventional cardiac care	Total
Dead	46	54	100
Alive	54	46	100
Total	100	100	200

Hazardous levels of alcohol use (Holman, English, Milne, & Winter, 1996)

Vital status at follow-up	Abstainers	"Hazardous drinkers"	Total
Dead	45	55	100
Alive	55	45	100
Total	100	100	200

Harmful levels of alcohol use (Holman, English, Milne, & Winter, 1996)

Vital status at follow-up	Abstainers	"Harmful drinkers"	Total
Dead	42	58	100
Alive	58	42	100
Total	100	100	200

Cholesterol-lowering drugs among high-risk patients (Smith, Song, & Sheldon, 1993)

Vital status at follow-up	Treated	Untreated	Total
Dead	46	54	100
Alive	54	46	100
Total	100	100	200

tude. Cholesterol-lowering drugs also have an effect on all-cause mortality among high-risk patients (Smith, Song, & Sheldon, 1993) that is of similar magnitude (54 treated patients still alive; 54 untreated patients dead). These comparisons suggest that religious involvement has a small but nontrivial association with all-cause mortality that is only slightly smaller than the associations of other behavioral, psychosocial, and medical variables (e.g., exercise-based cardiac rehabilitation, abstention from alcohol use, and cholesterol-lowering drugs) with all-cause mortality. Once again, it should be noted that our mean effect size estimate represents the *net association* of religious involvement and mortality after primary-study authors controlled for a variety of demographic, psychosocial, and physical health variables at the highest level of stringency that they saw fit.

The point of presenting these binomial effect size display data is not to argue that the association of religious involvement and mortality is important only to the extent that it is "large" or even "moderate" by conventional (arbitrary) rules of thumb. I do not even present these data to argue that the association between religious involvement and mortality is "as important as" any other predictor of mortality. Rather, I present these estimates for two reasons: first, to put the size of the association into perspective, and second, to show that even a "small" association can be important, regardless of size, if the association involves criterion variables that are important to individuals or society. Is the association of religious involvement and mortality an important one? Ultimately, I suppose one's answer depends on whether one is among the three additional persons in the "highly religious" group who would have survived to follow-up or the three additional persons in the "less religious" group who would have died as of follow-up!

ANSWERS AND MORE QUESTIONS

The association between religious involvement and mortality appears to be quite robust. Even the best studies reveal a favorable association between religious involvement and mortality, and this association cannot be explained away by appealing to the argument that the association is due to confounding. Moreover, an improbably large number of additional studies showing no relationship between religious involvement and mortality would be necessary to overturn the basic conclusion that religiousness is related to lower mortality. Given the robustness of this association, it is probably accurate to say that the religious involvement–mortality association is one of the most well-established findings in the religion and health literature. Additional studies are unlikely to overturn this basic conclusion, although they would certainly be welcome. Given this robustness, researchers investigating religious involvement and mortality in the future should probably focus less on "proving" or "disproving" whether such a link exists and instead should focus on addressing several ancillary questions.

Why Public Religious Involvement But Not Private?

Our meta-analytic review demonstrated that the means by which religious involvement was measured played a big role in the magnitude of the religious involvement–mortality association. The favorable association of religious involvement and mortality was most marked in studies that used public religious activity to assess religious involvement. This finding is consistent with speculations that the health-related effects of religious involvement are due partially to the psychosocial resources derived from frequent attendance at religious services, membership in religious groups, or involvement with other (religious) people (Goldbourt et al., 1993; Idler & Kasl, 1997). These psychosocial resources might include: (1) positive emotional states that are engendered by public religious worship and activities; (2) the pleasurable social interactions that people experience during religious activities; and (3) the formation of beneficial personal relationships. If it is true that public religious involvement exerts a causal influence on longevity but that subjective religiousness, prayer, meditation, and particular religious beliefs do not, then this finding has great theoretical significance. However, given the typically high correlation between public and private indicators of religious involvement, it will take some effort to determine why some measures of religious involvement (i.e., public measures) but not others (i.e., private measures) appear to be related to mortality.

The results of Krause's (1998) study may shed some light regarding this point. Krause examined the association of religious involvement and mortality in a sample of 819 older adults who were followed for 4 years. Krause measured three dimensions of religiousness: (1) organizational religiousness (a three-item scale assessing attendance at religious services or activities); (2) nonorganizational religiousness (a two-item scale assessing reading of religious texts and tuning in to religious broadcasting), and (3) use of religion for coping with stress (a three-item scale assessing reliance on religious support and guidance for dealing with difficulties and important decisions).

When controlling for age, sex, education, marital status, self-rated health, functional disability, and stress, Krause found that the three measures of religiousness had different relationships with the probability of dying during the 4-year follow-up period. Every standard unit change in organizational religiosity was associated with a 12% reduction in the odds of dying during the follow-up period. Every standard unit change in nonorganizational religiousness was associated with a nonsignificant 1% reduction in the odds of dying during the follow-up period. Every standard unit change in religious coping was associated with a 15% *increase* in the odds of dying during the follow-up period. Therefore, it appeared that the favorable association of religious involvement and mortality was confined only to organizational religious involvement, whereas nonorganizational religiousness had no appreciable association with mortality and using one's religion to cope with stress was related to *greater* probability of mortality. Future research conducted similar to Krause's (1998) study could help considerably to untangle the important dimensions and causal dynamics of religious involvement and mortality.

Why Is the Link Stronger for Women?

As noted previously, our meta-analysis revealed that the association of religious involvement and mortality is stronger for women than for men. Indeed, several studies that examined the associations of religious involvement and mortality for men and women separately (e.g., Clark, Friedman, & Martin, 1999; House, Robbins, & Metzner, 1982; Kark et al., 1996; Koenig et al., 1999; Strawbridge et al., 1997) revealed stronger associations for women than for men.

Why do women appear to receive more "protection" against early death by religious involvement than do men? Is it because religion replaces some health-promotive resource (i.e., social support) for women that men typically receive through other routes? Is it because religion provides unique health-promotive resources that men typically do not receive at all from religious involvement? Kirkpatrick, Shillito, and Kellas's (1999) study illustrates this possibility. Kirkpatrick et al. surveyed 123 female and 61 male students to examine the associations between perceptions of having a relationship with God and loneliness. Even after controlling for standard measures of perceived social support, women who reported a close relationship with God were less lonely than were those who did not report having a close relationship with God. For men, on the other hand, beliefs about having a strong relationship with God were either unassociated or *positively* associated with loneliness. Similarly, Idler and Kasl (1992) found that religious involvement has a stronger negative relationship to depression and disability among women than among men. In any case, because women live longer and are more religious than men in most cultures (Levin & Chatters, 1998; Levin & Taylor, 1997), researchers in the future would be wise to control statistically for gender or to estimate models separately for men and women to prevent confounding with gender.

Does Personality Play a Role?

Could the association of religious involvement and mortality be an artifact of the overlap of religious involvement with personality traits that are related to increased longevity? For example, Friedman and colleagues (1995) have shown that conscientious people live considerably longer than do less conscientious people. Conscientious people may obtain their survival advantage by virtue of less engagement in risky behaviors such as fast driving, dietary excesses, and physical inactivity, or of a tendency to respond early to bodily signs of physical health problems.

Interestingly, conscientiousness is one of the most robust correlates of religiousness. Researchers have employed measures of the constructs in the Big Five or Five Factor Model (John & Srivastava, 1999; McCrae & Costa, 1999)—a taxonomy of personality traits that accounts for major higher order dimensions of personality—to examine the association of religiousness and personality. Both Kosek (1999) and Taylor and MacDonald (1999) found that measures of Agreeableness and Conscientiousness were positively associated with religious involvement and religious orientation. Indirect evidence for the link between religiousness and conscientiousness also comes from research using Eysenck's (Eysenck & Eysenck, 1985) Big Three taxonomy of personality traits. Cross-sectional studies using measures of the Eysenckian Big Three indicate that religiousness (as measured by a variety of indicators including frequency of attendance at worship services, frequency of private prayer, and positive attitudes toward religion) is related inversely to Eysenckian Psychoticism (e.g., Francis, 1997; Francis & Bolger, 1997). Eysenckian Psychoticism appears to be a conflation of Big Five Conscientiousness and Agreeableness (Costa & McCrae, 1995). I have data also showing that conscientiousness but *not* agreeableness in childhood and adolescence predicts public religious involvement and subjective religiousness in adulthood (McCullough, 2000). Given the robust links of conscientiousness with longevity, conscientiousness with religiousness, and religiousness with longevity, more work is needed to explore whether the health-promotive effects of religiousness are attributable to the correlation of religious involvement with conscientiousness or other personality traits. The relationships among religiousness, hostility, and mortality also should be explored, as some research suggests that religious people are less hostile (for review see Koenig, McCullough, & Larson, 2000) and that hostile people live shorter lives (Miller, Smith, Turner, Guijarro, & Hallet, 1996).

How Can We Model the Dynamics of Religious Involvement and Mortality?

Most of the studies conducted on religious involvement and mortality to date have used one general analytic framework for testing hypotheses: A variety of potential predictors of mortality—including religious involvement—have been included in a logistic or Cox regression model to predict vital status at a discrete follow-up point or to predict differences in continuous survival functions. Such methods have helped to instill confidence that people who are more religious at baseline do live longer and that these effects cannot be attributed entirely to the overlap of religiousness with factors such as gender, age, socioeconomic status, health, social support, and health behaviors. Moreover, by examining the reductions in the religious involvement–mortality relationship with the successive addition of variables such as social support, smoking, and alcohol use, researchers have been able to infer that religious involvement might exert its effects on mortality partially via such variables as social support, smoking, and alcohol use.

As useful as such studies have been, they are not maximally helpful for testing dynamic hypotheses. Assuming that the association of religious involvement and mortality is a causal one, it is important to identify the health-promotive mechanisms that religious involvement might stimulate to influence mortality risk. For example, it would be enlightening to investigate whether the association of religious involvement and mortality is mediated by improvements in social support or changes in health behaviors that occur in the years between the assessment of religious involvement and the ascertainment of mortality. If researchers are interested in whether religious involvement truly is involved in a causal chain that eventuates in longer life, then the next step in research might be to conduct studies that allow us to observe the health-promotive or life-extending mechanisms that religious involvement might put into place.

In addition to finding that people frequently involved in public religious activities live longer lives, Strawbridge and his colleagues (1997) demonstrated that frequent church attenders were more likely to (1) quit smoking, (2) reduce their alcohol intake, (3) increase the frequency with which they exercised, (4) stay married to the same person, and (5) increase their number of social contacts over a 28-year period. The next step will be to integrate hypothesis tests regarding such health-promotive changes and hypothesis tests regarding religious involvement and mortality into a single statistical model. Of course, testing such dynamic models will call for multiple waves of panel data.

How Are Religious Cognitions, Emotions, and Actions Involved?

In a related vein, it would be fruitful to include a level of psychological theorizing that is too often absent from empirical examinations of the religious involvement–mortality phenomenon. Many if not most researchers have assumed that religious involvement influences mortality by building a tendency for cognitions, emotions, or actions that lead to healthy lifestyles or increased competence for coping with stress (Ellison & Levin, 1998; Hummer et al., 1999; Idler & Kasl, 1992; Kark et al., 1996; Koenig et al., 1999; Krause, 1998; Oman & Reed, 1998; Strawbridge et al., 1997). Most theorists seem to agree, for instance, that religious involvement can lead people to acquire (1) personal *norms* regarding food, alcohol, tobacco, and sexual behavior; (2) a *coherent world view* that helps to provide meaning in times of stress and suffering; and (3) social support.

But most researchers have lacked data for examining how religion might promote such life-extending psychological resources. Rather, they have focused on demonstrating that after nearly every conceivable risk factor for mortality is controlled, religious involvement still predicts mortality. These early research questions have been perfectly appropriate, but now we need studies of how static indicators of religious involvement get translated into religious cognitions, emotions, and actions that promote longer life.

Without including such a level of analysis, this line of research—no matter how statistically sophisticated the studies are—will be theoretically unsatisfying in the long run. Presumably, all researchers concur that simply getting out of bed on Wednesday, Friday, Saturday, or Sunday morning to get to a church, synagogue, or mosque probably does not make people live longer. However, if researchers do not begin to propose and test more interesting substantive mechanisms for the association of religious involvement and mortality, then I doubt that this line of research will be interesting enough to attract future researchers. To add more theoretical depth to these investigations, researchers might endeavor to make connections between the low-level behavior of religious attendance and mortality through more meaningful psychological constructs. If religion *qua* religion is exerting an influence on mortality, there must be something special going on inside of churches, synagogues, and mosques or in the heads of religious people that leads to reduced mortality. What health-relevant positive affects are stimulated by public religious involvement? What health-related beliefs does religious attendance engender? What sorts of health-relevant choices does religious involvement lead people to make? What cognitions, affects, behaviors, or social interactions does religion stimulate that help people to cope better with the longevity-compromising effects of stress?

Perhaps an analogy will help. It is well established that religious adolescents are less likely to use drugs, tobacco, and alcohol than are their less religious counterparts (e.g., see Willis, Wallston, & Johnson, Chapter 9, this volume). D'Onofrio and colleagues (1999) attempted to account for these associations with two constructs: (1) the number of religious peers each respondent had and (2) respondents' beliefs about drug use being a sin. D'Onofrio et al. (1999) demonstrated that the association of religious involvement and drug use could be accounted for completely by numbers of respondents' religious peers and the strength of their beliefs about drug use being a sin. In other words, these data suggested that religious adolescents refrain from drug use because they interact with a high number of religious peers and because they believe that drug use is sinful. Similar models could be tested to account for the associations of religious involvement and mortality. Researchers should consider adding measures of religious cognitions, emotions, and actions that would allow them to examine whether (1) religious involvement leads to (2) psychologically meaningful but nonetheless religious processes that (3) eventuate in health behaviors or mental states that (4) promote long life. Of course, in addressing such an agenda, researchers will need data bases that include measures for assessing such religious cognitions, emotions, and actions. An added methodological twist comes from the fact that religious involvement might begin to create these psychological structures (e.g., beliefs, norms, and coherent world views) in childhood or adolescence for most people. Therefore, religious involvement might have caused people to obtain these psychological resources long before they might be included, as adults, in a longitudinal study of religion and mortality. To tackle these thorny issues, researchers may need to adopt explicitly developmental theorizing about the nature of the relationships between religious involvement and mortality.

Life Worth Living?

Another question raised by the existing research on religion and mortality relates to quality of life. Evidently, religious people are living slightly longer lives, but what is the quality of those additional years of life? Are they characterized by fulfillment, peace, and love, or are they characterized by disability, pain, and isolation?

Researchers have developed methods for "quality-adjusting" the increments in lifespan that can be attributed to psychosocial factors or medical interventions. The Quality-Adjusted Life-Years (QALY) metric integrates longevity with quality of life in a single expression (Kaplan, 2000; Shen, Pulkstenis, & Hoseyni, 1999). Experts are beginning to view such measures as fairer appraisals of the benefits associated with a particular health factor because they account for the trade-off between length of life and quality of life. Researchers in religion and mortality could implement these methods profitably in future research.

What about the Mortality Burden of Religion?

A final question that is raised by the religion and mortality literature relates to the negative effects of religious involvement on length of life. The association of public religious involvement and mortality, at least among adults, is on balance a positive one. However, some conservative religious groups eschew standard medical care, and refusal of such care apparently can lead to untimely and unnecessary death. For example, in a recent study, Asser and Swan (1998) reviewed the medical records of 172 cases of children who died as a result of religion-motivated medical neglect. The parents of these 172 children typically belonged to isolated Christian sects that objected to the use of modern medical care. Asser and Swan found that 140 (80%) of the 172 children died of ailments that would have had more than a 90% likelihood of being cured if proper medical care had been received. Another 18% of the children had ailments with a greater than 50% likelihood of being cured. Only 3 of the 172 children died of conditions that would not have responded positively to medical care. These findings correspond to other studies documenting excess child and adult mortality among members of religious groups that forgo standard medical care (e.g., Kaunitz, Spence, Danielson, Rochat, & Grimes, 1984; Simpson, 1989; Wilson, 1965).

In all research areas, researchers typically go for the "Big Story" first. The study of religion and mortality has been no different: Researchers have been concerned primarily with the net association of religious involvement and mortality across the entire population. As a result of such studies, we now can say with some confidence that, on average, people who are actively involved in public expressions of religion live longer than people who are not. However, such "average" associations might be masking other trends, such as a trend toward higher child and perinatal mortality among members of religious groups that eschew standard medical care. It would be scientifically productive and socially valuable to pour more effort into examining the role that religious faith might play in interfering with adequate self-care and the receipt of proper medical care. By addressing such issues, researchers interested in religion can use their skills in greater service of the common good. They might also add more intrigue and complexity to a plot that otherwise could quickly become rather predictable.

CONCLUSION

People do not pursue religion in order to lengthen their lives. Indeed, for many people from many faiths, "keeping the faith" caused them to die early deaths. Also, much of the violence of world history has been religiously motivated. Moreover, some religions persuade people to eschew modern medical care. As a result of all these factors, it would be naïve not to acknowledge that some manifestations of religion can exact a toll in terms of longevity. Nonetheless, in the population, the net association of religious involvement and longevity appears to be a positive one. Religiously involved people—particularly those who are involved in public expressions of religion—gain a substantial survival advantage over people who are not involved in a religion. These associations are considerably larger for women than for men. We cannot conclude that these associations are causal, but they do persist even when researchers exert reasonable care in ruling out potential sources of spuriousness.

Although these findings answer many questions, they raise new ones: What specifically about public religious involvement causes it to be such a robust predictor of longevity, whereas the link is much less remarkable for private religiousness? Why would the religion–longevity link be so much stronger for women than for men? How do standard personality factors— particularly those that are robust correlates of religious involvement and mortality—play a role? How can we gain a better understanding of whether religious involvement actually puts health-promotive psychosocial resources into place? What happens at a psychological level that would cause religious people to embrace health-promotive behaviors or mental states? Are the extra years of life afforded to religious people worth the wait? Finally, how can we better integrate the robust association of religious involvement and mortality with the fact that religion also can cut life short for some people? Addressing these questions would help to enrich our understanding of the diverse connections between religious involvement and length of life. By doing so, the state of the science will improve, as will its potential contribution to prevention and health promotion.

ACKNOWLEDGMENTS

Parts of this chapter were presented as the 2000 Margaret Gorman Early Career Award Address of Division 36 (Psychology of Religion) at the 108th annual meeting of the American Psychological Association, Washington, DC. I gratefully acknowledge the assistance of William T. Hoyt in preparing the binomial effect size displays.

REFERENCES

Asser, S. M., & Swan, R. (1998). Child fatalities from religion-motivated medical neglect. *Pediatrics, 101*(4, Pt. 1), 625–629.

Berkman, L., & Syme, L. (1979). Social networks, host resistance, and mortality: A nine-year follow-up study of Alameda County residents. *American Journal of Epidemiology, 109*, 186–204.

Clark, K. M., Friedman, H. S., & Martin, L. R. (1999). A longitudinal study of religiosity and mortality risk. *Journal of Health Psychology, 4*, 381–391.

Cohen, J. (1988). *Statistical power analysis for the behavioral sciences* (2nd ed.). Hillsdale, NJ: Erlbaum.

Cohen, J. (1990). Things I have learned (so far). *American Psychologist, 45*, 1304–1312.

Comstock, G. W., & Partridge, K. B. (1972). Church attendance and health. *Journal of Chronic Disease, 25*, 665–672.

Comstock, G. W., & Tonascia, J. A. (1977). Education and mortality in Washington County, Maryland. *Journal of Health and Social Behavior, 18*, 54–61.

Cooper, H., & Hedges, L. V. (Eds.). (1994). *The handbook of research synthesis.* New York: Russell Sage Foundation.

Costa, P. T., & McCrae, R. R. (1995). Primary traits of Eysenck's P-E-N system: Three- and five-factor solutions. *Journal of Personality and Social Psychology, 69*, 308–317.

Davidoff, M. D., & Goheen, H. W. (1953). A table for the rapid determination of the tetrachoric correlation coefficient. *Psychometrika, 18*, 115–121.

D'Onofrio, B. M., Murrelle, L., Eaves, L. J., McCullough, M. E., Landis, J. L., & Maes, H. H. (1999). Adolescent religiousness and its influence on substance use: Preliminary findings from the Mid-Atlantic School Age Twin Study. *Twin Research, 2*, 156–168.

Durkheim, E. (1951). *Suicide: A study in sociology* (J. A. Spaulding & G. Simpson, Trans.). New York: Free Press. (Original work published 1897)

Ellison, C. G., & Levin, J. S. (1998). The religion–health connection: Evidence, theory, and future directions. *Health Education and Behavior, 25*, 700–720.

Eysenck, H. J., & Eysenck, M. W. (1985). *Personality and individual differences: A natural science approach*. New York: Plenum.

Francis, L. J. (1997). Personality, prayer, and church attendance among undergraduate students. *International Journal for the Psychology of Religion, 7*, 127–132.

Francis, L. J., & Bolger, J. (1997). Personality, prayer, and church attendance in later life. *Social Behavior and Personality, 25*, 335–337.

Friedman, H. S., Tucker, J. S., Schwartz, J. E., Tomlinson-Keasey, C., Martin, L. R., Wingard, D. L., & Criqui, M. H. (1995). Psychosocial and behavioral predictors of longevity: The aging and death of the "termites." *American Psychologist, 50*, 69–78.

Galton, F. (1872). Statistical inquiries into the efficacy of prayer. *Fortnightly Review, 12*, 125–135.

Goldbourt, U., Yaari, S., & Medalie, J. H. (1993). Factors predictive of long-term coronary heart disease mortality among 10,059 male Israeli civil servants and municipal employees. *Cardiology, 82*, 100–121.

Holman, C. D., English, D. R., Milne, E., & Winter, M. G. (1996). Meta-analysis of alcohol and all-cause mortality: A validation of the NHMRC recommendations. *Medical Journal of Australia, 164*, 141–145.

House, J. S., Robbins, C., & Metzner, H. L. (1982). The association of social relationships and activities with mortality: Prospective evidence from the Tecumseh Community Health Study. *American Journal of Epidemiology, 116*, 123–140.

Hummer, R. A., Rogers, R. G., Nau, C. B., & Ellison, C. G. (1999). Religious involvement and U.S. adult morality. *Demography, 36*, 273–285.

Idler, E. L., & Kasl, S. V. (1992). Religion, disability, depression, and the timing of death. *American Journal of Sociology, 97*, 1052–1079.

Idler, E. L., & Kasl, S. V. (1997). Religion among disabled and nondisabled persons II: Attendance at religious services as a predictor of the course of disability. *Journal of Gerontology: Social Sciences, 52B*, 5306–5316.

Janoff-Bulman, R., & Marshall, G. (1982). Mortality, well-being, and control: A study of a population of institutionalized aged. *Personality and Social Psychology Bulletin, 8*, 691–698.

John, O. P., & Srivastava, S. (1999). The Big Five trait taxonomy: History, measurement, and theoretical perspectives. In L. A. Pervin & O. P. John (Eds.), *Handbook of personality: Theory and research* (2nd ed., pp. 102–138). New York: Guilford Press.

Jolliffe, J. A., Rees, K., Taylor, R. S., Thompson, D., Oldridge, N., & Ebrahim, S. (2000). Exercise-based rehabilitation for coronary heart disease [computer file].

The Cochrane Database of Systematic Reviews, 4. CD001800. Cochrane Collaboration.

Kaplan, R. M. (2000). Two pathways to prevention. *American Psychologist, 55,* 382–396.

Kark, J. D., Shemi, G., Friedlander, Y., Martin, O., Manor, O., & Blondheim, S. H. (1996). Does religious observance promote health? Mortality in secular vs. religious kibbutzim in Israel. *American Journal of Public Health, 86,* 341–346.

Kaunitz, A. M., Spence, C., Danielson, T. S., Rochat, R. W., & Grimes, D. A. (1984). Perinatal and maternal mortality in a religious group avoiding obstetric care. *American Journal of Obstetrics and Gynecology, 150,* 826–831.

Kirkpatrick, L. A., Shillito, D. J., & Kellas, S. L. (1999). Loneliness, social support, and perceived relationships with God. *Journal of Social and Personal Relationships, 16,* 513–522.

Koenig, H. G., Larson, D. B., Hays, J. C., McCullough, M. E., George, L. K., Branch, P. S., Meador, K. G., & Kuchibhatla, M. (1998). Religion and survival of 1010 male veterans hospitalized with medical illness. *Journal of Religion and Health, 37,* 15–29.

Koenig, H. G., Hays, J. C., Larson, D. B., George, L. K., Cohen, H. J., McCullough, M. E., Meador, K. G., & Blazer, D. G. (1999). Does religious attendance prolong survival? A six-year follow-up study of 3968 older adults. *Journal of Gerontology: Medical Sciences, 54A,* M370–M376.

Koenig, H. G., McCullough, M. E., & Larson, D. B. (2001). *Handbook of religion and health.* New York: Oxford University Press.

Kosek, R. B. (1999). Adaptation of the Big Five as a hermeneutic instrument for religious constructs. *Personality and Individual Differences, 27,* 229–237.

Krause, N. (1998). Stressors in highly valued roles, religious coping, and mortality. *Psychology and Aging, 13,* 242–255.

Kune, G., Kune, S., & Watson, L. (1992). The effect of family history of cancer, religion, parity, and migrant status on survival in colorectal cancer. *European Journal of Cancer, 28A,* 1484–1487.

Levin, J. S., & Chatters, L. M. (1998). Religion, health, and psychological well-being in older adults. *Journal of Aging and Health, 10,* 504–531.

Levin, J. S., & Taylor, R. J. (1997). Age differences in patterns and correlates of the frequency of prayer. *Gerontologist, 37,* 75–88.

LoPrinzi, C. L., Laurie, J. A., Wieand, H. S., Krook, J. E., Novotny, P. J., Kugler, J. W., Bartel, J., Law, M., Bateman, M., Klatt, N. E., Dose, A. M., Etzell, P. S., Nelimark, R. A., Mailliard, J. A., & Moretel, C. G. (1994). Prospective evaluation of prognostic variables from patient-completed questionnaires. *Journal of Clinical Oncology, 12,* 601–607.

McCrae, R. R., & Costa, P. T. (1999). A five-factor theory of personality. In L. A. Pervin & O. P. John (Eds.), *Handbook of personality: Theory and research* (2nd ed., pp. 139–153). New York: Guilford Press.

McCullough, M. E. (2000). *Religiousness and the Big Five: A multimethod longitudinal study.* Unpublished manuscript, Southern Methodist University, Dallas, TX.

McCullough, M. E., Hoyt, W. T., Larson, D. B., Koenig, H. G., & Thoresen, C. E. (2000). Religious involvement and mortality: A meta-analytic review. *Health Psychology, 19,* 211–222.

McCullough, M. E., Larson, D. B., Koenig, H. G., & Lerner, R. (1999). The mismeasurement of religion: A systematic review of mortality research. *Mortality, 4*, 183–194.

Miller, T. Q., Smith, T. W., Turner, C. W., Guijarro, M. L., & Hallet, A. J. (1996). A meta-analytic review of research on hostility and physical health. *Psychological Bulletin, 119*, 322–348.

Oman, D., & Reed, D. (1998). Religion and mortality among the community-dwelling elderly. *American Journal of Public Health, 88*, 1469–1475.

Oxman, T. E., Freeman, D. H., & Manheimer, E. D. (1995). Lack of social participation or religious strength and comfort as risk factors for death after cardiac surgery in the elderly. *Psychosomatic Medicine, 57*, 5–15.

Reynolds, D., & Nelson, F. (1981). Personality, life situation, and life expectancy. *Suicide and Life-Threatening Behavior, 11*, 99–110.

Ringdal, G. (1996). Religiosity, quality of life and survival in cancer patients. *Social Indicators Research, 38*, 193–211.

Rosenthal, R. (1990). How are we doing in soft psychology? *American Psychologist, 45*, 775–777.

Rosenthal, R. (1991). Effect sizes: Pearson's correlation, its display via the BESD, and alternative indices. *American Psychologist, 46*, 1086–1087.

Shen, L. Z., Pulkstenis, E., & Hoseyni, M. (1999). Estimation of mean quality adjusted survival time. *Statistics in Medicine, 18*, 1541–1554.

Simpson, W. F. (1989). Comparative longevity in a college cohort of Christian Scientists. *Journal of the American Medical Association, 262*, 1657–1658.

Smith, G. D., Song, F., & Sheldon, T. A. (1993). Cholesterol lowering and mortality: The importance of considering initial level of risk. *British Medical Journal, 306*, 1648.

Strawbridge, W. J., Cohen, R. D., Shema, S. J., & Kaplan, G. A. (1997). Frequent attendance at religious services and mortality over 28 years. *American Journal of Public Health, 87*, 957–961.

Taylor, A., & MacDonald, D. A. (1999). Religion and the five factor model of personality: An exploratory investigation using a Canadian university sample. *Personality and Individual Differences, 27*, 1243–1259.

Wilson, G. E. (1965). Christian Science and longevity. *Journal of Forensic Science, 1*, 43–60.

Zuckerman, D., Kasl, S., & Ostfield, A. (1984). Psychosocial predictors of mortality among the elderly poor: The role of religion, well-being, and social contacts. *American Journal of Epidemiology, 119*, 410–442.

4

-◄{O}►-

RELIGIOUS INVOLVEMENT
AND HEALTH OUTCOMES
IN LATE ADULTHOOD

Findings from a Longitudinal Study
of Women and Men

PAUL WINK

MICHELE DILLON

In recent decades social scientists have learned a lot about the relation
between religiosity and health outcomes. Several studies document either a
direct or an indirect effect of religious participation on various indicators of
physical and mental health. As noted by the authors of one recent review
of research on the religion–health connection, notwithstanding variations
across studies, there tends to be statistically significant salutary effects of
religious involvement on health (Ellison & Levin, 1998). Although some
readers may chafe at the incorporation of what might appear to be a
nonscientific variable into analyses of medical processes, it should be
remembered that social scientists treat religious beliefs and practices as
external social facts (Durkheim, 1912/1976). In this view, religion is a
sociocultural phenomenon subject to empirical investigation in the same
way as are other everyday cultural processes. Social scientists are not interested in establishing the rational validity of beliefs; rather, they seek to
understand the contexts in which discrete beliefs and practices develop and
their social and psychosocial implications.

The relation between religion and health is complicated and there is still a lot of uncertainty as to the specific ways and life contexts in which religious involvement matters. The complexity is in part due to the multi-dimensional nature of the two concepts being investigated. Health status and religious involvement, moreover, are not stable over the life course. Rather, multiple shifts are possible in a person's ranking on either or both variables at any given stage in the life cycle. Studying the link between health and religion therefore involves, as Idler (1995) has pointed out, interrelated processes of aging and shifts in health and religious involvement.

This chapter uses longitudinal data from the intergenerational studies established at the Institute of Human Development (IHD), University of California, Berkeley, in the 1920s. We use data spanning early adulthood and old age from a random sample of men and women to examine the relation between religiosity and health in late adulthood. Because health and religious participation vary over the adult life course, long-term longitudinal research designs, as others have noted (e.g., Ellison & Levin, 1998; Markides, 1983), are necessary to illuminate the relation between these two constructs. A major strength of the IHD study is that it has followed the same people over virtually their entire life course, from adolescence to their late 60s and mid-70s, yielding self-report data on religion and health for the study participants at four points in adulthood.

Several studies have documented the positive impact of religious beliefs and church attendance on health, adaptation, and life satisfaction among the elderly (e.g., Blazer & Palmore, 1976; Hunsberger, 1985; Idler, 1987; Idler & Kasl, 1992; Levin, Markides, & Ray, 1996; Markides, 1983; Morse & Wisocki, 1988). Most of these studies, however, are either cross-sectional (e.g., Levin, Taylor, & Chatters, 1994) or short-term longitudinal, that is, spanning less than 12 years (e.g., Idler & Kasl, 1992; Markides, 1983; Levin, et al., 1996; Markides, Levin & Ray, 1987). We do not know, therefore, whether the positive relation observed is due to the late-adulthood effect of religiosity on health or of changing health status on religiosity or whether in fact the effect of religiosity is one that can be predicted from religiosity at adolescence or in early or middle adulthood. This is also the case with the first and second Duke University Longitudinal Studies of Aging. The median age of the sample in the first study (Blazer & Palmore, 1976) was 70.8 years at the time of the first round of interviews (1955-1959), and the sample in the second study ranged in age from 55 to 80, with a mean of 67 years (Koenig, Siegler, & George, 1989; Koenig, Siegler, Meador, & George, 1990). We thus lack firsthand prospective data concerning the status of the participants' health and religious involvement prior to late middle adulthood.

In addition to the IHD study's longitudinal design, the composition of the sample population is advantageous to understanding the complexity of the relation between religion and health. The sample was randomly drawn; its population comes from the West, a region of the country that tends to be underrepresented in studies of health and religion; and its participants are relatively healthy. Many existing studies use purposive rather than random samples. Some studies, for example, rely on volunteers (e.g., Blazer & Palmore, 1976) and people selected from community and senior centers (e.g., Koenig, Kvale, & Ferrel, 1988; Morse & Wisocki, 1988) or rehabilitation clinics (Idler, 1995). These sampling biases clearly attenuate the generalizability of the subsequent analyses of the relation between religiosity and health. There is also a tendency, especially on the part of medical researchers, to focus their investigations on nonhealthy populations and to, for example, tie postsurgical recovery rates to the patients' concurrent religious practices without paying attention to differences in patients' long-term, presurgery religious habits (e.g., Oxman, Freeman, & Manheimer, 1995). A further source of bias is the fact that many studies rely on samples drawn from Southern communities (e.g., Koenig, 1997; Larson et al., 1989). The greater religiosity, denominational homogeneity, and theological conservatism of the South relative to the West or to the Northeast may accentuate the positive relation observed between religiosity and various physical and mental health outcomes in Southern populations than in communities in which the public valence of religion is less pronounced.

We use the IHD data to investigate the concurrent implications of religious participation on health in late adulthood and to explore longitudinally whether religious involvement in early and middle adulthood bolsters health and well-being in later life. Most of the studies conducted on religion and health focus on physical health and on mental health operationalized by indicators of depression, adjustment, and affective and cognitive dimensions of life satisfaction (e.g., Courtenay, Poon, Martin, Clayton, & Johnson, 1992; Ellison, 1991; Ellison, Gay, & Glass, 1989; Koenig, 1997; Levin et al., 1996; Markides et al., 1987; Morse & Wisocki, 1988). In this study, we broaden the definition of mental health to include additional measures of social adaptation such as generativity, ego integrity, and social functioning. After we first describe our sample, we devote the remainder of this chapter to the presentation and discussion of our results. We begin by briefly discussing our findings on the study participants' patterns of religious involvement across the life course (Dillon & Wink, 2000). Following that, we present concurrent and longitudinal data on the relation between religiosity in late adulthood and (1) physical health, (2) mental health narrowly defined as life satisfaction, and (3) mental health broadly defined to include various measures of psychosocial adaptation.

SAMPLE AND DATA

The data come from the intergenerational studies established by the Institute of Human Development (IHD) at the University of California, Berkeley, in the 1920s. The original sample was a randomly generated representative sample of newborn babies in Berkeley, California, in 1928–1929 and of preadolescents (aged 10–12) selected from elementary schools in Oakland, California, in 1931 (and who were born in 1920–1921). Both cohorts were combined into a single IHD study in the 1960s. The current sample (N = 154) is thus differentiated by cohort: 36% born in the early 1920s (N = 56) and 64% born in the late 1920s (N = 98). The sample is also differentiated by gender: 52% are women (N = 80) and 48% are men (N = 74). All but two of the participants are white. Participants were studied intensively in childhood and adolescence and have been interviewed in depth four times in adulthood: in *early adulthood* (30s; interviews conducted in 1958–1959), *middle adulthood* (40s; 1969–1970), *late middle adulthood* (mid-50s/early 60s; 1982), and most recently in 1997–1999. At the last interview phase, the participants were in their late 60s or mid- to late 70s (*late adulthood*). At each interview phase the participants also completed self-administered questionnaires.

The current sample size (N = 154) represents 81% of the original participants who are available for follow-up (i.e., who are still alive and could be located). Overall, the attrition rates for each follow-up study conducted have been comparatively low (see Clausen, 1993; Wink & Dillon, in press). Attrition analyses comparing those individuals who participated in the latest follow-up (1997/1999) with those who participated in the prior assessment (1982) and who declined to participate in the latest study phase showed few differences on key social and personality variables. The two groups did not differ in health, well-being, extraversion, and impulse control. The main difference was greater introversion among participants who declined to participate in the 1997–1999 follow-up study.

CHARACTERISTICS OF THE SAMPLE
IN LATE ADULTHOOD

Of the 154 participants interviewed in 1997–1999, 71% were living with their spouses or partners, 5% were living with other relatives, and 24% were living alone. Women were significantly more likely than men to be living alone. One-third of the sample (33%) rated their life satisfaction as very high, and a further 57% rated it as moderately high. The median household income for the sample was $55,000, and the median value of the home was $225,000. Gender or cohort did not differentiate the economic status of the household. The majority of the sample are Protestant in religious origins (69%), and 22% come from Catholic family backgrounds. Eight percent of the respondents grew up in nonreligious families, and two (1%) of the participants grew up in Jewish households. In late adulthood, fifty-six percent of the study participants said that religion was important or very important in their lives.

RELIGIOSITY

Religiosity Measure

The multidimensional nature of religious belief and behavior is well established. In assessing religiosity in the IHD study, we had to take into account the fact that the data came from assessments conducted at different time periods. Although the study participants were asked about religion at each interview, there was some variation in the specific questions asked from one interview time to another. At Adult Time 1 (1958–1959), the older cohort were asked open-ended questions about the place of religion in their lives, their church attendance habits, and their beliefs about God and the afterlife, and the younger cohort were asked to talk about their religious attitudes, beliefs, and practices. Following the merger of the two cohorts into a single study, at Adult Time 2 (1969–1970) and Adult Time 3 (1982), all participants were asked about church membership and attendance, attitudes toward religion and their beliefs about God and the afterlife. The interview at Adult Time 4 (1997–1999) contained several detailed questions on religion. Respondents were asked open-ended questions about their religious affiliation, church attendance, spiritual practices (e.g., meditation, reading), and experiences, and beliefs about God and life after death (see Dillon & Wink, 2000).

The inconsistent use of different questions in the IHD study means that we did not have a straightforward indicator of church attendance or of strength of belief in God. At each of the assessments, however, it was possible to rate the *importance of religion* in the lives of the participants as reflected by either their attendance at a place of worship or by the centrality of religion in their lives or both. Therefore, the religiosity of the study participants at each of the four assessments conducted in adulthood was coded using a 5-point scale ranging from a low of 1 (religion not important in the life of the participant) to a high of 5 (religion central to the life of the participant). More specifically, a score of 1 meant that religion played no part in the life of the individual, as indicated by an absence of church attendance and/or private prayer and/or by an explicitly stated lack of belief in God or the afterlife. A score of 2 was given if religion played a peripheral or marginal role, as reflected by sporadic attendance at a place of worship (a couple of times a year at most), occasional prayer, and/or uncertainty about the existence of God or the afterlife. A score of 3 indicated that religion had some importance for the participant, as reflected in occasional (e.g., monthly) church attendance, private prayer, and belief in God and the afterlife. The person, however, did not see religion as playing a central role in making sense of his or her life. A score of 4 indicated frequent church attendance (weekly or almost weekly); belief in God and the afterlife and/or religion played an important role for the person in making sense of his or her daily life. A score of 5 indicated frequent church attendance; belief in God and the afterlife, and/or religion played a central role for the respondent in making sense of life.

Two trained coders used this 5-point scale to rate independently the importance of religion for every participant for whom we had data across each of the four assessments in adulthood. The ratings were based on the interview segments that contained open-ended questions on religion and that were photocopied and assigned a discrete, randomly generated number that did not identify the participant or the year in which the interview was conducted (N = 149 participants times 4 assessments conducted in 1958–1959 [30s]; 1969–1970 [40s]; 1982 [mid-50s and early 60s]; and 1997–1999 [late 60s and mid-70s]). The correlations between the ratings of the two coders ranged from a low of .87 for late middle adulthood (mid-50s and early 60s) to a high of .94 for late adulthood (late 60s and mid-70s). The kappas ranged from a low of .63 for late middle adulthood to a high of .69 in early adulthood.

A comparison of scores on our measure of religiosity in late adulthood with participants' self-reported answers to the Duke Religious Index (DRI; Koenig, Parkerson, & Meador, 1997) showed that they were significantly intercorrelated. Scores on our measure had an average correlation (for total sample and for men and women) with the DRI self-reported church attendance of .87. This strong correlation indicates that our religiosity measure is virtually indistinguishable from the DRI measure of church attendance.

Changes in Religious Involvement over Time

Table 4.1 displays the intercorrelation between scores on religiosity for the 149 participants for whom we had data across all four adult time periods. The correlations ranged from a low of .67 between religiosity in early (30s) and older (late 60s and mid-70s) adulthood to a high of .82 between religiosity in late middle and older adulthood. This means that participants in our study tended to preserve their rank ordering on religiosity over the course of adult life. That is, those individuals who tended to score high on the measure of the importance of religion in early adulthood also tended to score comparatively high on this measure at other time periods.

TABLE 4.1. Rank Order Stability of Religiosity
across Four Age Periods

| | Religiosity | | |
Age of participants	2	3	4
30s	.75	.68	.67
40s		.82	.80
Mid-50s and early 60s			.82
Late 60s and mid-70s			—

Note. N = 149. All correlations significant at the .001 level or below.

Our sample showed significant mean group changes in religiosity over the life course. As shown in Figure 4.1, the importance of religion decreased significantly between early (30s) and middle (40s) adulthood for women. Men retained a relatively low level of religious involvement throughout the first part of adult life. The importance of religion increased significantly for all the participants between late middle and late adulthood (Dillon & Wink, 2000). In sum, although the men and women in this study tended to preserve their rank order in terms of the importance of religion in their lives, the sample as a whole showed a U-shaped trajectory in terms of their mean scores on religiosity across the adult life cycle.

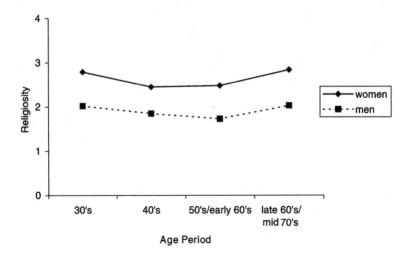

FIGURE 4.1. Mean levels of religiosity across four age periods for women and men.

RELIGIOSITY AND PHYSICAL HEALTH

In recent times, the relation between religion and physical health and mortality has been the object of much empirical investigation by both social scientists and epidemiologists (see Ellison & Levin, 1998; Hummer, Rogers, Nam, & Ellison, 1999; McCullough, Hoyt, Larson, Koenig, & Thoresen, 2000; Thoresen, Harris, & Oman, Chapter 2, this volume, for overviews). Notwithstanding diversity in conceptualization, sample populations, and methodological approaches used, many studies highlight the relevance of religion to the understanding of physical health outcomes. On closer examination, however, it is evident that there is still much ambiguity as to the pervasiveness, nature, and direction of this relationship. Some studies find a positive relationship between religiosity and *poor* health. For example, Courtenay et al. (1992) found a significant relationship between religiosity and some physical health problems in their study of 165 older Americans (aged 60 to over 100 years of age). In particular, they report that people with more severe health problems are likely to be more involved in the ritualistic dimension of religion.

Other cross-sectional studies of elderly populations find that there is a positive relationship between religiosity and *good* health (e.g., Ferraro & Albrecht-Jensen, 1991; Idler, 1987; Idler & Kasl, 1992; Levin & Markides, 1985). Idler (1987), for example, reports a positive association between greater religiosity and lower levels of functional disability. Although she cautions that a selection effect may be operating in that functional disability may prevent individuals from attending church, she also observes that functional disability is not entirely determinative of religious behavior. Other studies (e.g., Ainlay, Singleton, & Swigert, 1992; Levin & Markides, 1986) make a stronger case for attention to be given to the ways in which health impairments hinder church participation, especially that of the elderly, thus accentuating the positive association that may be found between religious involvement and good health.

Studies that have observed a direct positive effect of religion on physical health (e.g., Koenig, 1997; Levin, 1994; Strawbridge, Cohen, Shema, & Kaplan, 1997) point to the positive consequences that derive from the risk-averse lifestyle behaviors associated with frequent church attendance in general and specifically with membership in strict religious sects (e.g., Mormons and Seventh-Day Adventists) and denominations. Maintaining a low-fat diet, for example, or not smoking or drinking alcohol have a direct impact in protecting people from heart disease and cancer, the two major causes of death in the United States today. Researchers also emphasize the practical and social implications of religiously grounded values that emphasize moderation in personal habits (Ellison & Levin, 1998; Koenig, 1997). Thus some studies suggest that when confronted with stressful life events, elderly people who show higher levels of religiosity are less likely, for example, to drink alcohol than those who are less religious. In this view, religiosity rather than alcohol becomes the coping resource (Krause, 1991). Overall, there-fore, it may not be religiousness per se but the lifestyle practices and social consequences that stem from participation in a particular religion that, as first observed by Durkheim (1897/1951), provide sociocultural buffers against early mortality and the negative consequences of illness in general (cf. Idler, 1995; Idler & Kasl, 1992).

Measures of Physical Health in Late Adulthood

Several self-report and interview-based measures of physical health were available for the participants in late adulthood.

Self-Report Measures

The SF-36 Health Survey (Ware, 1993), a widely used self-report measure, includes seven scales assessing physical health and functioning (and two scales assessing emotional problems). The General Health scale evaluates the extent to which the respondent assesses his or her health as excellent. The Reported Health Transition scale measures the degree to which the individ-ual believes that his or her health is much better now than one year ago. The Physical Functioning scale assesses the ability to perform physical activities without limitations due to health. The Role-Physical scale measures the degree to which the person is free of problems in work or daily activity as a result of physical health. The Bodily Pain scale reflects the absence of pain or limitations due to pain. The Vitality scale measures the degree to which the person feels full of pep and energy. Finally, the Social Functioning scale reflects the degree to which the person is able to perform normal social activities without interference due to physical or emotional problems.

The Duke University Health Measure (DHM) is a self-report measure that uses a 5-point scale to assess both the presence and severity of a list of 22 major health problems (e.g., heart disease, diabetes, cancer, lung disease, and stroke).

Interview-Based Measures

As part of the in-depth interview, the study participants were asked several open-ended questions about their current state of health and health history. They were asked to list health problems and medications taken, to state the frequency of visits to a doctor and hospital or clinic within the past 12 months, and to describe their patterns of alcohol consumption and cigarette use. The participants used a 5-point scale to rate their subjective health compared with other people their age. The interview also included the Activities of Daily Living (ADL) measure that uses a 3-point scale to assess the level of difficulty that people have with such daily activities as dressing, walking, and remembering things.

The health section of the interview, along with the DHM, was used to rate reliably on a 4-point scale the participants' General Health Status (Belloc, Breslow, & Hochstim, 1971) by two trained coders (kappa = .68). The health status measure has been used to assess health functioning in relatively healthy populations in previous research (e.g., Adams, Cartwright, Ostrove, Stewart, & Wink, 1998). A score of 1 indicated no physical complaints; a score of 2 indicated the presence of minor physical illnesses (e.g. back pain, high levels of cholesterol, or high blood pressure controlled by medication); a score of 3 indicated the presence of one chronic illness (e.g., diabetes, heart disease, cancer diagnosed within the past 5 years); and a score of 4 indicated the presence of two or more chronic illnesses.

Health Findings in Late Adulthood

General Health of the Participants

The study participants were relatively healthy. During the interview, almost 9 out of 10 (89%) described their health as good or moderately good, and 93% described their energy levels as good. Sixty-five per cent evaluated their energy levels as being higher compared with others their age, and 29% rated their energy levels as average. Only 10% of the sample reported smoking regularly. By contrast, the majority of the respondents (77%) drank some alcohol, with 50% of these drinking on a daily basis. On the General Health Status scale, 25% of the participants were rated as having no health complaints; 39% were rated as having minor ailments (e.g., arthritis or blood pressure that was under control with medication); 31% had one chronic illness (e.g., diabetes, cancer, cardiovascular problem); and 5% had two or more chronic illnesses.

As expected, members of the younger cohort were rated as having better general health, $t(148) = 2.98$, $p < .01$. They also reported fewer problems with daily activities due to physical problems, $t(132) = 3.02$, $p < .01$, and less bodily pain, $t(132) = 2.30$, $p < .05$, than those in the older cohort. Men reported better physical functioning, $t(132) = 2.38$, $p < .05$, less impairment of social functioning due to health problems, $t(131) = 2.23$, $p < . 05$, and fewer problems in activities of daily living, $t(132) = 2.55$, $p < .05$, than women.

Relationship between Religiosity and Physical Health in Late Adulthood

Table 4.2 presents findings for the whole sample on the concurrent relationship between religiosity and various measures of physical health for late adulthood. (Note that the N is reduced to 132 participants for whom we had both ratings of religiosity and self-reported health data.) The main finding from these analyses is the virtual absence of a significant relationship between religiosity and either subjective or objective physical health measures. A similar pattern (not shown) emerged in analyses using the disaggregated measures of frequency of church attendance and of intrinsic religiosity taken from the Duke Religious Index (Koenig et al., 1997).

On the SF-36 Health Survey, the only significant finding was a positive relationship between religiosity and scores on the Reported Health Transition scale for the total sample and for women. In other words, highly religious women tended to report their current health as being better than it was a year ago. There was no relation between religiosity and the remaining six scales of the SF-36 Health Survey, subjective ratings comparing health

TABLE 4.2. Correlations between Religiosity and Physical Health in Late Adulthood

Physical health in late adulthood	Total	Women	Men
		Religiosity	
		Self-report measures	
SF-36 Health Study Survey			
General Health	−.00	.04	−.09
Reported Health Transition	.26***	.39**	.07
Physical Functioning	.00	.09	.00
Role-Physical	−.04	.08	−.12
Bodily Pain	−.07	.12	−.24
Vitality	.04	.19	−.08
Social Functioning	.04	.22	−.07
		Interview measures	
General Health Status	.04	−.01	.10
ADL	.01	−.19	.17
Subjective Health	.11	.20	.05
Alcohol Use	−.26***	−.28*	−.18

Note. N = 132 for the total sample; N = 71 for women and N = 61 for men. ADL, Activities of Daily Living scale.
*p ≤ .05; **p ≤ .01; ***p ≤ .001; two tailed.

with other same-age adults, or the ADL. As expected, highly religious individuals reported drinking less alcohol than nonreligious individuals. Religious involvement was also unrelated to the observer-based rating of general health status.

We repeated the correlational analyses reported in Table 4.2, breaking down our sample by cohort and denominational origins (Protestant or Catholic). Once again, we found few significant effects. For the older cohort, there was a significant negative correlation between religiosity and alcohol use, and there was a significant positive relationship with the SF-36's Reported Health Transition scale.

The Reported Health Transition scale was also significantly related to religiosity among both Protestants and Catholics. A significant negative effect of religiosity on alcohol use was true for the Protestants but not for the Catholics.

Predicting Health Outcomes in Late Adulthood from Religiosity in Early and Middle Adulthood

Although our analyses of the cross-sectional relationship between religiosity and physical health in late adulthood showed few significant effects, this does not preclude the possibility that an individual's investment in religious capital (e.g., Iannaccone, 1990) earlier in the life course has an impact on health in later adulthood. We now explore the relationship between physical health in late adulthood and religiosity earlier in life using the same set of self-report and interview-based health measures as used in the analyses described in the previous section. Our measure of religiosity consists of ratings of the construct taken from interview material obtained from assessments conducted in early (30s), middle (40s), and late middle (mid-50s and early 60s) adulthood.

Table 4.3 presents longitudinal analyses of the relation between religiosity in early (30s), middle (40s), and late middle (mid-50s and early 60s) adulthood and physical health in late adulthood (late 60s and mid-70s).

As in the case of the concurrent analyses, there were few significant longitudinal relationships between religiosity in early and middle adulthood and health outcomes in older age. For the total sample the only consistent finding was a positive relationship between religiosity at all three preceding time periods and scores on the SF-36's Reported Health Transition scale. This means that the tendency of participants in late adulthood to be optimistic about their health can be predicted from religious involvement as early as young adulthood (30s). There was also a consistent negative relation between religiosity and alcohol use.

Gender analyses revealed that the negative relationship between religiosity and alcohol use tended to be true of both men and women. The posi-

TABLE 4.3. Correlations between Religiosity in Early, Middle, and Late Middle Adulthood and Physical Health in Late Adulthood

Physical health in older age	Religiosity								
	Total			Women			Men		
	30s	40s	50s	30s	40s	50s	30s	40s	50s
Self-report measures									
SF-36 Health Survey									
General Health	−.04	−.00	.01	−.06	.07	.10	−.06	−.17	−.17
Reported Health Transition	.19*	.26**	.26**	.32**	.40**	.34**	.02	.02	.11
Physical Functioning	−.12	−.03	.04	−.04	.10	.22	−.09	−.13	−.10
Bodily Pain	−.12	−.07	−.03	.05	.10	.22	−.25*	−.24*	−.31*
Vitality	−.03	.07	.07	.16	.23	.27*	−.22	−.13	−.19
Role-Physical	−.02	−.02	.02	.11	.11	.19	−.08	−.14	−.15
Social Functioning	−.04	.07	.10	.16	.30*	.30*	−.20	−.20	−.07
Interview measures									
General Health Status	.08	.04	−.00	.04	−.06	−.14	.14	.17	.19
ADL	.22***	.06	.02	.06	−.11	−.15	.38***	.23	.20
Subjective Health	.04	.12	.10	.06	.26*	.25*	.05	.08	.11
Alcohol Use	−.19*	−.30**	−.25**	−.18	−.26*	−.22	−.16	−.33**	−.26*

Note. N ranges from 131 to 148 for the total sample; N ranges from 70 to 78 for women, and N ranges from 61 to 72 for men. ADL, Activities of Daily Living scale.
*$p \leq .05$; **$p \leq .01$; *** $p \leq .001$; two-tailed.

tive relationship over time between religiosity and scores on the Reported Health Transition scale was true only for women. There was also a positive relationship for women between religiosity in middle and late middle adulthood and the social functioning scale and ratings of subjective health in late adulthood. In the case of men, the absence of bodily pain in late adulthood was predicted by the degree of religiosity in early, middle, and late middle adulthood.

Supplemental analyses of the sample broken down by cohort and denomination (Protestant/Catholic) did not add to our understanding of the longitudinal relationship between health and antecedent religiosity already discussed. The only exception was the finding that lower levels of alcohol use in older age were predicted by antecedent religiosity for Protestants.

In sum, our longitudinal findings of a relationship between religiosity and lower consumption of alcohol and a positive outlook on health for women replicate over time the concurrent findings presented in Table 4.2. In the case of men there was a negative relationship between religious involvement and body pain longitudinally but not concurrently.

RELIGIOUS INVOLVEMENT
AND LIFE SATISFACTION

Empirical studies documenting a positive relationship between religion and mental health or life satisfaction are extensive (see Ellison & Levin, 1998; Levin & Chatters, 1998; Plante & Sharma, Chapter 10, this volume, for recent reviews). Overall, there is strong and compelling evidence that people who have higher levels of religiosity have higher levels of well-being and life satisfaction (e.g., Ellison, 1991; Koenig, 1997). Many studies document a strong positive relationship between religious involvement and some coping behaviors in response to negative life events (e.g., Courtenay et al., 1992; Koenig, Siegler, & George, 1989; Koenig, Siegler, Meador, & George, 1990; Pargament, 1997; Pargament et al., 1990; Sherman et al., 2001). Coping is clearly intertwined with personality differences and social circumstances. Yet it is also the case that trust in God, or openness to spiritual growth experiences, can enhance an individual's ability to manage traumatic events (Ellison, 1991), including life-threatening cancer (Sherman & Simonton, Chapter 7, this volume) and AIDS (Remle & Koenig, Chapter 8, this volume). It also appears that a strong religious sensibility can direct attention away from the physical self towards the nonphysical self and as a consequence nurture self-esteem and life satisfaction among those who have physical disabilities (Idler, 1995).

On the other hand, as Sherman and Simonton discuss (Chapter 7, this volume), some individuals may respond to a life-threatening illness by questioning or turning away from religion (negative religious coping). But as they also note, religious crises during times of adversity may have very different outcomes in the short term than in the long term. Other studies show that church attendance, independent of health status and other correlates of life satisfaction, has an increasingly positive effect on life satisfaction over time (Levin et al., 1996; Markides, 1983). Positive religious feelings, despite a decline in religious activities, have also been shown to have a strong impact on happiness and adjustment, especially for older people (Blazer & Palmore, 1976).

In spite of the robust findings linking religiosity to life satisfaction, there is ambiguity as to whether this effect is evident among all older adults or whether it is restricted to samples of individuals who have suffered some form of adversity. In other words, we are uncertain whether religion buffers life satisfaction both when things go well and when things go poorly in life or whether it is only in the latter eventuality. This uncertainty is due, in part, to the fact that several of the studies that report a positive effect of religiosity on mental health rely on data from purposive rather than random samples (e.g., Blazer & Palmore, 1976; Koenig et al., 1988; Morse & Wisocki, 1987; Pargament et al., 1990). For example, people who already have a physical disability and who attend a rehabilitation clinic (Idler, 1995) may be more primed than relatively healthy individuals to find new sources of self-esteem in religious involvement.

In the case of the IHD study participants, the relatively healthy nature of the sample may dampen the relevance of religiosity as a buffer of mental health simply because of a ceiling effect or because untroubled individuals do not need religion to feel good about themselves. If this is the case, then we may not find a direct relation between religiosity and measures of life satisfaction, but the two constructs may still be related in an indirect way. For example, religiosity may act as a buffer in protecting self-esteem only among individuals who have poor physical health. For these individuals, the feelings of meaninglessness or anomie that are triggered by adversity may be cushioned by the cognitive and social resources they have access to as part of their religious involvement. In this view, religious participation provides an external structure (Berger & Luckmann, 1966) from which participants derive personal meaning and communal solidarity in their adversity. If this is true, then we should expect significant interaction effects between physical health and religiosity as predictors of life satisfaction in older age.

It is also uncertain whether religiosity has the same effect on life satisfaction for men and women. Because women tend to be more religiously involved than men (Hout & Greeley, 1987; McFadden, 1996), it may be the case that they also derive more benefit from involvement in organized religion.

Measures of Religious Involvement and Life Satisfaction

Life Satisfaction Measures

We assessed life satisfaction with the Life Satisfaction Index (LSI; Neugarten, Havighurst, & Tobin, 1961). This 11-item self-report measure uses a 6-point scale to assess three dimensions of satisfaction with life (Liang, 1984). The Mood Tone subscale assesses the individual's current level of happiness with self; the Zest subscale measures the degree to which a person has an optimistic and positive outlook on life in the present and in the future; and the Congruence subscale assesses the extent to which a person thinks that he or she has attained desired goals. The LSI was available for 118 participants.

Measures of Religiosity and General Health Status

Religiosity in early, middle, late middle, and late adulthood and general health status in older adulthood were assessed with the measures discussed in the preceding sections. Physical health in middle adulthood, a covariate used in our longitudinal analyes, was assessed using a self-report scale that asked the participant to evaluate his or her own health on a 4-point scale (1 = severe impairment, restricting activities and behavior, 4 = no problems, excellent health).

Concurrent Relationship between Life Satisfaction, Religiosity, Physical Health, and Gender in Late Adulthood

To explore the hypothesis that religiosity had a differential effect on life satisfaction depending on level of physical health and gender, we conducted four 3-way ANOVAs with scores on the global LSI and its three subscales (Mood Tone, Zest, and Congruence) as dependent variables and religiosity, health status, and gender as the three independent factors. For the purpose of these analyses we grouped our participants into those who were either high (2.5 or above; $N = 53$) or low (below 2.5; $N = 65$) on the 5-point measure of religiosity. The second grouping comprised individuals who were either in good (score of 2 or below; $N = 77$) or poor (score above 2; $N = 41$) health on the 4-point General Health Status scale. The third grouping split the sample into men ($N = 59$) and women ($N = 59$). Our primary interest was in the main effect of religiosity on life satisfaction (an index of the direct relation between religiosity and life satisfaction in late adulthood), the two-way interactions between religiosity and physical health and religiosity and gender, and the three-way interaction between religiosity, physical health, and gender. (The interaction terms represent indices of an indirect relation between religiosity and life satisfaction as moderated by health status and gender).

In the case of the overall LSI, the three-way analysis of variance resulted in nonsignificant main effects of religiosity, $F(1,110) = 1.22$, physical health, $F(1,110) = 1.64$, and gender $F(1,110) = .014$. Among the two-way interactions, there was a significant joint effect of physical health and religiosity in predicting scores on the LSI, $F(1,110) = 6.11$. As shown in Figure 4.2, this interaction was due to a crossover effect, with nonreligious individuals who were in poor health showing the lowest levels of overall life satisfaction. Individuals high in religion and in poor health showed the highest levels of satisfaction. A follow-up t-test analysis revealed that there was a statistically significant difference, $t(39) = 2.31$; $p < .05$, in levels of life satisfaction among the two groups of individuals in poor physical health (but who differed in religion). Among individuals in good health, the difference in life satisfaction between the religious and nonreligious participants was not significant; $t(75) = .47$; n.s. The remaining two-way interactions between religiosity and gender and gender and health and the three-way interaction were all not significant.

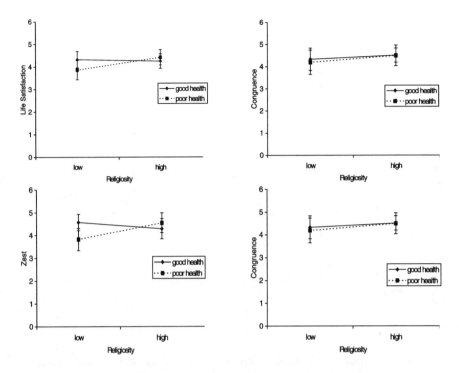

FIGURE 4.2. Levels of overall life satisfaction, mood tone, zest, and congruence in older age as functions of religiosity and health status in older age.

The same pattern of results was found for the Mood Tone and Zest subscales of the LSI. In both instances, there were no significant main effects, but there was a significant interaction between religiosity and physical health: $F(1,110) = 4.16$, $p < .05$, and $F(1,110) = 11.73$, $p = .001$, for Mood Tone and Zest, respectively (see Figure 4.2). Follow-up t-tests revealed that the interactions were due to differences in mood tone and zest between the highly religious and nonreligious participants who were in poor physical health: $t(39) = 1.81$, $p = .08$, and $t(39) = 2.47$, $p < .05$, for Mood Tone and Zest, respectively.

In the case of the Zest subscale, there was a significant interaction effect of religion and gender, $F(1,110) = 5.60$, $p < .05$ (see Figure 4.3). This interaction effect was due to the fact that highly religious women tended to score higher on the Zest subscale than women who were low in religiosity. The reverse pattern, however, was true for men.

For the Congruence subscale, there were no significant main effects or interactions.

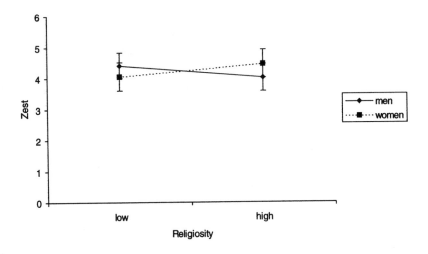

FIGURE 4.3. Levels of zest in older age as a function of religiosity in older age and gender.

In sum, these cross-sectional findings indicate that in our study religiosity did not have a direct effect on life satisfaction in late adulthood. Among individuals who were in poor physical health, however, those who were religious tended to be happier (more positive mood tone) and more optimistic (zestful) about the present and the future than those who were not religious. Religiosity did not have the same effect on life satisfaction for the majority of the participants in this study who were in good health and who showed high levels of life satisfaction irrespective of their religious status. Our results, therefore, support the hypothesis that religiosity may have a buffering effect on life satisfaction during times of personal adversity.

The findings also suggest that religiosity has a varied effect depending on the aspect of life satisfaction being measured. Thus, although religiosity appeared to have a buffering effect on levels of happiness and optimism about life among individuals who had to deal with physical illness, it did not have the same effect on feelings of congruence between one's expectations and goal attainment.

Finally, we found support for the hypothesis that religiosity may have a differential effect on life satisfaction among women and men. This was exemplified by the fact that it was highly religious women and, unexpectedly, nonreligious men who showed highest levels of optimism about the present and future.

Long-Term Effects of Religiosity on Life Satisfaction in Late Adulthood

Although we found a significant positive cross-sectional effect of religion on life satisfaction among individuals who suffered from physical problems in late adulthood, the concurrent nature of this finding renders its interpretation ambiguous. On the one hand, it could be argued that the findings described in the preceding section document a buffering effect of religion on life satisfaction in times of personal adversity (poor health). On the other hand, it could be the case that individuals who are highly satisfied with their lives in older adulthood tend to respond to major illnesses by becoming more religious. We now turn to the longitudinal data to obtain a better understanding of the temporal relation between religiosity and life satisfaction.

We repeated the three-way ANOVAs assessing the effect of religiosity (high vs. low) on life satisfaction among individuals who were either in good or poor physical health in older age and among men and women. This time we used measures of the importance of religion in middle (40s) and late middle (50s and early 60s) adulthood (as opposed to late adulthood) as our indices of religiosity. We also included subjective ratings of health in middle and late middle adulthood as covariates for two reasons. First, we wanted to make sure that we controlled for antecedent health status in interpreting the buffering effect of religiosity on life satisfaction among the group of participants who were in poor health in late adulthood. Second, because we used subjective ratings of health as covariates, we also hoped to control for the general sense of optimism or life satisfaction that is likely to be associated with feeling positively about one's health. The dependent variables were the LSI and its three subscales (Mood Tone, Zest, and Congruence). Again our interest was in the main effect of religiosity and the two-way and three-way interaction effects among religiosity and physical health and gender.

The three-way ANOVAs using religiosity in middle and late middle adulthood as predictors of life satisfaction in older age yielded the same results. We therefore only report the findings obtained using religiosity in middle adulthood as the independent variable. Our decision to do so was guided by the fact that predicting life satisfaction in late adulthood from data collected in middle adulthood involved a time interval of close to 30 years. The time span for analyses using measures of religiosity from late middle adulthood involves only 15 years.

In the three-way ANOVA using scores on the overall LSI as the dependent variable, there was a significant effect of the covariate, $F(1,95) = 5.12$, $p < .05$. In other words, as expected, life satisfaction in late adulthood was predicted by subjective ratings of health in middle adulthood. After controlling for the covariate, the main effects of religiosity in middle adulthood, health status in late adulthood, and gender were not significant. Among the two-way interactions, there was a significant joint effect of religiosity and health status on the LSI, $F(1,95) = 4.85$, $p < .05$. As shown in Figure 4.4, this interaction effect was due to the fact that among individuals who were physically ill in late adulthood, those who were rated as highly religious in middle age tended to score higher on the LSI than those individuals who were rated as low in religiosity, $t(38) = 1.87$, $p < .07$. Among individuals in good health, religiosity did not have an effect on levels of life satisfaction, $t(62) = .64$, n.s.

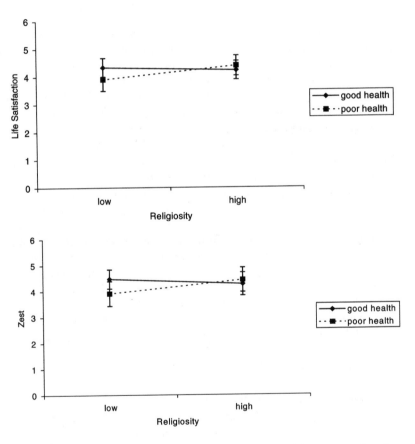

FIGURE 4.4. Level of overall life satisfaction and zest in older age as a function of religiosity in middle adulthood and health status in older age controlling for health in middle adulthood.

The same significant two-way interaction between religiosity and health status was found for the Zest subscale of the LSI, $F(1,95) = 5.87$, $p < .05$ (see Figure 4.4). As was the case with the overall LSI, the interaction effect was due to a marginally significant difference in zest or feelings of optimism between religious and nonreligious participants who were in poor physical health, $t(40) = 1.68$, $p = .10$, but there was no difference among participants who were in good physical health, $t(62) = 1.00$, n.s. The only other finding for the Zest subscale was a significant two-way interaction between religiosity and gender, $F(1,95) = 4.03$, $p < .05$ (see Figure 4.5). As was the case in the concurrent analysis described in the previous section, this interaction was due to a crossover between men and women, with highest levels of optimism being demonstrated by highly religious women and men who were low in religiosity.

The three-way ANOVAs using the Mood Tone and Congruence subscales of the LSI resulted in no significant main effects of religiosity, health status, or gender. None of the interactions was significant.

Finally, we repeated the four 3-way ANOVAs with LSI and its three subscales as dependent variables, using religiosity in early adulthood (30s), health status in late adulthood, and gender as independent variables. We were interested in finding out whether the buffering effect of religiosity on life satisfaction among individuals in poor health could be predicted over a time period of close to 40 years. The four ANOVAs did not result in any sig-

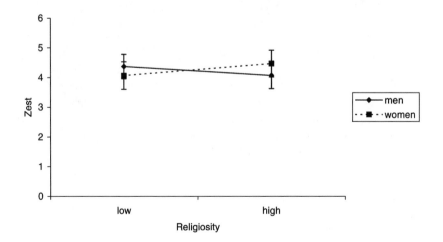

FIGURE 4.5. Level of zest in older age as a function of religiosity in middle adulthood and health status in older age, controlling for health in middle adulthood.

nificant main effects or interactions with the exception of the Zest subscale, for which was replicated the previously reported finding of a significant joint effect of religiosity and gender on feelings of optimism (zest) in older adulthood, $F(1,109) = 5.83$, $p < .01$.

In sum, our analyses using longitudinal data on religiosity to predict life satisfaction in late adulthood replicated very closely the findings we obtained using concurrent measures of religiosity and life satisfaction in older age. The analyses revealed two consistent sets of findings. First, the positive effect of religiosity on life satisfaction in general and feelings of zest in particular among individuals in poor physical health was not just a concurrent phenomenon. Rather, the buffering effect of religiosity on life satisfaction in late adulthood could be predicted from a time interval of close to 30 years even after controlling for the initial ratings of subjective health. Second, we also found a stable interaction effect between religiosity and gender, with women who were highly religious in early adulthood and men who were low in religiosity showing greater zest or optimism as older adults than other members in the study.

RELIGIOUS INVOLVEMENT
AND SOCIAL ADAPTATION

In the previous section, we investigated the concurrent and longitudinal implications of religiosity on feelings of life satisfaction in older age. Successful aging, however, does not revolve solely around issues of self-satisfaction. As argued by Erik Erikson (1982/1998), successful adaptation to old age includes the ability to maintain a vital involvement in life despite suffering multiple losses. It also involves, according to Erikson, the necessity to reintegrate identity in a way that will allow the individual to confront the inevitability of death with equanimity and the kind of trust that provides hope and meaning for members of the younger generations. The development of a sense of ego integrity and the ability to maintain a generative and vital involvement with others may lead to feeling cheerful and satisfied with self or it may not. In other words, a positive appraisal of one's status in older age can lead to feelings of contentment that may not be captured by scores on self-report measures of mental health and life satisfaction. In this section of our chapter, we extend the analyses of the role of religiosity in preserving a healthy outlook on life beyond the narrow issue of adjustment to include measures of the broader construct of psychosocial adaptation.

We argue that there are two distinct, albeit not necessarily unrelated, ways of successfully adapting to late adulthood or for that matter to any other stage of the life course (Wink, 1991). The first strategy involves an inner-focused process of self-exploration, personal growth, creativity, and reintegration of one's identity. We assume that this is what Erikson had in mind when he wrote about ego integrity as the task of successful adaptation to old age. The second path toward successful aging is more outer directed and focuses more on maintaining positive, harmonious, and empathic relations with others (Blatt & Shichman, 1983; Wink, 1991). It includes generative concerns about the welfare of future generations, involvement with communal undertakings, and maintaining close relations with family and friends. Because religious involvement tends to be a communal activity and assumes embracing, at least in part, an existing tradition or legacy, we assume that it is more likely to be associated with the more outer-directed and communal path of successful aging.

Measures of Psychosocial Adaptation

The two distinct types of psychosocial adaptation were assessed with self-report measures of ego development, sources of well-being, and engagement in daily life tasks.

Ego Development

The Ego Integrity Scale (Ryff & Heincke, 1983) assesses the extent to which individuals have come to terms with their successes and failures and whether they view their lives as meaningful and feel psychologically integrated. The Loyola Generativity Scale (McAdams, de St. Aubin, & Logan, 1993) assesses an individual's concern with the goal of providing for the next generation as reflected in teaching, creating things, commitment to others, and the desire to leave a legacy of some kind.

Sources of Well-Being

The Personal Growth Scale (Ryff, 1989) measures the extent to which an individual derives a sense of well-being from experiences of self as growing and expanding and continuing to develop (as contrasted with a sense of personal stagnation). The Positive Relations with Others Scale (Ryff, 1989) assesses the degree to which an individual derives a sense of well-being from having warm, satisfying, trusting relationships with others and the capacity to maintain a strong sense of affection and intimacy (as contrasted with feelings of isolation and mistrust).

Daily Life Tasks (Harlow & Cantor, 1996)

The Community Service Scale assesses how much an individual is involved in helping friends and neighbors and in community service. The Creative

Activities scale measures daily involvement in playing an instrument, painting, sculpting, and writing.

Among these six measures, the Ego Integrity, Personal Growth, and Creative Activities scales reflect the inner-directed mode of psychosocial adaptation. The Generativity, Positive Relations with Others, and Community Service scales assess the outer-directed way of psychosocial adaptation. In analyzing the relation between religiosity in early adulthood and the measures of outer-directed adaptation in older age, we used three control variables scored from the data in early adulthood (30s). Generative interests were measured with an observer-based index (Peterson & Klohnen, 1995) scored from the California Q-sort (Block, 1978). Personal sociability was measured with the California Psychological Inventory's Sociability scale (Gough & Bradley, 1996). Community involvement was coded from interview transcripts using a 0/1 dummy code.

Concurrent and Longitudinal Relations between Religiosity and Psychosocial Adaptation in Late Adulthood.

Table 4.4 presents the concurrent correlations between religiosity and measures of psychosocial adaptation in older age. The findings support our initial hypothesis that religiosity is related more closely to measures of outer directedness and an emphasis on relations with others than to measures of inner directedness and personal growth. For the total sample, religiosity was correlated positively with generativity, the attainment of well-being through positive relations with others, and an involvement in community-oriented activities. Among the measures of inner directedness, the only significant relation was that between religiosity and involvement in creative activities. For women, religiosity was correlated significantly with positive relations with others and with community service. For men, religiosity correlated positively with generativity and with involvement in creative activities and community service.

In Table 4.5 we present analyses involving the same psychosocial outcome variables as in Table 4.4, but we now use religiosity in early (30s), middle (40s), and late middle adulthood (mid-50s and early 60s) as our predictor measures. The overall pattern of findings for the total sample and for the subsample of men remained unchanged from that reported in Table 4.4. For the total sample, the only difference was an additional presence of marginally significant relations between personal growth and importance of religion from the 30s onward. In the case of women, however, the findings were quite different. Women who showed a lifelong involvement in religion, as opposed to an involvement only in late adulthood, were still more likely than their nonreligious counterparts to be

TABLE 4.4. Correlations between Religiosity and Measures of Psychosocial Adaptation in Late Adulthood

Measures of psychosocial adaptation	Religiosity		
	Total	Women	Men
Ego development			
Integrity	.05	.11	.05
Generativity	.20*	.14	.27*
Well-being			
Personal growth	.10	.12	−.01
Positive relationships with others	.26*	.27*	.08
Life tasks			
Creative activities	.24**	.14	.21[a]
Community service	.33***	.28*	.35**

Note. For the total sample, the N = 133, except for the Ego Integrity Scale for which N = 114. For women, the N = 70. For men, the N = 63.

[a]$p \leq .10$; *$p \leq .05$; **$p \leq .01$; ***$p \leq .001$; two-tailed.

TABLE 4.5. Correlations between Religiosity in Early, Middle, and Late Middle Adulthood and Psychosocial Adaptation in Late Adulthood

Measures of psychosocial adaptation	Religiosity								
	Total			Women			Men		
	30s	40s	50s	30s	40s	50s	30s	40s	50s
Ego development									
Integrity	.05	.04	.06	.19	.20	.19	−.06	−.15	−.06[a]
Generativity	.31***	.33***	.25**	.26*	.26*	.25*	.37**	.42***	.24[a]
Well-being									
Personal growth	.16[a]	.16[a]	.21*	.25*	.23*	.33*	−.04	−.03	−.05
Positive relationships with others	.27**	.31***	.27**	.25*	.36*	.30*	.11	.10	.03
Life tasks									
Creative activities	.34***	.29***	.31***	.29*	.24*[a]	.27*	.24[a]	.23[a]	.19
Community service	.35***	.30***	.33***	.20[a]	.22[a]	.28*	.48***	.36**	.34**

Note. For the total sample, the N ranges from 131 to 133, with the exception of the integrity scale, for which N = 114. For women, the N ranges between 70 and 71 (N = 60 for the integrity scale). For men, the N ranges from 61 to 62 (N = 53 for the integrity scale).

[a]$p \leq .10$; *$p \leq .05$; **$p \leq .01$; ***$p \leq .001$; two-tailed.

characterized by the outer-directed emphasis on maintaining positive relations with others and communal involvement. In addition, however, they also manifested an emphasis on generativity, personal growth, and involvement in daily creative activities. In other words, women who were religiously involved as young and middle-aged adults tended, as older adults, to develop a balanced pattern of adaptation involving a simultaneous concern for others and for personal growth. (The only exception was the consistent lack of relation between the importance of religion and the Ego Integrity scale, which means that any personal growth associated with religiosity does not include attempts at reorganization or reintegration of one's sense of identity.)

It is important to note the impressively consistent and stable life-course pattern of relations between religiosity and psychosocial outcomes in older age. In most instances, if we found a significant relation between a measure of psychosocial adaptation in older age and religiosity in late middle adulthood (a time interval of 15 years), then the same pattern was true for religiosity in early adulthood (a time interval of close to 40 years). In other words, knowing an individual's religious status in early adulthood (30s) served as an excellent predictor of psychosocial adaptation in late adulthood.

There are two possible explanations for the observed temporal consistency of the relationship between importance of religion and measures of outer-directed psychosocial adaptation in late adulthood. On the one hand, it could be argued that these findings make an important statement about the power of religious involvement in shaping human behavior. On the other hand, the findings could be interpreted as indicating something about the antecedent personalities and habits of individuals who tend to be religiously involved throughout the course of their adult lives. For example, it is uncertain whether the significant relationship between religiosity in early adulthood and communal involvement in late adulthood says something specifically about the lifelong implications of religious involvement or whether it reflects the more general stability over time of interest in community activities. In order to address this causal ambiguity, we performed three separate regression analyses predicting scores on measures of generativity, positive relations with others, and community service from religiosity in early adulthood while simultaneously controlling for generative interests, sociability, and community involvement in early adulthood (see the previous section on measures for the description of the control variables). As shown in Table 4.6, in all three instances, the relationship between religiosity in early adulthood and the outcome variables in older age remained significant even when generative interests, sociability, and community involvement in early adulthood were statistically controlled.

TABLE 4.6. Regression Analyses Predicting Three Aspects of Other Directedness in Late Adulthood from Religiosity and Control Variables in Early Adulthood

Measures	Beta weights
Regression predicting generativity in older age	
Generative interests in early adulthood	.03
Religiosity in early adulthood	.32**
R^2	.33**
(df)	(2, 109)
Regression predicting positive relations with others in older age	
Sociability in early adulthood	.17[a]
Religiosity in early adulthood	.24*
R^2	.32
(df)	(2, 100)
Regression predicting community service in older age	
Community involvement in early adulthood	.14
Religiosity in early adulthood	.30***
R^2	.37***
(df)	(2, 129)

Note. [a]$p \le .10$; *$p \le .05$; **$p \le .01$; ***$p \le .001$; two-tailed.

CONCLUSION

In this chapter, we use data from a longitudinal study of men and women to explore the relationship between religiosity and physical health and life satisfaction in older adulthood. Our sample consisted of a group of relatively healthy, older-aged persons born in California for whom we had data beginning with early adulthood. The comparatively small size of the sample and the fact that the majority of the participants still live in California limit the generalizability of the study's findings. Yet the longitudinal breadth of the study provides a unique perspective on the cross-sectional and long-term nature of the relationship between religiosity and health in late adulthood. Our findings can be summarized in three points.

First, we did not find evidence for a direct relationship between religiosity and physical health in either our concurrent or longitudinal analyses. The only exception was evidence of a tendency for religious women to have an optimistic attitude toward their health in late adulthood. The absence of a relationship between religiosity and physical health may be due to the overall good health of the study participants. It should be pointed out, of course, that whereas our health measures relied on self-report data, the use of clinicians' reports might have yielded different patterns in the data. Similarly, because our measure of religiosity collapsed across different dimensions of religiosity (church participation and importance of religion), more discrete measures of religiosity might show different correlates with physical health. On the other hand, our confidence in the reliability of our findings is enhanced by the fact that we also failed to find significant relationships between religiosity and physical health using measures of church attendance and intrinsic religiosity taken from the Duke Religious Index. Other studies similarly indicate that general patterns in research findings tend to be maintained regardless of the specific ways in which religiosity is measured (see Thoresen, 1999).

The lack of evidence for a direct relationship between religiosity and physical health may also stem from the impact that individuals' genetic profiles have in older age in obscuring the effect on health of the daily practices associated with religiosity (e.g., abstinence, prayer, family and community involvement). In any case, it is also important to note that the research literature on the relationship between religiosity and physical health is less consistent and compelling than the literature on the relationship between religion and mortality and religion and mental health.

Second, although we did not find a direct relationship between religiosity and physical health, we did find a pattern of significant interactions between religiosity and physical health in explaining overall levels of life satisfaction and zest (feelings of optimism) in particular. Our analyses indicated that religiosity did not have an influence on life satisfaction among physically healthy individuals. Among those individuals who had poor physical health, however, religiosity acted as a buffer of life satisfaction. In other words, our findings suggest that when confronted with personal adversity in late adulthood, such as poor health, nonreligious individuals showed a tendency to exhibit lower levels of optimism about the present and the future than those who were religious. This finding was true not just for older-aged individuals who were currently religious. The same pattern of salutary effects of religion on life satisfaction among older age individuals who were in poor physical health could be predicted using measures of religiosity scored from interview data in middle adulthood (a time interval of close to 30 years), even after controlling for antecedent levels of general health. Although one should be cautious in making causal inferences, it would seem that the positive relationship between religion and life satisfaction in times of adversity goes beyond the mere possibility that psychologically healthy individuals acquire faith in times of stress. It seems, rather, that, as many social theorists have argued (e.g., Berger & Luckmann, 1966; Durkheim 1897/1951), religious participation is a critical, although somewhat latent, social anchor and that long-term investment in religious capital yields dividends that can compensate for subsequent declines in other human stock (e.g., declining health). Finally, it is important to note that our findings suggest that religiosity has a selective effect on life satisfaction. In particular, it appears to buffer against feelings of pessimism, but it does not have the same effect on feelings of congruence between expectations and goal attainment.

We also found evidence of gender differences in the relationship between religion and life satisfaction. In particular, feelings of optimism about the present and the future (zest) were particularly true of religious women and nonreligious men. This interaction effect of religion and gender in predicting feelings of zest in old age was obtained using measures of religious involvement starting from early adulthood onward.

Third, in this chapter we have argued for the importance of broadening the concept of psychological well-being in late adulthood to include not only measures of adjustment (life satisfaction) but also of psychosocial adaptation. There is more to life than subjective feelings of happiness (cf. Ryff, 1989; Ryff & Singer, 1998), even though self-satisfaction has an impact on the quality of one's life. We found that among older-aged individuals, religious involvement has important implications for how one relates to oneself and to others. Not unexpectedly, religious individuals were more generative and more involved in community activities and tended to derive more satisfaction from personal relations with others as older adults. Once again this pattern of results was not only obtained with a concurrent measure of religiosity scored from interview material in late adulthood but also was evident in our analyses using measures of religiosity scored from interviews obtained at earlier time periods. These relations held true even when we controlled for antecedent levels of generativity, community involvement, and sociability. In the case of women, religious involvement early on in life also predicted an interest in personal growth and engagement in creative activities in older age. Thus the importance of religion for well-being in older adulthood extends beyond the confines of life satisfaction and feelings of optimism to include a much broader pattern of psychosocial adaptation.

ACKNOWLEDGMENTS

Our research was supported by a grant from the Project on Death in America of the Open Society Institute to Paul Wink and by Grant No. 1998039 from the Louisville Institute's program on religion supported by the Lilly Foundation to Paul Wink and Michele Dillon. We thank Tom Plante and Allen Sherman and participants in the Santa Clara University conference on Faith and Health (May 2000) for helpful comments and suggestions.

REFERENCES

Adams, S., Cartwright, L., Ostrove, J., Stewart, A., & Wink, P. (1998). Psychological predictors of good health in three longitudinal samples of educated midlife women. *Health Psychology, 17,* 412–420.

Ainlay, S., Singleton, R., & Swigert, V. (1992). Aging and religious participation: Reconsidering the effects of health. *Journal for the Scientific Study of Religion, 31,* 175–188.

Belloc, N., Breslow, L., & Hochstim, J. (1971). Measurement of physical health in a general population survey. *American Journal of Epidemiology, 93,* 328–336.

Berger, P., & Luckmann, T. (1966). *The social construction of reality.* Garden City, NY: Doubleday.

Blatt, S. J., & Shichman, S. (1983). Two primary configurations of psychopathology. *Psychoanalysis and Contemporary Thought, 6,* 187–254.

Blazer, D., & Palmore, E. (1976). Religion and aging in a longitudinal panel. *Gerontologist, 16,* 82–85.

Block, J. (1978). *The Q-sort method in personality assessment and psychiatric research.* Palo Alto, CA: Consulting Psychologists Press.

Clausen, J. (1993). *American lives: Looking back at the children of the great depression.* New York: Free Press.

Courtenay, B., Poon, L., Martin, P., Clayton, G., & Johnson, M. (1992). Religiosity and adaptation in the oldest-old. *International Journal of Aging and Human Development, 34,* 47–56.

Dillon, M., & Wink, P. (2000, August). *Religious involvement over the life-course: Evidence from a longitudinal study.* Paper presented at the annual meeting of the American Sociological Association, Washington, DC.

Durkheim, E. (1951). *Suicide: A study in sociology* (J. A. Spaulding & G. Simpson, Trans.). New York: Free Press. (Original work published 1897)

Durkheim, E. (1976). *The elementary forms of the religious life.* London: Allen & Unwin. (Original work published 1912)

Ellison, C. G. (1991). Religious involvement and subjective well-being. *Journal of Health and Social Behavior, 32,* 80–99.

Ellison, C. G., Gay, D., & Glass, T. (1989). Does religious commitment contribute to individual life satisfaction? *Social Forces, 68,* 100–123.

Ellison, C. G., & Levin, J. (1998). The religion–health connection: Evidence, theory, and future directions. *Health Education and Behavior, 25,* 700–720.

Erikson, E. (1998). *The life-cycle completed.* New York: Norton. (Original work published 1982)

Ferraro, K., & Albrecht-Jensen, C. (1991). Does religion influence adult health? *Journal for the Scientific Study of Religion, 30,* 193–202.

Gough, H. G., & Bradley, P. (1996). *CPI manual* (3rd ed.). Palo Alto, CA: Consulting Psychologists Press.

Harlow, R., & Cantor, N. (1996). Still participating after all these years: A study of life task participation in later life. *Journal of Personality and Social Psychology, 71,* 1235–1249.

Hout, M., & Greeley, A. (1987). The center doesn't hold: Church attendance in the United States, 1940–1984. *American Sociological Review, 52,* 325–345.

Hummer, R. A., Rogers, R. G., Nam, C. B., & Ellison, C. G. (1999). Religious involvement and U.S. adult mortality. *Demography, 36,* 273–285.

Hunsberger, B. (1985). Religion, age, life satisfaction, and perceived sources of religiousness: A study of older persons. *Journal of Gerontology, 40,* 615–620.

Iannaccone, L. (1990). Religious practice: A human capital approach. *Journal for the Scientific Study of Religion, 29,* 293–314.

Idler, E. (1987). Religious involvement and the health of the elderly: Some hypotheses and an initial test. *Social Forces, 66,* 226–238.

Idler, E. (1995). Religion, health, and non-physical senses of self. *Social Forces, 74,* 683–704.

Idler, E., & Kasl, S. (1992). Religion, disability, depression, and the timing of death. *American Journal of Sociology, 97,* 1052–1079.

Koenig, H. (1997). *Is religion good for your health?* Binghamton, NY: Haworth Press.

Koenig, H., Kvale, J., & Ferrel, C. (1988). Religion and well-being in later life. *Gerontologist, 28,* 18–28.

Koenig, H., Parkerson, G., & Meador, K. (1997). Religion index for psychiatric research. *American Journal of Psychiatry, 153,* 885–886.

Koenig, H., Siegler, I., & George, L. (1989). Religious and non-religious coping: Impact on adaptation in later life. *Journal of Religion and Aging, 5,* 73–84.

Koenig, H., Siegler, I., Meador, K., & George, L. (1990). Religious coping and personality in later life. *International Journal of Geriatric Psychiatry, 5,* 123–131.

Krause, N. (1991). Stress, religiosity, and abstinence from alcohol. *Psychology and Aging, 6,* 134–144.

Larson, D., Koenig, H., Kaplan, B., Greenberg, R., Logue, E., & Tyroler, H. (1989). The impact of religion on men's blood pressure. *Journal of Religion and Health, 28,* 265–278.

Levin, J. (1994). Investigating the epidemiologic effects of religious experience. In J. Levin (Ed.), *Religion in aging and health* (pp. 3–17). Thousand Oaks, CA: Sage.

Levin, J. S., & Chatters, L. M. (1998). Research on religion and mental health: An overview of empirical findings and theoretical issues. In H. Koenig (Ed.), *Handbook of religion and mental health* (pp. 33–50). San Diego, CA: Academic Press.

Levin, J., & Markides, K. (1985). Religion and health in Mexican Americans. *Journal of Religion and Health, 24,* 60–69.

Levin, J., & Markides, K. (1986). Religious attendance and subjective health. *Journal for the Scientific Study of Religion, 25,* 31–40.

Levin, J., Markides, K., & Ray, L. (1996). Religious attendance and psychological well-being in Mexican Americans: A panel analysis of three-generations data. *Gerontologist, 36,* 454–463.

Levin, J., Taylor, R., & Chatters, L. (1994). Race and gender differences in religiosity among older adults: Findings from four national surveys. *Journal of Gerontology: Social Sciences, 49,* S137–S145.

Liang, J. (1984). Dimensions of the Life Satisfaction Index: A structural formulation. *Journal of Gerontology, 39,* 613–622.

Markides, K. (1983). Aging, religiosity, and adjustment: A longitudinal analysis. *Journal of Gerontology, 38,* 621–625.

Markides, K., Levin, J., & Ray, L. (1987). Religion, aging, and life satisfaction: An eight-year, three-wave, longitudinal study. *Gerontologist, 27,* 660–665.

McAdams, D., de St. Aubin, E., & Logan, R. (1993). Generativity among young, midlife, and older adults. *Psychology and Aging, 8,* 221–230.

McCullough, M. E., Hoyt, W. T., Larson, D. B., Koenig, H. G., & Thoresen, C. E. (2000). Religious involvement and mortality: A meta-analytic review. *Health Psychology, 19,* 211–222.

McFadden, S. (1996). Religion, spirituality, and aging. *Handbook of the psychology of aging* (pp. 162–177). San Diego, CA: Academic Press.

Morse, C., & Wisocki, P. (1988). Importance of religiosity to elderly adjustment. *Journal of Religion and Aging, 4,* 15–26.

Neugarten, B. L., Havighurst, R. J., & Tobin, S. (1961). The measurement of life satisfaction. *Journal of Gerontology, 16,* 134–143.

Oxman, T. E., Freeman, D. H., & Manheimer, E. D. (1995). Lack of social participation or religious strength and comfort as risk factors for death after cardiac surgery in the elderly. *Psychosomatic Medicine, 57,* 5–15.

Pargament, K. I. (1997). *The psychology of religion and coping: Theory, research, practice.* New York: Guilford Press.

Pargament, K., Ensing, D., Falgout, K., Olsen, H., Reilly, B., Van Haitsma, K., & Warren, R. (1990). God help me: I. Religious coping efforts as predictors of the outcomes to significant negative life events. *American Journal of Community Psychology, 18*(16), 793–824.

Peterson, B. E., & Klohnen, E. C. (1995). Realization of generativity in two samples of women at midlife. *Psychology and Aging, 10,* 20–29.

Ryff, C. (1989). Happiness is everything, or is it? Explorations on the meaning of psychological well-being. *Journal of Personality and Social Psychology, 57,* 1069–1081.

Ryff, C., & Heincke, S. (1983). Subjective organization of personality in adulthood and aging. *Journal of Personality and Social Psychology, 44,* 807–816.

Ryff, C. D., & Singer, B. (1998). The contours of positive human health. *Psychological Inquiry, 9,* 1–28.

Sherman, A., Plante, T., Simonton, N., Moody, V., & Wells, P. (2001). *Impact of religiousness and religious coping on quality of life outcomes for multiple myeloma patients receiving bone marrow transplantation.* Manuscript under review.

Strawbridge, W. J., Cohen, R. D., Shema, S. J., & Kaplan, G. A. (1997). Frequent attendance at religious services and mortality over 28 years. *American Journal of Public Health, 87,* 957–961.

Thoresen, C. E. (1999). Spirituality and health: Is there a relationship? *Journal of Health Psychology, 4,* 291–300.

Ware, J. (1993). *SF-36 Health Survey: Manual and interpretation guide.* Boston: New England Medical Center.

Wink, P. (1991). Self and object-directedness in adult women. *Journal of Personality, 59,* 769–791.

Wink, P., & Dillon, M. (in press). Spiritual development across the adult life course: Findings from a longitudinal study. *Journal of Adult Development.*

5

◄◦►

UNFORGIVENESS, FORGIVENESS, RELIGION, AND HEALTH

EVERETT L. WORTHINGTON, JR.
JACK W. BERRY
LES PARROTT III

For the past 20 years, researchers have investigated the connection between religious faith and mental and physical health (Koenig, 1999; Koenig, McCullough, & Larson, 2000; Larson, Swyers, & McCullough, 1998; Levin, 1994; Thoresen, 1999; see also McCullough, Chapter 3; Plante & Sharma, Chapter 10; and Thoresen, Harris, & Oman, Chapter 2, this volume). Data have accumulated to show a positive association. Some have urged caution (i.e., Sloan, Bagiella, & Powell, 1999; also Chapter 14, this volume).

Researchers have begun to parse the different reasons why religion might be expected to produce better mental or physical health than might non-religion. Three explanatory mechanisms are thought to mediate the connection between religion and health. First, religion promotes a pro-virtue constellation of personality traits, which affects health. This effect has not been well researched (Thoresen et al., Chapter 2, this volume). Second, the social support that comes about through organized religion affects health. This has been well researched (McCullough, Hoyt, Larson, Koenig, & Thoresen, 2000). Third, religion equips a person to cope more effectively with stress. This too has been well researched (Pargament, 1997).

In this chapter, we explore the simple model that connects these mediators and hypothesizes some possible physiological mechanisms relating psychosocial variables (e.g., religious beliefs and values, culture, pro-virtue personality characteristics, interpersonal stress, and social support) with health outcomes. We suggest that this hypothesized chain can work through the ways people deal with transgressions and unforgiveness. Namely, we propose that religion and perhaps prosocial (even though nonreligious) world views can lead to a core of pro-virtue characteristics, which affect people's experiences of unforgiveness and perhaps forgiveness, which are in turn related to illness or health. We emphasize the negative effects of chronic unforgiveness on health and happiness. In contrast, the virtues are thought to lead to mental, physical, and social health. Harmonious social interaction leads to positive health outcomes through reducing stress and hostility and promoting positive emotions. We argue that forgiveness is one of many ways of overcoming unforgiveness. Our hypotheses can be summarized in a linear model (see Figure 5.1, below), which will be elaborated in the following pages.

THEORETICAL EXPLORATIONS OF UNFORGIVENESS, FORGIVENESS, AND RECONCILIATION

Definitions

Unforgiveness

Unforgiveness is a complex of related emotions, consisting of resentment, bitterness, hatred, hostility, residual anger, and fear (Worthington & Wade, 1999), which are experienced after ruminating about a transgression. A transgression is perceived as a mixture of hurt and offense. To the extent that a transgression is perceived as hurt, the person responds immediately with fear (Worthington, 1998). To the extent that a transgression is perceived as an offense, the person will respond immediately with anger (Fitzgibbons, 1986; Thoresen, Luskin, & Harris, 1998). Fear and anger are not unforgiveness. Unforgiveness occurs when people ruminate about the event, its consequences, their own reactions to it, the transgressor's motives, and potential responses from the self or the transgressor. Rumination *can* produce the emotions of resentment, bitterness, hatred, hostility, residual anger, and fear, which we call *unforgiveness*.

People do not like to feel unforgiveness. Although the anger and the revenge motive can energize and empower, people usually try quickly to reduce, eliminate, or avoid unforgiveness. People avoid or reduce unforgiveness in many ways (Worthington, in press). These involve pursuing justice (seeking civil justice, seeking restitution, turning judgment over to God), resolving conflicts, working for social justice, denying unforgiveness, projecting blame, telling a different story about the transaction involving justification or excuse, and forbearing (i.e., accepting) transgressions. All such efforts tend to inhibit aggressive, antisocial, vengeful, or hostile emotions and acts. Another way to reduce unforgiveness involves increasing warm, prosocial, affiliative emotions—that is, by forgiving. Forgiving reduces unforgiveness by concurrently promoting positive emotional states.

Forgiveness

Forgiveness is the contamination or prevention of unforgiving emotions by experiencing strong, positive, love-based emotions as one recalls a transgression. The positive, love-based emotions can be empathy, sympathy, compassion, agape love, or even romantic love for the transgressor. Such emotions motivate a reconciliation or conciliation with the transgressor if it is safe, prudent, and possible to do so (Worthington, 1998). Other positive emotions, such as humility over one's own culpability and past transgressions and gratitude for one's own experiences of forgiveness, might intermix to contaminate the emotions of unforgiveness, replace the emotions of anger and fear, or merely facilitate the emotional replacement.

We are not talking about subjective *feelings* when we say that unforgiveness and forgiveness are emotions. Although emotions involve feelings (i.e., our ways of labeling emotions; Damasio, 1999), emotions also involve thoughts, memories, associations (Lazarus, 1999), neurochemicals in the brain (Damasio, 1999), pathways through various brain structures (LeDoux, 1996), hormones in the bloodstream (Sapolsky, 1994, 1999), "gut feelings" (Damasio, 1999), facial musculature (Plutchik, 1994), gross body musculature (Plutchik, 1994), and acts of emotional expression (Damasio, 1999).

Reconciliation

Reconciliation is the restoration of trust in a relationship in which trust has been violated, sometimes repeatedly (Worthington & Drinkard, 2000). Reconciliation can involve forgiveness or other ways of reducing unforgiveness. Reconciliation always occurs within a relationship (Worthington & Drinkard, 2000).

Forgivingness and Unforgivingness as Personality Dispositions

Research in basic social psychology and intervention research aimed at promoting forgiveness have focused almost exclusively on individual acts of forgiveness (see Worthington & Wade, 1999, for a review). Individual differences in the disposition to forgive have gone largely unstudied. Roberts (1995) suggested the term *forgivingness* to refer to "an enduring disposition to the act or process of forgiveness" (p. 289) to distinguish the personal disposition or virtuous trait from specific instances of forgiveness. A person high in forgivingness is, *ceritus paribus*, more likely than a person low in forgivingness to forgive a particular transgression.

Much discussion of the desirability of forgiveness for health and well-being is, at least implicitly, about forgivingness. Most religious traditions attempt to foster beliefs and teach methods that can facilitate forgivingness (Pargament & Rye, 1998). A secondary goal of secular interventions for promoting transgression-related forgiveness is to teach people how to forgive more effectively and consequently to foster dispositional forgivingness. Dispositional forgivingness that persists for years—not forgiveness of a particular transgression—is thought to promote health.

We will employ the term *unforgivingness* to refer to the enduring disposition to states of unforgiveness, that is, the proneness to experience the emotions of hostility, hatred, bitterness, and resentment in response to interpersonal transgressions. Chronic unforgivingness is thought to promote ill health. We wish to emphasize that unforgivingness is not synonymous with low forgivingness, and forgivingness is not synonymous with low unforgivingness.

A Discrete Systems View of Forgiveness and Unforgiveness

In our model, forgiveness and unforgiveness are not the opposite poles of a single continuum. Overcoming unforgiveness does not imply forgiveness. We propose that forgiveness and unforgiveness reflect the activation of two related but relatively independent adaptive systems. This perspective bears many similarities with recent research and theory on emotion, personality, and evolved adaptive strategies. In Table 5.1, we provide examples of discrete systems and discrete social adaptation strategies that might be involved in forgiveness and unforgiveness.

The systems involved in forgiveness support adaptive strategies for achieving affiliation, cooperation, and warm emotional bonds between people. Buss (1996) refers to such social strategies as "strategic facilitation." The systems involved in unforgiveness support adaptive strategies for self-promotion, dominance, and self-protection against external and internal threats. In Buss's (1996) terminology, these systems contribute to solving problems of "strategic interference," which are essentially problems of conflicts of interest with others.

Our model of forgiveness and unforgiveness is compatible with a number of discrete-emotion theories. There is much evidence that positive and

TABLE 5.1. Examples of Discrete Systems That Parallel Our Hypothesized Distinction between Unforgiveness and Forgiveness Systems

Forgiveness	Unforgiveness	Author
Social adaptation strategies		
Strategic facilitation	Strategic interference	Buss (1996)
Structure of affect		
Positive affect	Negative affect	Watson & Tellegen (1985)
Personality		
Agreeableness	(Low) Conscientiousness/ neuroticism	John (1990)
Affiliation	Control	Kiesler (1983)
Intimacy motivation	Power motivation	McAdams (1994)
Biological systems		
Expectancy circuits	Fear and rage circuits	Panksepp (1982)
Behavioral activation system	Behavioral inhibition system	Gray (1994)

negative emotions reflect discrete, separate systems (Watson & Tellegen, 1985; Watson, Wiese, Vaidya, & Tellegen, 1999). In this view, the positive and negative emotions form two bipolar dimensions rather than opposite poles of a single dimension. Biological research has also provided evidence that positive and negative emotions are associated with separate neurological and biochemical systems (Panksepp, 1982; Plutchik, 1994). Witvliet and Vrana (1995) have mapped physiological responses onto an organization of emotions that is bipolar. Typically, emotions have been conceptualized along two dimensions of valence (positive to negative) and arousal (high to low). Researchers have had difficulty differentiating negative and high-arousal emotions (such as anger and fear) physiologically using EMG, startle reflexes, and sympathetic indicators (such as skin conductance). Witvliet and Vrana (1995) showed, however, that if the axes were rotated 45°, two independent dimensions that they called negative affect and positive affect were produced. In such a mapping, the axis of high pleasant affect (such as joy) versus low pleasant affect (such as sadness) is distinctly different from the axis of high negative affect (such as fear) versus low negative affect (such as pleasant feelings). Such rotation is consistent with historic theories (Lang, Bradley, & Cuthbert, 1990; Schnierla, 1959). Witvliet and Vrana showed which peripheral physiological indicators differentiate such negative and positive affective states.

Saying that such systems are "independent" does not mean they cannot be antagonistic. For example, if people were exposed to a fear-producing stimulus and a joy-producing stimulus, one emotion would likely predominate. A convenient example is a horror movie that has a happy ending.

Despite the presence of many states of fear throughout the movie, if the movie also produces joy and has a satisfactory ending, the predominant affect produced by the movie would be joy, not fear.

That unforgiveness is associated with the negative emotions is intuitively obvious. It is perhaps less obvious that forgiveness is associated with the positive emotions rather than with the absence of negative emotions. Yet terms that loaded highly on the high pole of positive affects in the studies analyzed by Watson and Tellegen (1985) include "warmhearted," "affectionate," "friendly," "kindly," "sociable," "good natured," and "forgiving."

At the level of personality dispositions, our perspective on trait forgivingness and trait unforgivingness has parallels with several recent theories of personality. As shown in Table 5.1, many theories of personality include a trait dimension or type associated with warmth and affection. An example is the Agreeableness factor in the Big Five model of personality (John, 1990). Each theory also includes a dimension or type assumed to be relatively independent of the other dimension associated with self-protection or the detection of threats. In the Big Five model, high Neuroticism reflects a general tendency to worry and to experience negative affect, such as anxiety, hostility, and depression (John, 1990). Low Conscientiousness appears to be associated with lack of conscience and with unsocialized aggression.

As MacDonald (1992) argues, the test of a discrete systems approach is whether people can be simultaneously high and low on traits in a manner that would be incompatible with a single-dimension approach. In our view, it is theoretically possible to be high in trait unforgivingness and simultaneously high in trait forgivingness, low in each, or high in one but low in the other. For example, a person high in unforgivingness would quickly, in many situations, develop a sense of unforgiveness in which rumination brought about the cold emotions of hatred, hostility, bitterness, and resentment. Such a person might or might not be likely eventually to forgive these transgressions. A person who is high in forgivingness would, once unforgiveness is detected, wrestle with it and, in most cases, successfully forgive the transgression. Someone low in forgivingness might never work through many transgressions to forgive them.

A person might be low in unforgivingness and thereby rarely develop unforgiveness over transgressions. Such a person might avoid ruminating or might simply be relatively nonreactive to provocations. In most people's lives, though, occasional transgressions occur that result in some unforgiveness. So even the person low in unforgivingness will have some occasions to consider forgiveness. Such a person could be either high or low in forgivingness.

These two illustrations demonstrate that people can fill out any one of four cells of a 2 × 2 matrix of high versus low trait forgivingness and trait unforgivingness. We have found that there is generally a high negative correlation between unforgivingness and forgivingness.

Using the Trait Forgivingness Scale (TFS; Berry, Worthington, O'Connor, Parrott, & Wade, 2001), which has items assessing both trait forgivingness and trait unforgivingness, we found in three studies of college students that the correlations between forgivingness and unforgivingness ranged from −.40 to −.59 (Worthington et al., 1999). We combined the three data sets consisting of 320 student-participants. All participants completed the TFS scale. We cast each participant into a 2 × 2 matrix using a median split. Participants were not distributed randomly in the categories, $\chi^2(1) = 62.1$, $p < .0001$. Of the 320 participants, 59 (18%) were high in both variables and 32 (10%) were low in both variables. Of the 320, 121 (38%) were high in unforgivingness and low in forgivingness; 108 (34%) were low in unforgivingness and high in forgivingness.

THE HEALTH CORRELATES AND CONSEQUENCES OF UNFORGIVINGNESS

Thus far we have focused mostly on the aspect of our model labeled "Responses to Transgressions" (see Figure 5.1 below). We now turn our attention to the potential link between those responses and health effects. The link is "potential" because prospective longitudinal research is needed to firmly establish the link, and the scientific study of forgiveness has not existed long enough to accumulate such data.

Typically, an individual transgression will have few health consequences. An obvious exception involves a trauma, which can have lasting mental and physical consequences. However, the large majority of transgressions are not traumatic.

Health consequences of unforgiveness are expected to show up most starkly in people who are chronically unforgiving—that is, those who have personality characteristics of unforgivingness (especially if they are also low in trait forgivingness). Trait unforgivingness is expected to be associated with trait anger, trait hostility, a tendency to ruminate, and perhaps (at the temperament level) neuroticism (see Berry, Worthington, O'Connor, Parrott, & Wade, 2001; Berry, Worthington, Parrott, O'Connor, & Wade, in press).

At present, we can array a fairly massive amount of circumstantial evidence that there are biological correlates of traits associated with unforgivingness. Unforgivingness has been defined as being part of a constellation of emotions, thoughts, and behaviors that have negative effects on health. However, at present, research has not demonstrated conclusively that unforgivingness is empirically related to such well-studied experiences. Furthermore, even if found to be related, unforgivingness might not stimulate anger, hostility, stress, or fear in such intensity that it becomes clinically relevant. In order of likelihood of involvement, that constellation involves (1) anger and hostility, (2) stress, and (3) fear. We examine the health correlates and consequences of chronic exposure to each of these, all of which are presumed to be part of unforgiveness. However, validity of our analyses awaits empirical investigation of unforgivingness.

Health Correlates and Consequences of Unforgivingness Arising from Anger and Hostility

Unforgivingness is an emotional complex, and part of that complex presumably includes trait anger and hostility. Trait anger is cross-situational. Hostility is a generalized negativity toward others, the world, and the future.

Chronic anger and hostility have been found to adversely affect health (Kaplan, 1992; Kaplan, Munroe-Blum, & Blazer, 1993; Smith & Christensen, 1992; Williams, 1989). Chronic anger has been associated with health-compromising behaviors and conditions such as high blood pressure, depression, increased substance abuse, and general poor health status (e.g., Hecker, Chesney, Black, & Frautschi, 1989; Perini, Muller, & Buhler, 1991). Anger has also been implicated in the decreased functioning of the immune system (see Herbert & Cohen, 1993, for a meta-analysis). However, there is some evidence that appropriate anger can enhance immune system functioning (Weiss et al., 1996).

Research in Type A behavior has shown that chronic hostility is related to poor cardiovascular health (Rhodewalt & Morf, 1995). Because chronic hostility is part of an unforgiving disposition, the implication is that chronic unforgiveness might be related to poor cardiovascular health. In addition, Thoresen and Powell (1992) have found that narcissism has been related conceptually to Type A behavior. Narcissism is characterized by a difficulty in empathizing with others (Emmons, 2000; Sandage, Worthington, Hight, & Berry, 2000), which might be a core process in forgiving (McCullough, Worthington, & Rachal, 1997) and in being willing to seek forgiveness (Sandage et al., 2000). These findings suggest that being low in trait forgivingness might permit unforgiveness to be experienced unchecked, resulting in cardiovascular difficulties.

Unforgiveness as Acute Stress, Unforgivingness as Chronic Stress

A stressor is an environmental change that makes a demand for the organism to adjust. When a stressor occurs, the body responds. Sapolsky (1994) has argued that human bodies are intended to respond to acute stressors and that stress-related illnesses occur primarily because we structure our lives so that we experience a multitude of chronic stressors. The concept that describes the body's adjustment to a stressor is *allostasis* (McEwen & Stellar, 1993). The cumulative effects of allostasis on biological systems is referred to as *allostatic load*. Under conditions of chronic environmental demand, the allostatic load on biological systems can produce a long-term negative impact on physical and mental health (McEwen, 1998).

Sapolsky (1994, 1999) summarizes hundreds of studies on chronic stress, including its effects on hormones, cardiovascular system, metabolic system, elimination system, growth-regulating systems, sexual and reproductive systems, immune system, and pain-control system. He examines many negative health effects of chronic stress (including aging, death, and psychological disorder). The immune system is particularly affected in chronic stress (Futterman, Kemeny, Shapiro, Polonsky, & Fahey, 1992). Thoresen, Harris, and Luskin (2000) have hypothesized that transgressions that are responded to with unforgiveness can increase allostatic load.

Chronic unforgiveness can occur in three primary ways. First, a person could live in an environment characterized by numerous transgressions—for example, a negative work environment, a conflictual family situation, or a war-torn society. Second, when a transgression occurs, people can habitually turn the reactive emotions of anger or fear into the delayed emotions of unforgiveness through ruminating (Worthington & Wade, 1999). In effect, through ruminating, the person is exposing himself or herself to multiple experiences with the stressor. Thus rumination can create a type of chronic stress. Unforgiveness places strains on existing relationships, or it can involve memories from relationships that are no longer active. Third, when relationships go sour, negative feelings are often generalized to the entire relationship rather than being localized to memories of specific relational events. Once generalization occurs, the person reexperiences a stressor almost every time the person thinks of the relationship or the partner, which is considerably more often than the frequency with which the person recalls (or experiences) a specific transgression in the relationship. In extreme cases, generalization beyond the relationship can occur.

Newberg, d'Aquili, Newberg, and deMarici (2000) also argue that stress is involved with unforgiveness. They begin by assuming that a person has a sense of self, which is damaged when a transgression occurs. The brain senses the discrepancy between the former and posttransgression sense of self and responds by activating sympathetic nervous system responses.

Salovey, Rothman, Detweiler, and Steward (2000) argue that negative emotions reduce the release of secretory immunoglobulin A, an antibody that fights bacteria and viruses (such the common cold). Immune system functioning has been found to be compromised by negative emotions (Stone, Marco, Cruise, Cox, & Neale, 1996). Negative moods are related to many physical disorders (Cohen & Rodriguez, 1995).

Unforgiveness, like stress, is a reaction to an event that makes a demand on the person to adjust. It is likely to act on the body like any stressor, producing allostasis. Unforgiveness, if it becomes chronic, is similar to chronic stress and may have the same health correlates and consequences as chronic stress.

Health Correlates and Consequences of Unforgiveness Arising from Fear

A Fear-Conditioning Model

Previously, Worthington (1998) hypothesized that fear conditioning is the primary mechanism of unforgiveness. Recently, though, he has advocated that either anger or fear (or both) might trigger the development of unforgiveness, which is brought to fruition by rumination (Worthington, 2000, in press). Fear conditioning is thought to occur but is seen as less frequent than anger in triggering unforgiveness. A fear-conditioning model of unforgiveness accounts for some of the fear, anger, stress, depression, and loss of control experienced in unforgiveness. It is thus possible to consider potential health correlates and consequences of unforgiveness within such a model.

When people are hurt, they may become fear conditioned in a classical conditioning sense. A person receives a hurt, offense, injustice, or rejection (unconditioned stimulus) from an offender (conditioned stimulus). Unforgiveness responses are associated with the offender. If the unforgiving person encounters the offender, responses occur. First, he or she gets tense, which is the vestige of orienting and freezing. Second, the stress-response system is activated. Third, the person may try to avoid or withdraw from the offender. Fourth, if withdrawal or cognitive avoidance is not possible, then anger, retaliation, or defensive fighting may occur. (Recall that most transgressions generate anger *directly*. Here we are talking about fear-conditioning hurts, which constitute a minority of offenses.) Fifth, if such fighting is unwise, self-destructive, or futile, the person might give the human equivalent of a submissive gesture—depression, which declares that the person is weak and helpless. Depression usually elicits help and inhibits aggression.

Based on this model, unforgiveness is thought to have predictable concomitants. The health effects of chronic fear in its various forms—fear, anxiety, anxiety disorders, posttraumatic stress disorder, panic attacks, and the like—have been investigated. We examine the potential effects of three fear-related factors: (1) cognitive avoidance, denial, and defensiveness, (2) loss of control, and (3) chronic fear or anxiety. (Note: We have already described the potential effects of anger and stress, which are also subsumed within a fear-conditioning model of unforgiveness.)

Potential Health Effects of Cognitive Avoidance, Denial, and Defensiveness

When people successfully avoid a threatening stimulus, they may be unaware of the effects of the stimulus on their lives. Consequently, they do not present themselves to mental or physical health specialists for treatment, nor do they identify themselves as candidates for research. Little is known about successful avoidance, denial, and defensiveness against threats.

Only when unconscious defenses are unsuccessful do people manifest psychosomatic symptoms or psychological or relationship problems. The understanding of the effects of denial, repression, suppression, and other defenses is necessarily skewed by sampling. Nonetheless, by studying psychosomatic disorders and psychotherapy patients, we can discover the effects of failed cognitive defensiveness. Some research evidence suggests that individuals who are high in repression and defensiveness are at greater risk for health problems (Brown et al., 1996; Sapolsky, 1994). Some examples of the effects of chronic unexpressed anger on health include greater vulnerability to essential hypertension (Perini, Muller, & Buhler, 1991); heart disease and stroke (Williams, 1989); depression (Bromberger & Matthews, 1996); rheumatoid arthritis (Solomon, 1985); migraines (Grothgar & Scholz, 1987); and the common cold (Evans & Edgerton, 1991).

Potential Health Correlates and Consequences of Loss of Control

For more than 20 years, researchers have detailed the neurobiology of lack of control (e.g., Laudenslager et al., 1983; Weiss, Sundar, & Becker, 1989). Hundreds of articles have described the neurobiology of loss of control, documenting neural pathways, neural and chemical mechanisms, and physiological effects on and correlates with health and immune-system functioning. Such findings could be extended to create hypotheses about chronic unforgiveness.

Potential Health Correlates and Consequences of Chronic Fear and Anxiety

Chronic anxiety, worry, and fearfulness may have an adverse impact on health (Friedman & Booth-Kewley, 1987). According to Sapolsky (1999), physical and mental health status are related to basal hypersecretion of cortisol. There is research evidence that people high on trait anxiety or social distress have elevated basal cortisol levels (Bell et al., 1993; Sapolsky, 1994) and show signs of decreased immune functioning (Esterling, Antoni, Kumar, & Schneiderman, 1993). Research has also found basal hypersecretion of stress hormones among anxiety-disordered individuals (see Sapolsky, 1999), in addition to Type A individuals (Williams, 1989).

In summary, chronic unforgivingness—especially when it is not accompanied by high forgivingness—has a variety of potential health correlates and consequences. These include (1) anger and hostility, (2) stress, and (3) fear and anxiety. The web of research demonstrating this "potential" is complex but thin. Whereas innumerable studies have demonstrated links of anger, stress, and fear to changes in bodily functioning (e.g., immune system, cardiovascular system, etc.), fewer studies have related anger, stress, and fear to discrete diseases. It is thus tentatively that we suggest that if these negative health effects are to be avoided, mitigated, or ameliorated, a person needs to combat the constellation of emotions that make up unforgivingness.

THE PRO-VIRTUE CONSTELLATION OF PERSONAL QUALITIES AS WAYS OF OVERCOMING UNFORGIVENESS

Two Types of Virtues

We now turn our attention to the connection between dispositional characteristics that are virtuous and ways in which people respond to transgressions (see Figure 5.1). We have argued that unforgiveness and forgiveness are contrasting emotions. Because each set of emotions involves *embodied* experiences (e.g., hormones, brain pathways, visceral responses, gross behavior, facial musculature contractions), one set of emotions—unforgiveness or forgiveness—will "win out" when juxtaposed. When a person practices unforgiveness until it becomes the disposition of unforgivingness or practices forgiveness until it becomes the disposition of forgivingness, the person will

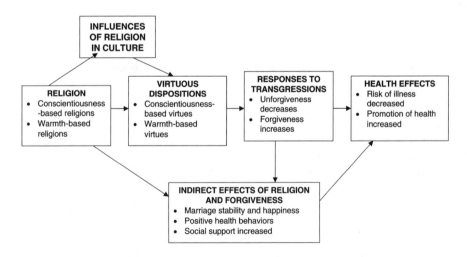

FIGURE 5.1. Simplified model for relating religion, virtuous dispositions, responses to transgressions, and health effects.

likely develop a constellation of personality dispositions or traits associated with unforgivingness or forgivingness.

We have also argued that people can reduce unforgiveness through many ways other than forgiveness. For example, a person could reduce unforgiveness through pursuing justice, resolving conflicts, working for social justice, telling a more prosocial story about a transgression, or forbearing a transgression. Each effort involves inhibiting unforgiving emotions. It is conceivable that practicing these means of overcoming unforgiveness could result in personality dispositions (McCrae, 1999).

We suggest, therefore, that two sets of pro-virtue characteristics can lessen or overcome unforgiveness. The first set of virtues, which we call the *conscientiousness-based virtues*, either (1) decrease the likelihood of antisocial, destructive, self-protective motivations or (2) increase the likelihood of self-control and restraint in responding to interpersonal transgressions. These virtues involve either the reduction of the emotions of unforgiveness through a variety of interactional or intrapersonal means or the rechanneling of potentially destructive behaviors in a socially appropriate fashion.

The second set of virtues, which we call the *warmth-based virtues*, increases the likelihood of the prosocial, affiliative emotions and consequent motivations linked to forgiveness. The warmth-based virtues result in emotional replacement or superimposition of unforgiving emotions with warm, loving emotions. Emotions associated with warmth compete with the emotions associated with unforgiveness.[1]

Conscientiousness–Based Virtues

Self-control is an important conscientiousness-based virtue. Baumeister and Exline (1999) have argued that self-control may be the overarching virtue, a necessary component of all other virtues. Self-control may involve restraint of one's impulses to do harm to self or others, or it may involve delay of gratification.

Integrity involves the pursuit of truth and the faithful sculpting of one's behavior in conformity to the way one perceives truth and goodness. Integrity is another conscientiousness-based virtue. A sense of justice and the desire for peace can be aspects of one's conception of goodness, and integrity can be a motive for self-control.

A *sense of justice* is a conscientiousness-based virtue that can promote behavior and alter perceptions that reduce unforgiveness. Justice is necessary when the social scales have been put out of balance by a crime, a wrong, an injustice, or a transgression. A sense of justice may be restored if a victim (1) exacts revenge, (2) pursues legal justice (Worthington, 2000), (3) receives personal restitution (Zehr, 1995), (4) acknowledges Divine justice, and, (5) in Eastern religions, attends to a belief in karma, a sense of immutable justice that suggests that all wrongs will be ultimately balanced (Rye et al., 2000). Perpetrators can contribute to the victim's sense of justice if perpetrators (1) engage in esteem-lowering acts (Baumeister, Exline, & Sommer, 1998) or (2) perform ceremonial acts of repentance, apology, confession, and public asking for forgiveness (Exline & Baumeister, 2000; Shriver, 1998).

Whereas both punitive and restorative justice seek to deal after the fact with transgressions, seeking *social justice* involves establishing conditions in which transgressions are less likely to occur in the future. In society, this might involve establishing agreed-upon norms for behavior toward an offending group, reforming a justice system to incorporate fair laws, or establishing social structures that are just. Between two partners, establishing social justice means agreeing on fair norms for continued interaction. Working for social justice can prevent future transgressions or at least make them less likely, rendering the experience of unforgiveness also less likely. However, working for social justice can also reduce one's feelings of unforgiveness because one diverts the negative energy aimed at emotions of unforgiveness into a sublimated positive energy for social good.

A *desire for peace* that promotes a sincere effort toward conflict resolution is also a conscientiousness-based virtue. When a conflict has existed for a substantial period, emotions of anger, fear, anxiety, and distress can color a person or society's world view. If hostilities are brought to an end through a truce or an agreement, people experience a sense of relief, some mitigation of unforgiveness, and an increased willingness to compromise. A compromise involves giving up some favored point, making a concession when it seems to be commensurate with a concession made by the other side. By compromise, the person or society feels more positive toward the other side and thereby reduces some of the unforgiveness felt toward the other side. Finally, beyond compromise, individuals or elements in society might negotiate agreement in which principles govern their joint solution to problems (Ury & Fisher, 1981). Negotiated agreement of a "win-win" solution can reduce the negative emotions that make up unforgiveness.

Warmth-Based Virtues

At the center of the warmth-based virtues is a sense of *other-oriented love* aimed primarily at blessing others rather than blessing oneself. Much research on other-oriented love has centered on the existence of altruistic acts. We view forgiveness as an altruistic gift based on love. Love involves passion, intimacy, and commitment (Sternberg, 1986). Depending on the mix of the three elements, Sternberg (1986) posits that there are different types of love.

Empathy for others is an important component of the warmth-based constellation. Empathy is at the root of many altruistic behaviors (Batson, Bolen, Cross, & Neuringer-Benfiel, 1986). For example, for a gift giver, empathy is needed to know what gift the recipient might like. For a gift recipient, empathy is needed to respond appropriately. The connection between empathy and forgiveness has been empirically established by McCullough, Worthington, and Rachal (1997), who demonstrated that (1) empathy mediates the apology–forgiveness connection; (2) empathy-based forgiveness interventions result in more forgiveness than do interventions not based on empathy (or than no intervention); and, (3) regardless of type of intervention, more successful forgiveness was related to more empathy.

Another element of the warmth-based constellation is *humility* (Tangney, 2000). Humility involves not merely defeating pride (partly by acknowledging the value of others) but also embracing a sense of one's existence as it is and being grateful to God or some other outside source for what gifts one has received. Humility can facilitate forgiveness because, by acknowledging one's own real or potential transgressions and imperfections, a victim can experience empathy for the transgressor.

Gratitude or thanksgiving for what others have done or for what one has received is part of the pro-virtue constellation (Emmons, 1999). Gratitude is likely to grow out of interpersonal relationships characterized by other-oriented love. Forgiveness is an act of love for which one can be grateful.

Forgiveness is one of the warmth-based virtues. It often occurs because love, empathy, humility, and gratitude work together with it.

These warmth-based virtues have been described and elaborated by Templeton (1997). He has relied on literature, religion, and the humanities to derive "world-wide laws of life" that suggest an intercorrelation of warmth-based virtues across religions and cultures. Such speculations have as yet received scant empirical attention.

RELIGIOUS FAITH AND ITS CONNECTION TO UNFORGIVENESS, FORGIVENESS, AND HEALTH

Because this book is focused on religion and health, we now describe ways in which religion might enter into our model (see Figure 5.1). Religious faith is composed of beliefs, values, and behaviors. Beliefs are statements of propositional truth that one endorses. Values describe the relative importance given to beliefs in one's value hierarchy (Rokeach, 1973). For example, one could believe that Jesus is God and is Lord of one's life yet place very little value on those beliefs, and therefore one would rarely act on that belief. Religious behaviors usually spring, to some degree, from religious beliefs that are valued. For example, one might believe that one should pray. If a person indeed values that belief and values the act of prayer, then the person will be more likely to pray.

Worthington (1988) has suggested that one's commitment to one's religious values is a key variable in understanding the centrality of religion in a person's life. He suggested that if people scored one standard deviation or more above the mean on a standard religious commitment inventory, they would tend to see their world through a religious perspective (see Worthington, Kurusu, McCullough, & Sandage, 1996, for an evaluation of some research on this hypothesis). They would likely embrace the pro-virtue constellation and act consistently with that constellation. On the other hand, people who scored lower than one standard deviation above the mean on religious commitment might still endorse religious beliefs, but their value of religion would not be high enough in their value hierarchy to shape their world view. Worthington (1988) suggested that a nonlinear transformation in perception occurs with very high religious commitment.

Religion Is Related to the Pro-Virtue Constellation

How is religion related to the pro-virtue constellation of personality characteristics in general and forgivingness in particular? The effects are thought to be direct (for those who are highly religious) and also indirect through the impact of religions on cultural and subcultural norms. The indirect pathway could affect people who are not highly religious (and even those opposed to religion) to the extent that culture reflects religious values. The pro-virtue constellation involves conscientiousness-based virtues (e.g., self-control, integrity, sense of justice, and desire for peace) and warmth-based virtues (e.g., love, humility, gratitude, empathy, and forgiveness). Such a constellation might involve beliefs that come from one's religious world view or from one's secular world view. Either conscientiousness-based or warmth-based virtues might predominate, or both might be (nearly) equally powerful. This is a direct effect of one's religion on one's personality.

Often friends, family, and culture will reinforce each other to support such pro-virtue attitudes and qualities. Sometimes only one or two elements reinforce those qualities. For example, one's peers, but not one's parents or one's work setting, might support one's religious beliefs. People might embrace a pro-virtue constellation of personal qualities without being highly religious or without being religious at all. Such a constellation would be activated under certain conditions, such as powerful religious stimuli or when facing a dilemma that forced a person to think about the religious implications of actions. Personal characteristics consistent with religion might be developed indirectly because one adheres to cultural norms that were influenced by religion.

The Cultural Context of Religion

Most societies are, to some degree, religious. In most societies, substantial majorities of people might embrace a variety of different religions. For example, in Singapore, which is a politically secular country, there are substantial numbers of traditional Chinese folk religions, Buddhists, Hindus, Christians, and Muslims. Although the government does not support one religion over any others, most people in Singapore subscribe to one of the religions.

Because culture is a container for many religious beliefs, even people who do not embrace a religion formally are often exposed to its belief and value systems. They may develop pro-virtue characteristics consistent with those religious belief and value systems even though they do not endorse the religion per se. Even in cultures that are very little influenced by religion, the people might develop pro-virtue characteristics because many of those are simply consistent with peaceful survival of the community. Thus religion might directly, indirectly, or not at all lead to the development of pro-virtue personal characteristics.

Direct Effects of Religion on the Person: For Highly Religious Individuals

Highly religious individuals presumably incorporate the main beliefs and values of their religion into their lives. That incorporation also presumably affects the development of character virtues. The beliefs of various religions become important.

Some religions, or subgroups within the religions, are more aimed at promoting conscientiousness than are others. One might suggest that fundamentalist Islam is, in general, more aimed at promoting conscientiousness-based virtues than is (for example) theologically liberal Christianity.

Differences within Religions

There are notable differences in emphasis within religions. A person might be a highly committed Christian and place a high value on conscientiousness-based virtues such as righteousness and justice, advocating strict behavior control and laws to enforce positive behavior. Although the person might doctrinally affirm the importance of love and other warmth-based virtues, the person might not frequently manifest that belief in his or her life. On the other hand, another Christian might highly value love but value justice less. That person might be lenient toward establishing and enforcing laws and might be highly involved in compassionate social activities and personal behaviors. A third Christian might highly value both love and justice.

Given that important variations *within* religions occur, there are also some broad differences *between* religions. These are described in the following sections.

Forgiveness in Christianity

The specific beliefs important in various religions differ, and the centrality of forgiveness as a part of a religious belief system differs among the religions as well (see Rye et al., 2000, for a review). For Christianity, forgiveness is the central cornerstone of the religion (Marty, 1998).

This centrality of forgiveness operates on two levels. One level is divine forgiveness—that is, forgiveness by God of humans. In Christian theology, Jesus, being God, voluntarily died a substitutionary death available to all but effective for those who believe. Such a death fulfills some of the demands of justice but also moves God the Father to an emotional forgiveness of humans on whose behalf God's son died. Because divine forgiveness and a Christian believer's acceptance of it are crucial to Christianity, forgiveness holds a central part in Christian theology.

At the second level, the interpersonal level, many commands within the Christian New Testament admonish Christians to extend forgiveness to those who transgress against them, whether Christians or non-Christians. In fact, some Christian scriptures argue that divine forgiveness can be conditional on interpersonal forgiveness (e.g., see Matthew 6 and 18).

Forgiveness in Judaism

For Jewish believers (Dorff, 1998), forgiveness is more of an imbedded concept than in Christianity. Forgiveness is imbedded in the word *teshuvah,* which suggests that a transgressor return to the path of God (Dorff, 1998). Christians use the word "repentance" to capture this notion. For Jewish believers, forgiveness is conditional on a perpetrator's *teshuvah.* If the perpetrator does not make an effort to return to the path of God, the Jewish believer is not obligated to forgive. However, if the person attempts to return to the path of God, then forgiveness is necessary. If a person who has been wronged does not offer forgiveness to a returned (repentant) perpetrator, then the unforgiving person has sinned.

Forgiveness in Islam

In Muslim theology, forgiveness is understood more within the concept of justice than it is in Jewish or Christian theology (Rye et al., 2000). God is seen to administer justice but also to meet out divine forgiveness. Interpersonal forgiveness is not thought to be compelled, as it is in Christianity.

Forgiveness in Hinduism and Buddhism

For Eastern religions, the concept of divine justice is meaningless, especially for Hinduism and Buddhism, in which the doctrine of karma exists (Rye et al., 2000). Karma implies that justice will happen eventually—if not in the present life, then in a future life. If justice is immutable, then there is no place for the concept of divine justice. In addition, ontological assumptions hold that reality as humans know it is illusory or *Maya* and that ultimately all of existence will be aimed at a reunification of oneness. Such assumptions make the interpersonal recede in ultimate importance. Nonetheless, Hinduism and Buddhism (especially Buddhism) emphasize compassion as a central virtue. Part of interpersonal compassion is not to seek revenge or hold grudges.

Forgiveness in Folk Religions

Folk religions might involve spiritism or ancestor worship. In Chinese folk religions, shame has a distinct negative connotation, and loss of face is seen as greatly shameful. Shame can be mitigated by forgiveness. Many folk religions rely on collections of wise sayings that are often paradoxical. Many wise sayings in Chinese folk religion advocate revenge or an eventual balancing of the scales of justice through a fateful intervention. Other sayings advocate forgiveness and mercy.

Varying Emphasis on Forgiving

The belief systems of the various world religions, some of which we have briefly sampled, place forgiveness in different light. In most religions, interpersonal forgiveness is esteemed. Therefore, to the extent that people are committed to their religion, they often embrace and value interpersonal forgiveness. However, different religions might advocate conscientiousness-based virtues more than warmth-based virtues, or vice versa. Even within each religion, some theological variations will occur (as illustrated for Christianity). Thus the emphasis on interpersonal forgiveness necessarily varies widely between and within religions.

   If we consider religious commitment to be one of the virtues, it is unclear whether it would be a conscientiousness-based or warmth-based virtue. It depends on the emphasis of the particular religious beliefs and behaviors. For highly religiously committed people, religious commitment (and thus beliefs and values) could be a master virtue, which organizes and empowers other virtues within the pro-virtue constellation (Worthington, 1988). For moderately to mildly religiously committed people, religious commitment might be a virtue, but not a master virtue.

Religion and Health

The research on religion and health (including mental health) has accumulated over a century. It has accumulated especially rapidly during the past 30 years (see Larson et al., 1998). The possible benefits of religion to physical health have been documented in several extensive reviews (Koenig, 1997; Larson et al., 1998; see also Thoresen et al., Chapter 2, this volume). Although there is much debate over issues of causality and possible mechanisms linking religion to health (Thoresen, 1999), a positive relationship between the two appears to be a robust finding across diverse studies. Religious commitment has been shown to predict longevity (see McCullough et al., 2000 and McCullough, Chapter 3, this volume, for a meta-analysis and discussion). Religion has also been associated with positive outcomes for many specific physical health problems (Idler & Kasl, 1992; see also Remle & Koenig, Chapter 8, and Sherman & Simonton, Chapter 7, this volume).

Research has also established the benefits of religion for psychological adjustment (Gartner, Larson, & Allen, 1991; Larson et al., 1998; see also Plante & Sharma, Chapter 10, this volume). There is evidence that religion is associated with lower rates of depression (Pressman, Lyons, Larson, & Strain, 1990), suicide (Stack, 1983), and divorce (Larson, 1985) and with higher self-esteem and subjective well-being (Jones, 1993).

To the extent that religious commitment is a person's master virtue, it might be responsible for activating health benefits of the conscientiousness-based virtues (which might also reduce unforgiveness) and the warmth-based virtues (which might also reduce unforgiveness through promoting forgiveness). Benefits to physical and mental health would thus be additive across the two dimensions of the pro-virtue constellation.

The Pro-Virtue Constellation and Health

Religion can directly affect the development of character virtues, which can directly affect whether people forgive or reduce unforgiveness in other ways, which might be related differentially to health outcomes. The literature on the health-compromising effects of unforgiveness or related emotions is far more developed than is the literature on the health-promoting effects of conscientiousness-based and warmth-based virtues (Salovey et al., 2000). Given the abundant research linking chronic anger and hostility to negative health consequences, we can hypothesize that the reduction of these affects (through the conscientiousness-based virtues) or the replacement of these affects (through the warmth-based virtues) will likely yield long-term benefits to health and well-being. Next we review research on the health correlates and consequences of each virtue constellation.

Conscientiousness-Based Virtues and Health

Several studies have provided evidence that certain personality traits associated with low conscientiousness, such as lack of self-control, impulsivity, and carelessness, may be risk factors for poor health behaviors (Seeman, Kaplan, Knudsen, Cohen, & Guralnik, 1987; Vingerhoets, Croon, Jeninga, & Menges, 1990). Baumeister, Heatherton, and Tice (1994) reviewed a large body of research linking self-control to a number of variables related to psychological and social adjustment.

There are quite a few studies that directly assess the impact of conscientiousness on physical health outcomes (see Aspinwall, 1998; Salovey et al., 2000, for reviews). In a 70-year longitudinal study based on data from Terman and Oden (1947), Friedman et al. (1993) found that Conscientiousness/Social Dependability (measured by parent ratings of participants' prudence, conscientiousness, truthfulness, and freedom from vanity/egotism at age 11) was a significant predictor of longevity into middle and old age among 1,178 male and female participants.

Salovey et al. (2000) review the literature and describe five contributions that conscientiousness-based emotion states might make to health. (They do not conceptualize the emotions as conscientiousness based, but that concept appears to fit with the contributions they identify.) For example, mood affects (1) reports of symptoms (Watson, 2000), (2) perception of personal vulnerability (Weinstein, 1993), (3) perception of risk (Mayer, Gaschke, Braverman, & Evans, 1992), (4) self-efficacy (Salovey, Rothman, & Rodin, 1998), and (5) delay in seeking health care (Schwartz & Clore, 1996).

Forgiveness (and Other Warmth-Based Virtues) and Health

A lifestyle characterized by forgivingness is often thought to be also characterized by love, empathy, humility, and gratitude. Although no research has explicitly tested the link between forgivingness and health outcomes, studies have identified health benefits with traits associated with forgiveness.

Other-oriented love, which we think of as often being the central warmth-based virtue, has been studied in many guises. Luks and Payne (1992) summarized evidence that altruism is a powerful healing force. Kalliopuska (1992) found that highly empathic students, compared with the least empathic students, had more positive attitudes toward health behaviors and were less likely to smoke and consume alcohol.

There have been few studies on the health effects of gratitude. Gratitude appears to be associated with positive emotions and psychological well-being (Overwalle, Mervielde, & De Schuyter, 1995; Walker & Pitts, 1998).

From an evolutionary perspective, gratitude is thought to promote recipro-cal altruism and thus help maintain social ties and cooperation. Through this means, gratitude could have an indirect positive impact on health by strengthening social support (see the next section). In an experimental study of gratitude and well-being, Emmons (1999) has shown that, over a semes-ter, college students who were instructed to write about five things they were grateful for each week had positive health consequences (e.g., had fewer physical complaints, spent more time exercising) relative to students who wrote about five complaints each week or those who wrote about five events that happened in their lives.

Forgiveness (and Other Warmth-Based Virtues), Social Support, and Health

The presence of forgiveness and other warmth-based virtues is likely to be related to better interpersonal functioning and therefore to promote better marriages, a higher quality of family life, and a wider, more fulfilling social network. Therefore, additional health benefits might accumulate through these indirect pathways. Religion promotes social interactions (and therefore social support) directly (see Figure 5.1). A substantial literature has accumu-lated investigating the relationships between various types of social support and health (see Salovey et al., 2000, for a review). Emotional social support has particularly been associated with reducing cardiovascular reactivity (Kamarck, Manuck, & Jennings, 1990), promoting healing after a heart attack (Fontana, Kerns, Rosenberg, & Colonese, 1989), and reducing other risk factors (Amick & Ockene, 1994). Social support, particularly emotional social support, has also been involved in reduction of stress (Kennedy, Kiecolt-Glaser, & Glaser, 1988; Steinglass, Weisstub, & De-Nour, 1988). Social support has also been related to increased survival rates from different types of cancer (Ell, Mantell, Hamovitch, & Nishimoto, 1989; Fawzy et al., 1993).

Forgiveness (and Other Warmth-Based Virtues), Marriage, and Health

Religion also affects the value people place on marriage and can act through relationship behaviors to affect marriage (see Figure 5.1 for the two path-ways). Forgiveness is related to reconciliation after conflicts during marriage (Worthington, 1998; Worthington & Drinkard, 2000). To the extent that happy marriages are fostered in couples characterized by one or both part-ners who manifest high trait forgivingness, we might expect positive health consequences and correlates associated with long-term marriage stability and satisfaction to accrue to the married partners. Marriage has been shown to be associated with longevity (Burman & Margolin, 1992) and divorce with health hazards (Hu & Goldman, 1990). Divorce has been found to have fewer health risks than has unhappy marriage (Sarason, Sarason, & Pierce, 1990).

There are competing explanations for this relationship between marriage and health (Hahn, Brooks, & Hartsough, 1993; Wyke & Ford, 1992). Possible explanations are that married people (1) have an economic advantage relative to unmarried people (but the relationship between unhappy marriage and ill health suggests that such an explanation is not likely to be causal); (2) are happier, which is related to better health; (3) experience more emotional social support; (4) experience more concern by a close family member that prompts regular medical care; and (5) have better eating habits. Marriage has been related to lower incidences of coronary heart disease, lower blood pressure (Medalie & Goldbourt, 1976), better survival rates from cancer (Goodwin, Hunt, Key, & Samet, 1987), and better immune system functioning (Kiecolt-Glaser & Glaser, 1989).

CONCLUSIONS

This chapter focuses on the potential health consequences and correlates of unforgiveness, the reduction of unforgiveness, and forgiveness. Religion is treated as a variable that affects a pro-virtue constellation of personality characteristics (both directly through individual beliefs and values and indirectly through culture), and its effects on unforgiveness and forgiveness have been particularly considered. Religion also affects health through individual behavior in relationships and through the value religions place on relationships.

Specifically, the ways in which people deal with the multitude of emotional transgressions with which they must cope—through holding onto unforgiveness, through reducing unforgiveness by any of a variety of ways other than forgiving, and through forgiving—is thought to play a large part in health or illness. We suggest that the pivotal nature of unforgiveness and forgiveness can (1) explain some of the religion–health connections and (2) suggest physiological mechanisms for this connection (e.g., those dealing with emotional experience and expression).

We believe that the road map of research suggested in Figure 5.1 could be especially attractive to health psychology researchers. The field of health psychology has focused on three primary areas: (1) health-related behaviors and their physical and mental health consequences, (2) stress and its health consequences, and (3) health care (Smith, Chapter 15, this volume). Researchers from the first two focal areas certainly would find a ready home investigating unforgiveness and the varieties of ways to reduce unforgiveness. With the report of the Institute of Medicine (1999) that suggested that up to 98,000 medical errors occur annually in the United States, the field of health care also seems to be ripe for the investigation of unforgiveness. We believe that researchers in health psychology—those who study religion and those who do not—can find many stimulating questions to investigate within the study of unforgiveness, how it is dealt with, and its effects on health.

For example, prospective longitudinal research is needed that examines unforgivingness and forgivingness and that carefully delineates the contribution of each to health outcomes and the processes that lead to those outcomes. In addition, outcomes and processes of the many alternatives to forgiving must be determined. Religion might be an important mediator or moderator for various of these health outcomes. The various roles of religion, and especially of conscientiousness-based versus warmth-based religions, should be studied. Finally, another priority for research involves interventions to promote the reduction of unforgiveness and the granting of forgiveness, both in religious and secular communities.

ACKNOWLEDGMENTS

We wish to express our gratitude to and acknowledge support from Virginia Commonwealth University's General Clinical Research Center, which is supported by NIH Grant No. M01 RR00065, and from the John Templeton Foundation (Grant No. 239). Portions of this chapter were supported by each.

NOTE

1. This dual classification of virtues that deal prosocially with antisocial tendencies bears a resemblance to two mechanisms underlying socialization: the capacity for inhibitory control and the capacity for warmth (MacDonald, 1997). The capacity for inhibitory control is associated with conscientiousness, planning, delaying gratification, and inhibiting impulsive antisocial behaviors. The capacity for warmth involves giving and receiving affection. It is important for maintaining parent–child bonds, friendships, and romantic relationships. Research on parental socialization has identified two systems that parallel our dual classification of means of reducing unforgiveness. Many factor analytic studies of socialization practices among parents have found two dimensions that are thought to contribute to the development of conscience and to the internalization of values. These dimensions have been variously labeled warmth/hostility versus dominance/ submission (Symonds, 1939); love/hostility versus control/autonomy (Schaefer, 1959); warmth/hostility versus restrictiveness/ permissiveness (Becker, 1964); and accepting–responsive/rejecting–unresponsive versus demanding–controlling/

undemanding–low controlling (Maccoby & Martin, 1983). We can make distinctions between parents who tend to practice warmth-based virtues toward their children, those who practice conscientiousness-based virtues, and those who practice neither or both.

REFERENCES

Amick, T. L., & Ockene, J. K. (1994). The role of social support in the modification of risk factors for cardiovascular disease. In S. A. Shumaker & S. M. Czajkowski (Eds.), *Social support and cardiovascular disease* (pp. 259–278). New York: Plenum.

Aspinwall, L. G. (1998). Rethinking the role of positive affect in self-regulation. *Motivation and Emotion, 22,* 1–32.

Batson, C. D., Bolen, M. H., Cross, J. A., & Neuringer-Benfiel (1986). Where is the altruism in the altruistic personality? *Journal of Personality and Social Psychology, 50,* 212–220.

Baumeister, R. F., & Exline, J. J. (1999). Virtue, personality, and human relations. *Journal of Personality, 67,* 1165–1194.

Baumeister, R. F., Exline, J. J., & Sommer, K. L. (1998). The victim role, grudge theory, and two dimensions of forgiveness. In E. L. Worthington, Jr. (Ed.), *Dimensions of forgiveness: Psychological research and theological perspectives* (pp. 70–104). Philadelphia: Templeton Foundation Press.

Baumeister, R. F., Heatherton, T. F., & Tice, D. M. (1994). *Losing control: How and why people fail at self-regulation.* San Diego, CA: Academic Press.

Becker, W. C. (1964). Consequences of different kinds of parental discipline. In M. L. Hoffman & W. L. Hoffman (Eds.), *Review of child development research* (Vol. 1, pp. 169–208). New York: Sage Foundation.

Bell, I. R., Martino, G. M., Meredith, K. E., Schwartz, G. E., Siani, M. M., & Morrow, F. D. (1993). Vascular disease factors, urinary free cortisol, and health histories in older adults: Shyness and gender interactions. *Biological Psychology, 35,* 37–49.

Berry, J. W., Worthington, E. L., Jr., O'Connor, L. E., Parrott, L., III, & Wade, N. G. (2001). *The measurement of trait forgivingness.* Manuscript submitted for publication.

Berry, J. W., Worthington, E. L., Jr., Parrott, L., III, O'Connor, L. E., & Wade, N. G. (in press). Dispositional forgivingness: Construct validity and development of the Transgression Narrative Test of Forgivingness (TNTF). *Personality and Social Psychology Bulletin.*

Bromberger, J. T., & Matthews, K. A. (1996). A "feminine" model of vulnerability to depressive symptoms: A longitudinal investigation of middle-aged women. *Journal of Personality and Social Psychology, 70,* 591–598.

Brown, L. L., Tomarken, A. J., Orth, D. N., Loosen, P. T., Kalin, N. H., & Davidson, R. J. (1996). Individual differences in repressive-defensiveness predict basal salivary cortisol levels. *Journal of Personality and Social Psychology, 70,* 362–371.

Burman, B., & Margolin, G. (1992). Analysis of the association between marital relationships and health problems: An interactional perspective. *Psychological Bulletin, 112,* 39–63.

Buss, D. M. (1996). Social adaptation and the five major factors of personality. In J. S. Wiggins (Ed.), *The five-factor model of personality: Theoretical perspectives* (pp. 180–207). New York: Guilford Press.

Cohen, S., & Rodriguez, M. S. (1995). Pathways linking affective disturbances and physical disorders. *Health Psychology, 14,* 374–380.

Damasio, A. R. (1999). *The feeling of what happens: Body and emotion in the making of consciousness.* New York: Harcourt Brace.

Dorff, E. N. (1998). The elements of forgiveness: A Jewish approach. In E. L. Worthington, Jr. (Ed.), *Dimensions of forgiveness: Psychological research and theological perspectives* (pp. 29–55). Philadelphia: Templeton Foundation Press.

Ell, K. O., Mantell, J. E., Hamovitch, M. B., & Nishimoto, R. H. (1989). Social support, sense of control, and coping among patients with breast, lung, or colorectal cancer. *Journal of Psychosocial Oncology, 7,* 63–89.

Emmons, R. A. (1999). *The psychology of ultimate concerns: Motivation and spirituality in personality.* New York: Guilford Press.

Emmons, R. A. (2000). Personality and forgiveness. In M. E. McCullough, K. I. Pargament, & C. E. Thoresen (Eds.), *Forgiveness: Theory, research, and practice* (pp. 156–175). New York: Guilford Press.

Esterling, B. A., Antoni, M. H., Kumar, M., & Schneiderman, N. (1993). Defensiveness, trait anxiety, and Epstein–Barr viral capsid antigen antibody titers in healthy college students. *Health Psychology, 12,* 132–139.

Evans, P. D., & Edgerton, N. (1991). Life-events and mood as predictors of the common cold. *British Journal of Medical Psychology, 64,* 35–44.

Exline, J. J., & Baumeister, R. F. (2000). Expressing forgiveness and repentance: Benefits and barriers. In M. E. McCullough, K. I. Pargament, & C. E. Thoresen (Eds.), *Forgiveness: Theory, research, and practice* (pp. 133–155). New York: Guilford Press.

Fawzy, F. I., Fawzy, N. W., Hyun, C. S., Elashoff, R., Guthrie, D., Fahey, J. L., & Morton, D. L. (1993). Malignant melanoma: Effects of an early structured psychiatric intervention, coping, and affective state on recurrence and survival 6 years later. *Archives of General Psychiatry, 50,* 681–689.

Fitzgibbons, R. P. (1986). The cognitive and emotive uses of forgiveness in the treatment of anger. *Psychotherapy, 23,* 629–633.

Fontana, A. F., Kerns, R. D., Rosenberg, R. L., & Colonese, K. L. (1989). Support, stress, and recovery from coronary heart disease: A longitudinal causal model. *Health Psychology, 8,* 175–193.

Friedman, H. S., & Booth-Kewley, S. (1987). The "disease-prone personality": A meta-analytic view of the construct. *American Psychologist, 42,* 539–555.

Friedman, H. S., Tucker, J. S., Tomlinson-Keasey, C., Schwartz, J. E., Wingard, D. L., & Criqui, M. H. (1993). Does childhood personality predict longevity? *Journal of Personality and Social Psychology, 65,* 176–185.

Futterman, A. D., Kemeny, M. E., Shapiro, D., Polonsky, W., & Fahey, J. L. (1992). Immunological variability associated with experimentally-induced positive and negative affective states. *Psychological Medicine, 22,* 231–238.

Gartner, J., Larson, D. B., & Allen, G. D. (1991). Religious commitment and mental health: A review of the empirical literature. *Journal of Psychology and Theology, 19,* 6–25.

Goodwin, J. S., Hunt, W. C., Key, C. R., & Samet, J. M. (1987). The effect of marital status on stage, treatment, and survival of cancer patients. *Journal of the American Medical Association, 258,* 3125–3130.

Gray, J. A. (1994). Three fundamental emotion systems. In P. Ekman & R. J. Davidson (Eds.), *The nature of emotion* (pp. 243–247). New York: Oxford University Press.

Grothgar, B., & Scholz, D. B. (1987). On specific behavior of migraine patients in an anger provoking situation. *Headache, 27,* 206–210.

Hahn, W. K., Brooks, J. A., & Hartsough, D. M. (1993). Self-disclosure and coping styles in men with cardiovascular reactivity. *Research in Nursing and Health, 16,* 275–282.

Hecker, M., Chesney, M., Black, G., & Frautschi, N. (1989). Coronary-prone behaviors in the Western Collaborative Group Study. *Psychosomatic Medicine, 50,* 153–164.

Herbert, T., & Cohen, S. (1993). Stress and immunity in humans: A meta-analytic review. *Psychosomatic Medicine, 55,* 364–379.

Hu, Y., & Goldman, N. (1990). Mortality differentials by marital status: An international comparison. *Demography, 27,* 233–250.

Idler, E. L., & Kasl, S. V. (1992). Religion, disability, depression and the timing of death. *American Journal of Sociology, 97,* 1052–1079.

Institute of Medicine. (1999). *To err is human: Building a safer health system.* Washington, DC: Author.

John, O. P. (1990). The "Big Five" factor taxonomy: Dimensions of personality in the natural language and in questionnaires. In L. A. Pervin (Ed.), *Handbook of personality: Theory and research* (pp. 66–100). New York: Guilford Press.

Jones, J. W. (1993). Living on the boundary between psychology and religion. *Religion Newsletter, 18*(4), 1–7.

Kalliopuska, M. (1992). Attitudes towards health, health behavior, and personality factors among school students very high on empathy. *Psychological Reports, 70,* 1119–1122.

Kamarck, T. W., Manuck, S. B., & Jennings, J. R. (1990). Social support reduces cardiovascular reactivity to psychological challenge: A laboratory model. *Psychosomatic Medicine, 52,* 42–58.

Kaplan, B. H. (1992). Social health and the forgiving heart: The Type B story. *Journal of Behavior Medicine, 15,* 3–14.

Kaplan, B. H., Munroe-Blum, H., & Blazer, D. G. (1993). Religion, health, and forgiveness: Traditions and challenges. In J. S. Levin (Ed.), *Religion in aging and health: Theoretical foundations and methodological frontiers* (pp. 52–77). Thousand Oaks, CA: Sage.

Kennedy, S., Kiecolt-Glaser, J. K., & Glaser, R. (1988). Immunological consequences of acute and chronic stressors: Mediating role of interpersonal relationships. *British Journal of Medical Psychology, 61,* 77–85.

Kiecolt-Glaser, J. K., & Glaser, R. (1989). Interpersonal relationships and immune function. In L. Carstensen & J. Neale (Eds.), *Mechanisms of psychological influence on physical health* (pp. 43–59). New York: Plenum Press.

Kiesler, D. J. (1983). The 1982 Interpersonal Circle: A taxonomy for complementarity in human transactions. *Psychological Review, 90,* 185–214.

Koenig, H. G. (1997). *Is religion good for your health? Effects of religion on mental and physical health.* Binghamton, NY: Haworth Press.

Koenig, H. G. (1999). *The healing power of faith: Science explores medicine's last great frontier.* New York: Simon & Schuster.

Koenig, H. G., McCullough, M. E., & Larson, D. (2000). *Handbook of religion and health: A century of research reviewed.* New York: Oxford University Press.

Lang, P. J., Bradley, M. M., & Cuthbert, B. N. (1990). Emotion, attention, and the startle reflex. *Psychological Bulletin, 97,* 377–395.

Larson, D. B. (1985). Religious involvement. In G. Rekers (Ed.), *Family building* (pp. 121–147). Ventura, CA: Regal.

Larson, D. B., Swyers, J. P., & McCullough, M. E. (1998). *Scientific research on spirituality and health: A consensus report.* Rockville, MD: National Institute for Healthcare Research.

Laudenslager, M. L., Ryan, S. M., Drugan, R. C., Hyson, R. L., & Maier, S. F. (1983). Coping and immunosuppression: Inescapable but not escapable shock suppresses lymphocyte proliferation. *Science, 221,* 568–571.

Lazarus, R. S. (1999). *Stress and emotion: A new synthesis.* New York: Springer.

LeDoux, J. (1996). *The emotional brain: The mysterious underpinnings of emotional life.* New York: Simon & Schuster.

Levin, J. S. (1994). Religion and health: Is there an association, is it valid, and is it causal? *Social Sciences and Medicine, 38,* 1475–1482.

Luks, A., & Payne, P. (1992). *The healing power of doing good: The health and spiritual benefits of helping others.* New York: Fawcett Columbine.

Maccoby, E., & Martin, J. (1983). Socialization in the context of the family. In E. M. Hetherington (Ed.), *Handbook of child psychology: Vol. 4. Socialization, personality, and social development* (pp. 1–101). New York: Wiley.

MacDonald, K. B. (1992). Warmth as a developmental construct: An evolutionary analysis. *Child Development, 63,* 753–773.

MacDonald, K. B. (1997). The coherence of individual development: An evolutionary perspective on children's internalization of parental values. In J. Grusec & L. Kuczynski (Eds.), *Parenting and children's internalization of values: A handbook of contemporary theory* (pp. 362–397). New York: Wiley.

Marty, M. E. (1998). The ethos of Christian forgiveness. In E. L. Worthington, Jr. (Ed.), *Dimensions of forgiveness: Psychological research and theological perspectives* (pp. 9–28). Philadelphia: Templeton Foundation Press.

Mayer, J. D., Gaschke, Y. N., Braverman, D. L., & Evans, T. W. (1992). Mood-congruent judgement is a general effect. *Journal of Personality and Social Psychology, 63,* 119–132.

McAdams, D. P. (1994). *The person: An introduction to personality psychology* (2nd ed.). Fort Worth, TX: Harcourt Brace.

McCrae, R. R. (1999). Mainstream personality psychology and the study of religion. *Journal of Personality, 67,* 1209–1218.

McCullough, M. E., Hoyt, W. T., Larson, D. B., Koenig, H. G., & Thoresen, C. E. (2000). Religious involvement and mortality: A meta-analytic review. *Health Psychology, 19,* 211–222.

McCullough, M. E., Worthington, E. L., Jr., & Rachal, K. C. (1997). Interpersonal forgiveness in close relationships. *Journal of Personality and Social Psychology, 75*, 321–326.

McEwen, B. S. (1998). Protective and damaging effects of stress mediators. *New England Journal of Medicine, 338*, 171–179.

McEwen, B. S., & Stellar, E. (1993). Stress and the individual: Mechanisms leading to disease. *Archives of Internal Medicine, 153*, 2093–2101.

Medalie, J. H., & Goldbourt, U. (1976). Angina pectoris among 10,000 men. II. Psychosocial and other risk factors as evidenced by a multivariate analysis of a five-year incidence study. *American Journal of Medicine, 60*, 910–921.

Newberg, A. B., d'Aquili, E. G., Newberg, S. K., & deMarici, V. (2000). The neuropsychological correlates of forgiveness. In M. E. McCullough, K. I. Pargament, & C. E. Thoresen (Eds.), *Forgiveness: Theory, research, and practice* (pp. 91–110). New York: Guilford Press.

Overwalle, F. V., Mervielde, I., & de Schuyter, J. (1995). Structural modeling of the relationship between attributional dimensions, emotions, and performance of college freshmen. *Cognition and Emotion, 9*, 59–85.

Panksepp, J. (1982). Toward a general psychobiological theory of emotions. *Behavioral and Brain Sciences, 5*, 407–468.

Pargament, K. I. (1997). *The psychology of religion and coping: Theory, research, practice.* New York: Guilford Press.

Pargament, K. I., & Rye, M. S. (1998). Forgiveness as a method of religious coping. In E. L. Worthington, Jr. (Ed.), *Dimensions of forgiveness: Psychological research and theological perspectives* (pp. 59–78). Philadelphia: Templeton Foundation Press.

Perini, C., Muller, F., & Buhler, F. (1991). Suppressed aggression accelerates early development of essential hypertension. *Journal of Hypertension, 9*, 499–503.

Plutchik, R. (1994). *The psychology and biology of emotion.* New York: HarperCollins.

Pressman, P., Lyons, J. S., Larson, D. B., & Strain, J. J. (1990). Religious belief, depression, and ambulation status in elderly women with broken hips. *American Journal of Psychiatry, 147*, 758–760.

Rhodewalt, F., & Morf, C. C. (1995). Self and interpersonal correlates of the Narcissistic Personality Inventory: A review and new findings. *Journal of Research in Personality, 29*(1), 1–23.

Roberts, R. C. (1995). Forgivingness. *American Philosophical Quarterly, 32*, 289–306.

Rokeach, M. (1973). *The nature of human values.* New York: Free Press.

Rye, M. S., Pargament, K. I., Ali, M. A., Beck, G. L., Dorff, E. N., Hallisey, C., Narayanan, V., & Williams, J. G. (2000). Religious perspectives on forgiveness. In M. E. McCullough, K. I. Pargament, & C. E. Thoresen (Eds.), *Forgiveness: Theory, research, and practice* (pp. 17–40). New York: Guilford Press.

Salovey, P., Rothman, A. J., Detweiler, J. B., & Steward, W. T. (2000). Emotional states and physical health. *American Psychologist, 55*, 110–121.

Salovey, P., Rothman, A. J., & Rodin, J. (1998). Health behavior. In D. T. Gilbert, S. T. Fiske, & G. Lindzey (Eds.), *The handbook of social psychology* (4th ed., Vol. 2, pp. 633–683). New York: McGraw-Hill.

Sandage, S. J., Worthington, E. L., Jr., Hight, T. L., & Berry, J. W. (2000). Seeking forgiveness: Theoretical context and an initial empirical study. *Journal of Psychology and Theology, 28,* 21–35.

Sapolsky, R. M. (1994). *Why zebras don't get ulcers: A guide to stress, stress-related diseases, and coping.* New York: Freeman.

Sapolsky, R. M. (1999). Hormonal correlates of personality and social contexts: From non-human to human primates. In C. Panter-Brick & C. M. Worthman (Eds.), *Hormones, health, and behavior: A socio-ecological and lifespan perspective* (pp. 18–46). Cambridge, England: Cambridge University Press.

Sarason, I. G., Sarason, B. R., & Pierce, G. R. (1990). Social support, personality, and performance. *Journal of Applied Sport Psychology, 2,* 117–127.

Schaefer, E. S. (1959). A circumplex model for maternal behavior. *Journal of Abnormal and Social Psychology, 59,* 226–235.

Schneirla, T. C. (1959). An evolutionary and developmental theory of biophasic process underlying approach and withdrawal. In M. Jones (Ed.), Current theory and research on motivation. *Nebraska Symposium on Motivation: Vol. 7* (pp. 1–42). Lincoln: University of Nebraska Press.

Schwartz, N., & Clore, G. L. (1996). Feelings and phenomenal experiences. In E. T. Higgins & A. W. Kruglanski (Eds.), *Social psychology: Handbook of basic principles* (pp. 433–465). New York: Guilford Press.

Seeman, T. E., Kaplan, G. A., Knudsen, L., Cohen, R., & Guralnik, J. (1987). Social network ties and mortality among the elderly: The Alameda County Study. *American Journal of Epidemiology, 126,* 714–723.

Shriver, D. W. J. (1998). Is there forgiveness in politics? Germany, Vietnam, and America. In R. D. Enright & J. North (Eds.), *Exploring forgiveness* (pp. 131–149). Madison, WI: University of Wisconsin Press.

Sloan, R. P., Bagiella, E., & Powell, T. (1999). Religion, spirituality, and medicine. *Lancet, 353,* 664–667.

Smith, T. W., & Christensen, A. J. (1992). Hostility, health, and social contexts. In H. S. Friedman (Ed.), *Hostility, coping, and health* (pp. 33–48). Washington, DC: American Psychological Association.

Solomon, G. F. (1985). The emerging field of psychoneuroimmunology. *Advances, 2,* 6–19.

Stack, S. (1983). The effect of religious commitment on suicide: A cross-national analysis. *Journal of Health and Social Behavior, 24,* 362–374.

Steinglass, P., Weisstub, E., & De-Nour, A. K. (1988). Perceived personal networks as mediators of stress reactions. *American Journal of Psychiatry, 145,* 1259–1264.

Sternberg, R. (1986). A triangular theory of love. *Psychological Review, 93,* 119–135.

Stone, A. A., Marco, C. A., Cruise, C. E., Cox, D. S., & Neale, J. M. (1996). Are stress-induced immunological changes mediated by mood? A closer look at how both desirable and undesirable daily events influence s Ig A antibody. *International Journal of Behavioral Medicine, 3,* 1–13.

Symonds, P. M. (1939). *The psychology of parent–child relationships.* New York: Norton.

Tangney, J. P. (2000). Humility: Theoretical perspectives, empirical findings and directions for future research. *Journal of Social and Clinical Psychology, 19,* 70–82.

Templeton, J. M. (1997). *The world-wide laws of life.* Radnor, PA: Templeton Foundation Press.

Terman, L. M., & Oden, M. H. (1947). *Genetic studies of genius: IV. The gifted child grows up: Twenty-five year follow-up.* Stanford, CA: Stanford University Press.

Thoresen, C. E. (1999). Spirituality and health: Is there a relationship? *Journal of Health Psychology, 4,* 291–300.

Thoresen, C. E., Harris, A. H. S., & Luskin, F. (2000). Forgiveness and health: An unanswered question. In M. E. McCullough, K. I. Pargament, & C. E. Thoresen (Eds.), *Forgiveness: Theory, research, and practice* (pp. 254–280). New York: Guilford Press.

Thoresen, C. E., Luskin, F., & Harris, A. H. S. (1998). Science and forgiveness interventions: Reflections and recommendations. In E. L. Worthington, Jr. (Ed.), *Dimensions of forgiveness: Psychological research and theological speculations* (pp. 163–192). Philadelphia: Templeton Foundation Press.

Thoresen, C. E., & Powell, L. H. (1992). Type A behavior pattern: New perspectives on theory, assessment, and intervention. *Journal of Consulting and Clinical Psychology, 60,* 595–604.

Ury, R., & Fisher, W. (1981). *Getting to yes: Negotiating agreement without giving in.* New York: Penguin Books.

Vingerhoets, A. J., Croon, M., Jeninga, A. J., & Menges, L. J. (1990). Personality and health habits. *Psychology and Health, 4,* 333–342.

Walker, L. J., & Pitts, R. C. (1998). Naturalistic conceptions of moral maturity. *Developmental Psychology, 34,* 403–419.

Watson, D. (2000). *Mood and temperament.* New York: Guilford Press.

Watson, D., & Tellegen, A. (1985). Toward a consensual structure of mood. *Psychological Bulletin, 98,* 219–235.

Watson, D., Wiese, D., Vaidya, J., & Tellegen, A. (1999). The two general activation systems of affect: Structural findings, evolutionary considerations, and psychological evidence. *Journal of Personality and Social Psychology, 76,* 820–838.

Weinstein, N. D. (1993). Testing four competing theories of health-protective behavior. *Health Psychology, 12,* 324–333.

Weiss, D., Hirt, R., Rarcic, N., Berxon, Y., Ben-Zur, H., Breznitz, S., Glaser, B., Baras, M., & O'Dorision, T. (1996). Studies in psychoneuroimmunology: Psychological, immunological, and neuroendocrinological parameters in Israeli civilians during and after a period of Scud missile attacks. *Behavioral Medicine, 22,* 5–14.

Weiss, J. M., Sundar, S. K., & Becker, K. J. (1989). Stress-induced immunosuppression and immunoenhancement: Cellular immune changes and mechanisms. In E. J. Goetz & N. H. Spector (Eds.), *Neuroimmune networks: Physiology and diseases* (pp. 193–206). New York: Liss.

Williams, R. (1989). *The trusting heart.* New York: Times Books.

Witvliet, C. & Vrana, S. R. (1995). Psychophysiological responses as indices of affective dimensions. *Psychophysiology, 32,* 436–443.

Worthington, E. L., Jr. (1988). Understanding the values of religious clients: A model and its application to counseling. *Journal of Counseling Psychology, 35,* 166–174.

Worthington, E. L., Jr. (1998). The Pyramid Model of Forgiveness: Some interdisciplinary speculations about unforgiveness and the promotion of forgiveness. In E. L. Worthington, Jr. (Ed.), *Dimensions of forgiveness: Psychological research and theological perspectives* (pp. 107–137). Philadelphia: Templeton Foundation Press.

Worthington, E. L., Jr. (2000). Is there a place for forgiveness in the justice system? *Fordham Urban Law Journal, 27,* 1401–1414.

Worthington, E. L., Jr. (in press). Forgiveness and reconciliation: Religion, public policy, and conflict transformation. In R. Petersen & R. Helmick (Eds.), *Forgiveness in international relations.* Philadelphia: Templeton Foundation Press.

Worthington, E. L., Jr., & Drinkard, D. T. (2000). Promoting reconciliation through psychoeducational and therapeutic interventions. *Journal of Marital and Family Therapy, 26,* 93–101.

Worthington, E. L., Jr., Kurusu, T. A., McCullough, M. E., & Sandage, S. J. (1996). Empirical research on religion and psychotherapeutic processes and outcomes: A ten-year review and research prospectus. *Psychological Bulletin, 119,* 448–487.

Worthington, E. L., Jr., Berry, J. W., Parrott, L., O'Connor, L., Gramling, S., & Nicholson, R. (1999). *Studies in trait unforgiveness and states of unforgiveness.* Paper presented at the annual meeting of the American Psychological Association, Boston.

Worthington, E. L., Jr., & Wade, N. G. (1999). The social psychology of unforgiveness and forgiveness and implications for clinical practice. *Journal of Social and Clinical Psychology, 18,* 385–418.

Wyke, S., & Ford, G. (1992). Competing explanations for associations between marital status and health. *Social Science and Medicine, 34,* 523–532.

Zehr, H. (1995). *Changing lenses: A new focus on crime and justice.* Scottsdale, PA: Herald Press.

6

◄○►

ASSESSMENT
OF RELIGIOUSNESS
AND SPIRITUALITY
IN HEALTH RESEARCH

ALLEN C. SHERMAN
STEPHANIE SIMONTON

Religion is one of the most deeply held and profoundly personal aspects of human life; it encompasses some of our grandest mysteries and most ineffable experiences. Little wonder then that assessing spiritual or religious involvement is a challenging enterprise. A recent editorial on this subject in the journal *Psycho-Oncology* was aptly titled, "Can You Measure a Sunbeam with a Ruler?" (Lederberg & Fitchett, 1999). The task for health professionals is to remain firmly anchored in sound methodology without losing sight of the sunbeam—not an easy feat. Nevertheless, over the past few decades scholars of religion have developed a multitude of instruments to assess various aspects of religious and spiritual involvement. Regrettably, many health professionals are unaware of these resources, a situation that results in a certain amount of redundant labor (Hill & Hood, 1999). Several recent reviews may help health investigators become more familiar with these tools and their current stage of development (e.g., Fetzer Institute/National Institute on Aging, 1999; Gorsuch & Miller, 1999; Hill & Hood, 1999). Still, the interests and constraints of health researchers are not always the same as those of students of religion working in other areas. In this chapter we review several *quantitative* measures that are particularly relevant for use in health settings. In Chapter 11 (this volume), Chirban discusses *qualitative* assessment in the psychotherapy setting.

There are a number of guiding principles that may help health professionals navigate this terrain. Religiousness and spirituality are complex, multidimensional constructs, so investigators need to be thoughtful about which facets they are interested in pursuing. Different dimensions of faith seem to have distinct health correlates. Assessment instruments should avoid obscuring important differences among these dimensions—for example, by combining them arbitrarily into a total score (Fetzer Institute/National Institute on Aging, 1999). Typically, health research requires measures that are brief in order to minimize patient burden and instruments that are sufficiently broad to accommodate individuals from diverse religious and cultural backgrounds. There also has been a growing call to move from a reliance on descriptive measures—which examine the practices and beliefs that people profess—to more functional measures, which highlight how individuals actually make use of their faith in their daily lives (Ellison & Levin, 1998; Gorsuch & Miller, 1999). Knowing that a cancer patient goes to the synagogue three times a week (a descriptive indicator) is less informative than knowing why she goes, what she seeks from the experience, whom she looks forward to seeing there, and for whom she prays. Finally, the value of a particular instrument also depends on whether the items are confounded with the health outcomes one is interested in exploring, and whether the time frame of assessment is appropriate for the purposes at hand. Measures of religiousness that include questions about peacefulness and well-being may not be especially helpful in predicting emotional distress; similarly, measures that inquire if the respondent has *ever* had a particular type of spiritual experience may not be very sensitive in assessing changes over time (Gorsuch & Miller, 1999).

In this review, we focus on (1) published measures that are (2) brief and practical for use with medical or psychiatric patients and (3) whose psychometric properties in health settings are established or at least promising. In addition, we (4) emphasize instruments that are applicable to non-Christian as well as Christian individuals from varied age and ethnic groups. This review is not exhaustive—new measures are being developed rapidly. Moreover, our criteria resulted in the omission of a great many scales that are very appealing conceptually but that lack sufficient data on reliability and validity, that are too lengthy and burdensome to be readily incorporated within health research, or that are restricted to individuals from Christian traditions. Measures of general religiousness, religious coping, spiritual well-being, and other related constructs are discussed separately. Although most of these instruments are short questionnaires, in the final section we briefly note several alternate approaches to assessment.

MEASURES OF GENERAL RELIGIOUSNESS

These instruments assess an individual's typical involvement in religion or spirituality—such as religious commitment, spiritual experiences, strength of faith, or religious motivation. Collectively, these different facets of experience are sometimes referred to as "subjective" religiousness or spirituality (Chatters, Levin, & Taylor, 1992). Public or "organizational" and private or "nonorganizational" religious practices are also important dimensions of general religious orientation.

Santa Clara Strength of Religious Faith Questionnaire (SCSORF)

The SCSORF (Plante & Boccaccini, 1997a) is a brief instrument designed to assess a dimension of religious involvement that has received relatively little attention in health research—strength of religious faith (e.g., "I look to my faith as a source of inspiration"). This 10-item questionnaire demonstrated high internal consistency and good convergent validity in several studies with community civic group members, students (Plante & Boccaccini, 1997a, 1997b; Plante, Yancey, Sherman, Guertin, & Pardini, 1999) and substance abusers (Pardini, Plante, & Sherman, 2000). To examine its psychometric properties with medical patients, the instrument was administered to 175 women receiving care at a gynecology clinic and to 104 cancer patients receiving treatment in a bone marrow transplantation program (Sherman et al., 1999). In both medical samples, the SCSORF demonstrated high internal consistency (alphas = .96–.97) and strong associations with other measures of religious involvement (e.g., intrinsic religiosity, organizational religious practice, nonorganizational religious practice, strength and comfort derived from religion, and perception of self as religious). In addition, it displayed only modest associations with conceptually related measures used in health research, such as optimism, social support, hardiness, and purpose in life, indicating that the SCSORF contributes unique information. The instrument was not significantly associated with social desirability response bias or with other theoretically unrelated constructs (e.g., relationship cohesion, negative affect), demonstrating good divergent validity. Consistent with other research concerning religious orientation, scores were influenced by gender and income.

A subsequent study with breast cancer patients ($N = 95$) and healthy young adults ($N = 53$) was designed to examine the test–retest reliability of the SCSORF and to obtain additional information about convergent validity (Sherman, Simonton, et al., in press). In both samples, the measure demonstrated good test–retest reliability ($r = .82–.93$) and internal consistency (alphas = .95–.97). Convergent validity was demonstrated by moderately high correlations with intrinsic religiosity and moderate correlations with other measures of religiousness. Cancer patients further along in recovery scored higher than more recently diagnosed patients.

Results of these studies suggest that the SCSORF holds promise as a brief, practical measure of religious faith. However, the relatively high mean scores that have been obtained among medical patients in a Bible Belt region of the country suggest possible ceiling effects (i.e., religious participants score near the high end of the scale), and this possibility should be monitored in future studies. An abbreviated version of the scale is under development.

Systems of Belief Inventory—Revised (SBI-15R)

The SBI-15R (Holland et al., 1998) is a 15-item questionnaire that includes two subscales: (1) religious beliefs and practices and (2) social support from a religious community. It is one of the few instruments to focus explicitly on social aspects of spiritual life, which represents an important contribution. Item content seems to include elements of general religiousness (e.g., "religion is important in my everyday life"), religious coping with illness (e.g., "I pray for help during bad times"), and religious outcomes or well-being (e.g., "I have experienced peace of mind through my prayers and meditation"). Thus some items may be somewhat confounded with psychological adjustment. Research among medically healthy individuals ($N = 301$) provided evidence of test–retest reliability ($r = .95$) and internal consistency (alphas = .93 for the Total score, .92 for Beliefs and Practices, and .89 for Social Support; Holland et al., 1998). Construct validity was supported by factor analysis and by the instrument's high correlations with measures of intrinsic religiosity (Religious Orientation Inventory; Allport & Ross, 1967) and of spiritual experiences (Index of Core Spiritual Experience; Kass, Friedman, Leserman, Zuttermeister, & Benson, 1991). In addition, religious participants (e.g., ministers, nuns, rabbis) received significantly higher scores than lay participants. However, little information was provided about the validity of the two subscales as opposed to the total score. Nor was information available about social desirability bias or overlap with conceptually related measures such as optimism, nonreligious social support, or purpose in life.

In two subsequent studies with malignant melanoma patients, one involving American participants ($N = 117$; Holland et al., 1999) and the other involving an Israeli sample ($N = 100$; Baider et al., 1999), an earlier version of the instrument (SBI-54) was significantly associated with retrospective reports of changes in religious practice since childhood. The total score was not associated with nonreligious social support. No information was provided about the subscales.

More recently, an international study examined a Spanish version of the brief instrument (SBI-15R) among medical patients and staff members in Mexico, Uruguay, and Chile (Almanza et al., 1999). The investigators reported high internal consistency for the total score and for each subscale. A factor analysis using data from the combined sample supported the two subscales, but the factor structure varied across countries (yielding three rather than two factors in the Mexican sample).

These studies provide support for use of the SBI-15 among medical patients. Additional information is needed about the psychometric properties of the subscales as opposed to the total score. Data concerning relationships with conceptually related constructs and with social desirability would also be helpful.

Duke Religious Index (DUREL)

The DUREL (Koenig, Meador, & Parkerson, 1997) is a brief measure designed to assess three dimensions of religious involvement: (1) organizational or public religious expression (e.g., church attendance), (2) nonorganizational or private religious expression (e.g., prayer or meditation), and (3) intrinsic religiosity (e.g., incorporation of religious convictions into one's daily life). The Organizational and Nonorganizational scales are composed of one item each, and the Intrinsic scale is composed of three items drawn from the Intrinsic Religious Motivation Scale (Hoge, 1972). In large studies with elderly medical patients and community residents, organizational religiosity was significantly inversely associated with measures of depression, functional impairment, illness severity, and mortality (Koenig et al., 1997). In addition, this scale was significantly correlated with social support, as might be expected. Conversely, nonorganizational religiosity was associated with poorer physical health. These findings support the construct validity of the DUREL, and illustrate how different dimensions of religious involvement may have different health correlates. However, no information was provided about the reliability of the instrument as a whole, its associations with other measures of religious involvement (i.e., convergent validity), or its correlations with social desirability (i.e., divergent validity).

Additional data concerning the psychometric performance of the DUREL were provided by the study of bone marrow transplant and gynecology clinic patients noted previously (Sherman, Plante, et al., 2000). Results provided support for the internal consistency (alphas = .90–.94 for the Intrinsic scale; alphas = .87–.90 for the Total score) and convergent validity of the instrument. Among the cancer patients, there was a small but significant association with social desirability for the Intrinsic and Total scores (r_s = .21 for both scales). Modest correlations with related measures used in health research (e.g., optimism, social support, emotional control) supported the divergent validity of the instrument. Contrary to expectations, the Organizational Religiosity scale was not associated with a measure of perceived social support. Some of the DUREL scales were related to age, income, and education. Overall, these findings support the value of the DUREL for use with medical patients. A limitation is that the Organizational and Nonorganizational scales each contain only a single item, which contributes to the brevity of the instrument but may detract from its reliability.

Index of Core Spiritual Experience (INSPIRIT)

The INSPIRIT (Kass et al., 1991) was designed to assess core spiritual experiences, defined as (1) a distinct spiritual event that resulted in a personal conviction of the existence of God or a Higher Power and (2) which evoked feelings of closeness to God and the perception that God dwells within. The INSPIRIT contains 7 items (though the 7th item is actually a checklist of 12 items, with scoring based on the highest response to any of those items). Psychometric properties were examined in a sample of 83 outpatients with a variety of medical conditions who were participating in a relaxation/meditation training program. A principal-components factor analysis suggested a single underlying factor. The instrument demonstrated high internal consistency (alpha = .90). Construct validity was demonstrated by significant associations with a measure of intrinsic religiosity and with length of time participants had been practicing meditation. Moreover, responses were significantly associated with increases in a measure of Life Purpose and Satisfaction (Kass et al., 1991) and with decreases in frequency of medical symptoms over the course of the meditation program. Women scored higher than men.

A subsequent study evaluated the instrument in a sample of 247 ambulatory cancer patients and a sample of 124 family members recruited from a surgical waiting room (VandeCreek, Ayres, & Bassham, 1995). Estimates of internal consistency were high in both settings (alphas = .79–.85). The questionnaire was significantly correlated with a measure of intrinsic religiousness (Intrinsic Religious Motivation Scale; Hoge, 1972), and the factor structure was consistent with that obtained by Kass et al. (1991). However, VandeCreek and colleagues advocated a different approach to scoring the final item on the instrument; they suggest that each of the questions on this 12-part checklist should be scored, not only the one with the highest score. This type of scoring resulted in high internal consistency but a different factor structure and greater discrimination among groups.

In a more recent study with medically healthy individuals ($N = 301$), Holland and colleagues (1998) found that the INSPIRIT was highly correlated with intrinsic religiosity (Religious Orientation Inventory; Allport & Ross, 1967), providing further support for the instrument's construct validity (using the original scoring). Other investigators have reported significant relationships with pain and health ratings among patients treated in a family practice clinic (McBride, Arthur, Brooks, & Pilkington, 1998). As yet, however, we are not aware of any data concerning social desirability response bias (divergent validity) or associations with other, more diverse measures of religious or spiritual involvement (convergent validity). Moreover, despite the broad appeal of a measure of "spiritual experiences," the references to God in this scale may limit its applicability to individuals from theistic traditions.

Intrinsic/Extrinsic Religiosity Measures

Some of the oldest and most widely used instruments in the field of psychology of religion are measures of religious motivation. Derived from Gordon Allport's pioneering work (Allport, 1950; Allport & Ross, 1967), these measures focus on underlying religious motivation rather than overt practices or beliefs. Intrinsic religious motivation refers to internalized attitudes that guide the respondent's life, whereas extrinsic motivation involves pursuing religion for utilitarian purposes, such as emotional comfort or social benefits. Several related instruments have been developed based on this conceptual model, the most famous of which is the Religious Orientation Scale (ROS; Allport & Ross, 1967). These measures have enjoyed widespread use in behavioral science research, but they have not been free from criticism. Some writers have expressed reservations about methodological shortcomings (e.g., uncertain factor structure), implicit value judgments about "good" (intrinsic) and "bad" (extrinsic) religiousness, and questionable applicability for nonreligious respondents (Kirkpatrick & Hood, 1990). In addition, these scales may be somewhat confounded by social desirability (Burris, 1999a) and by liberal versus conservative religious beliefs (Wulff, 1999).

One of several measures of religious motivation is the Intrinsic Religious Motivation Scale (IRMS; Hoge, 1972). In contrast to Allport and Ross' (1967) original questionnaire (ROS), with which it shares several items, this 10-item measure focuses more purely on motivation rather than on religious behavior (e.g., "My religious beliefs are what really lie behind my whole approach to life"). It also appears to be more applicable to non-Christian respondents. This instrument has demonstrated high internal consistency and construct validity in community and medical samples (Hoge, 1972; Koenig, Moberg, & Kvale, 1988; Sherman, Plante, et al., 2000). In our own work with gynecology and oncology patients, alphas ranged from .89 to .91 (Sherman, Plante, et al., 2000).

Another measure of religious motivation is the Age Universal Religious Orientation Scale (AUROS; Gorsuch & Venable, 1983). This 20-item measure was drawn directly from the Allport and Ross (1967) instrument but was reworked to accommodate younger respondents and those with lower levels of reading comprehension. Unlike the IRMS, it yields separate scales for Intrinsic and Extrinsic motivation, consistent with research indicating that these orientations are orthogonal rather than opposite poles of a single dimension. In our own work with medical patients, we found good internal consistency for the Intrinsic scale (alphas = .86–.91) but poor reliability for the Extrinsic scale (alphas = .57–.61; Sherman, Plante, et al., 2000). A more recent revision of this questionnaire (Gorsuch & McPherson, 1989) further divides the Extrinsic dimension into a Personal Orientation subscale (i.e., turning to religion for comfort, protection, or peacefulness) and a Social Orientation subscale (i.e., using religion for social purposes; see Kirkpatrick, 1989, for additional support for this distinction). Research with college students (Gorsuch & McPherson, 1989; Schaefer & Gorsuch, 1991) and elderly cancer patients (Fehring, Miller, & Shaw, 1997) supported the construct validity of this 14-item version, but the internal consistency of the two extrinsic scales was low.

Although measures of intrinsic and extrinsic motivation have commanded most of the spotlight in psychological research on religion, a third dimension of religious motivation has also generated growing interest. The "quest" orientation focuses on an appreciation for the complexity of life's fundamental questions, and on an openness to doubt and change of religious convictions as one searches for answers (Batson & Schoenrade, 1991a; Batson, Schoenrade, & Ventis, 1993). This emphasis on open-ended questioning, on avoidance of easy answers to difficult existential dilemmas, was an important part of Allport's (1950) early theorizing about religious maturity but was not incorporated within measures of intrinsic and extrinsic motivation (Batson, 1976). The Quest Scale has gone through several revisions, with early versions criticized due to poor internal consistency (see Burris, 1999b, for a review). Others have argued that religious doubt is a less appropriate indicator of religious maturity than is open-mindedness (Dudley & Cruise, 1990). The most recent version is a 12-item measure that has demonstrated acceptable internal consistency, test–retest reliability, and preliminary evidence of construct validity in college student samples (Batson & Schoenrade, 1991a, 1991b; Burris, 1999b; Burris, Jackson, Tarpley, & Smith, 1996). However, we are not aware of research with medical or psychiatric populations.

Overall, given their central role in social science research, measures of religious motivation have seen relatively little use in health settings. These instruments merit further consideration, notwithstanding the limitations noted previously (Kirkpatrick & Hood, 1990). The I/E-Revised Scale (Gorsuch & McPherson, 1989), which differentiates between social and personal extrinsic orientation, and the Quest Scale (Batson & Schoenrade, 1991a, 1991b), which assesses a tentative search for existential meaning, may be especially useful.

Additional Measures of General Religious or Spiritual Involvement

Several other brief instruments may be alluring to health researchers; we note these only briefly because they have rarely or never been used in health settings. More complete reviews can be found in Hill and Hood (1999). The Structure of Prayer Scale (Luckow, Ladd, Spilka, McIntosh, Parks, & Laforett, cited in David, 1999; Luckow, McIntosh, Spilka, & Ladd, 2000) is a 43-item instrument that assesses seven different types of prayer (e.g., Material Petition, Confession-Closeness, Ritualistic, etc.). Preliminary research supported the internal consistency and construct validity of the scales. The current version (Luckow et al., 2000) is an expanded questionnaire, which eliminates some items from an earlier form that might have been confounded by psychological well-being (David, 1999). It has not yet been used with medical patients. The Religious Doubts Scale (Altemeyer, 1988) is one of several measures of religious doubt, which is an area of growing interest in social scientific research on religion. The 10-item measure demonstrated good internal consistency and construct validity among college students and their parents (Altemeyer, 1988); apparently, however, it has yet to be employed in health settings. The Religious Experience Questionnaire (Edwards, 1976) is a 12-item measure of personal, subjective religious experience. In contrast to measures that focus on cognitive aspects of religious involvement, such as attitudes and beliefs, this scale was designed to reflect an emotional connection with a personal, caring, forgiving God. No information was provided about reliability. Evidence of construct validity was obtained in several diverse samples, including hospitalized patients (see Hall, 1999, for a review). Finally, the Mysticism Scale (Form D; Hood, 1975) is a well-established measure of self-reported mystical experiences. An advantage of this instrument is that it is one of only a few measures that are applicable to individuals who do not belong to theistic religious traditions. The instrument is based on eight theoretical components of mystical experience (Stace, 1960). Its 32 items yield a total score, as well as scores for three factor-derived subscales (i.e., a sense of unity with the outside world, unity with "nothingness," and a religious interpretation of these experiences). Internal consistency for the subscales is adequate, and there is evidence for construct validity across a number of settings, including psychiatric samples (see Burris, 1999c, for a review). We are not aware of its use with medical patients.

MEASURES OF RELIGIOUS COPING

In contrast to measures of general religiousness, measures of religious coping are intended to capture how individuals draw on religion in response to a specific stressor, such as cancer diagnosis or treatment for multiple sclerosis. Exploring religious coping provides information that is distinct from general religiousness. We begin to see how faith is colored by context. Adjustment to difficult circumstances appears to be better predicted by religious coping than by general religiousness (Pargament, 1997; Pargament et al., 1999; see also Sherman & Simonton, Chapter 7, this volume). Several widely used multidimensional measures of coping, such as the Ways of Coping Questionnaire (Folkman & Lazarus, 1988), the Coping Responses Inventory (Moos, 1993), and the Dealing with Illness Inventory—Revised (Fawzy et al., 1990), include individual items that are relevant to religious coping (i.e., "found new faith," "prayed for guidance or strength," "trusted my belief in God"). However, these items are embedded within other scales and do not provide a separate religious coping score. More recent instruments are beginning to rectify this omission (e.g., Vanderbilt Multidimensional Pain Coping Inventory; Smith, Wallston, Dwyer, & Dowdy, 1997; Revised Ways of Coping Checklist; Vitaliano, 1991). Below we discuss some of the measures that may be especially useful to health investigators.

Coping Orientations to Problems Experienced (COPE)

The COPE (Carver, Scheier, & Weintraub, 1989) yields scores for 15 coping patterns (e.g. Active Coping, Planning, Acceptance). The 4-item Religion scale inquires about putting trust in God, seeking God's help, finding comfort in religion, and prayer. Studies have demonstrated good psychometric properties for the instrument among healthy college students (Carver et al., 1989), and it has subsequently been widely used in research with medical patients (e.g., Carver et al., 1993). In our own work using an abbreviated version of the COPE, the internal consistency of the three-item Religion scale was .81 among head and neck cancer patients ($N = 120$; Sherman et al., 2000). Despite the broad use of the COPE, there have been few systematic efforts to establish the construct validity of the Religion scale.

RCOPE

More recently, several instruments have been developed that focus exclusively on religious approaches to coping. The RCOPE is the most comprehensive of these measures (Pargament, Koenig, & Perez, 2000). It offers information about 17 factor-derived religious coping strategies (e.g., Benevolent Religious Reappraisal, Seeking Spiritual Support, Spiritual Discontent, Religious Purification/Forgiveness). This measure provides a much richer, more nuanced picture of religious coping than has previously been available. Research among elderly medical patients and among college students provided support for the internal consistency, factor structure, and concurrent validity of the instrument (Pargament et al., 2000). However, the length of the questionnaire may be prohibitive in many settings. The standard form contains 105 items, and an abbreviated form includes 63 items.

Brief RCOPE

Examining specific coping strategies through measures such as the RCOPE provides a wealth of information. However, coping responses also tend to cluster together in patterns. The Brief RCOPE (Pargament, Smith, Koenig, & Perez, 1998) was developed to assess broader constellations of religious coping. The instrument assesses two global dimensions: (1) Positive Religious Coping (i.e., movement toward religious resources in response to stress) and (2) Negative Religious Coping (i.e., conflict or movement away from religious resources). In our view, the names of these scales are perhaps unfortunate, in that they may imply that the former mode of coping is adaptive and the latter is not. The value of these coping approaches in particular contexts is an empirical question, and *a priori* judgments are best avoided. Nevertheless, these scales address an intriguing dimension of religious coping.

Several versions of this instrument have been developed. An initial 21-item version was evaluated among church members in the aftermath of the bombing of the Oklahoma City federal building; the findings supported the instrument's reliability (alphas = .78–.87) and construct validity (Pargament et al., 1998). We adapted this measure for use with cancer patients, eliminating items that were specific to the bombing (Sherman et al., 2001). Data from multiple myeloma patients suggested acceptable reliability (alphas = .91 for Positive Religious Coping and .70 for Negative Religious Coping) and construct validity. Pargament and colleagues (1998) developed another version of the instrument, with items drawn directly from the more comprehensive RCOPE (Pargament et al., 2000) described previously. This 14-item measure demonstrated acceptable internal consistency (alphas = .69–.90), factor structure, and concurrent validity in samples of college students and elderly, hospitalized medical patients (Pargament et al., 1998). A more abbreviated version of these scales showed good internal consistency for the three-item Positive Religious Coping scale (alpha = .81) but poorer reliability for the two-item Negative Coping scale (alpha = .54) in a large random national survey (1997–1998 General Social Survey, cited in Fetzer Institute/ National Institute on Aging, 1999).

Ways of Religious Coping Scale (WORCS)

The WORCS (Boudreaux, Catz, Ryan, Amaral-Melendez, & Brantley, 1995) offers another approach to assessing broad patterns of religious coping. This 40-item instrument provides a total score, as well as separate scores for Internal/Private coping (e.g., "I pray for strength") and External/Social coping (e.g., "I get help from clergy"). In a sample of college students, the measure demonstrated good internal consistency (alphas = .93–.97) and significant correlations with other measures of religious coping and general religiousness. A factor analysis generally provided further support for construct validity. Each of the scales displayed a small, significant correlation with social desirability (r = .21–.26). In subsequent research with undergraduates, Willis, Wallston, and Johnson (Chapter 9, this volume) found significant associations between coping scores and health-compromising behaviors such as smoking and alcohol use. Additional information was provided by a study in an inner-city municipal hospital, which provided norms for family practice patients, general medical outpatients, hemodialysis patients, and patients with HIV (O'Hea et al., 2000); most participants were African Americans with limited incomes. Scores were influenced by race, gender, age, and religious affiliation. Although the WORCS has been used with individuals from diverse religious backgrounds (Boudreaux et al., 1995), item content suggests that a few of the items are inappropriate for non-Christian respondents (e.g., "I think about Jesus as my friend") and that an additional one or two items may be somewhat confounded by psychological well-being.

Religious Problem-Solving Scales

The process of coping is closely related to problem solving, which concerns how people define difficulties, generate solutions, and establish a sense of control. The Religious Problem-Solving Scales (Pargament et al., 1988) include 36 items that measure three approaches to solving problems in life within a religious framework. These approaches differ in whether the individual assumes an active or passive posture toward the problem and whether primary responsibility is attributed to self or to God. The Self-Directing style emphasizes the freedom God provides to solve difficulties on one's own. The Deferring style involves turning to God for solutions, and the Collaborative style involves a sense of partnership and shared responsibility with God. Research with college students supported the test–retest reliability of the scales, and studies with church members demonstrated internal consistency and construct validity (Pargament et al., 1988). This instrument has subsequently been used in a number of health settings (e.g.,

Friedel & Pargament, 1995; Harris & Spilka, 1990; Pargament et al., 1999). It is worth noting that religious problem-solving styles also were incorporated within the RCOPE (Pargament et al., 2000), discussed previously, but that the two instruments assess these constructs in somewhat different ways.

These various measures of religious coping and problem solving are tied to more general concepts of stress and coping that play an important role in health research; consequently, these instruments are apt to become widely used over the next few years. The functional orientation of these measures is a notable advantage; they offer information about how individuals make use of their faith when confronted by difficult circumstances. Moreover, Pargament's coping measures (Pargament et al., 2000; Pargament et al., 1998) include an explicit focus on some of the painful aspects of religion, such as ambivalence and perceived abandonment, in addition to the more positive dimensions that are usually emphasized. Finally, these measures offer tools to assess specific types of religious coping (e.g., RCOPE), as well as broader, more global patterns of coping (Brief RCOPE, WORCS). However, information is limited concerning how Pargament's scales are related to other measures of religiousness (convergent validity). Moreover, the extent to which these instruments are influenced by social desirability (divergent validity) is unclear.

MEASURES OF SPIRITUAL WELL-BEING

These measures assess religious or existential aspects of well-being. A number of investigators have argued that commonly used measures of health-related quality of life provide a narrow picture because they do not include a spiritual or existential dimension, which many patients report is important to them and which is conceptually distinct from other aspects of quality of life (Brady, Peterman, Fitchett, Mo, & Cella, 1999; Cohen, Mount, Strobel, & Bui, 1995). Measures of spiritual well-being were developed to fill this gap. Evidence supports the notion that spirituality is an important aspect of well-being. However, there has been ambiguity regarding how spiritual well-being is best conceptualized, with some investigators regarding it as a resource that patients draw on rather than an outcome that changes in response to the demands of illness or stress. Consistent with its inclusion in broader quality of life (i.e., outcome) measures, we suspect that spiritual well-being is best viewed as an outcome. In our view, these measures provide information about spiritual responses to illness, presumably influenced by but distinct from the spiritual resources that patients bring to the experience (general religious/spiritual orientation) or their efforts to cope with it (religious/spiritual coping).

Functional Assessment of Chronic Illness Therapy (FACIT) Spiritual Well-Being Scale

One of the most widely used multidimensional measures of quality of life in oncology and AIDS research is the FACIT (Cella, 1997). The FACIT is a modular instrument that incorporates a general questionnaire, designed to be used with patients across different types of illnesses, as well as a series of disease- and treatment-specific modules, which provide information about concerns that are unique to particular types of illness or treatment. Recently, a module that assesses spiritual well-being was added to the instrument (Rush Spiritual Belief Module). A large international study of patients with cancer and HIV infection (N = 1,120) demonstrated high internal consistency for the module (alpha = .87; Fitchett, Peterman, & Cella, 1996). Principal components factor analysis yielded two factors: (1) Faith and Assurance (e.g., "I find comfort in my faith or spiritual beliefs" and (2) Meaning and Purpose (e.g., "I feel peaceful"). Moderate correlations with the total quality-of-life scores and with the separate Emotional, Functional, Social, and Physical Well-Being scales suggested that the Spiritual Well-Being scale was reliably related to other aspects of quality of life, but offered unique information. Compared with the Faith and Assurance factor, the Meaning and Purpose factor was more strongly associated with the other dimensions of quality of life. Scores on the total Spiritual Well-Being scale were influenced by gender, marital status, ethnicity, religious affiliation, and, more weakly, by age. Patients with no symptoms or functional disability obtained higher scores than those with more extensive symptoms or disability.

In subsequent research with cancer and HIV-infected patients (N = 131), the Spiritual Well-Being scale demonstrated significant, moderate correlations with measures of organizational religiosity (r = .34), nonorganizational religiosity (r = .31), and intrinsic religiosity (r = .41; Peterman, 2000). These findings offer support for the convergent validity of the scale. The instrument showed a small but significant correlation with social desirability (Peterman, Fitchett, Brady, & Cella, 2000). As expected, spiritual well-being was associated with adjustment to cancer (Cotton, Levine, Fitzpatrick, Dold, & Tang, 1999). As yet, however, little information has been presented regarding its association with other measures of well-being, life satisfaction, or existential meaning (aside from other FACIT scores).

McGill Quality of Life Questionnaire (MQOL)

Another multidimensional measure of health-related quality of life, the MQOL, includes a scale designed to assess existential well-being (e.g., "My life has been utterly meaningless and without purpose/very purposeful and meaningful"; Cohen et al., 1997; Cohen et al., 1995). The scale draws items from the Purpose in Life Test (Crumbaugh & Maholick, 1968), which has been used for several decades. Research with Canadian cancer patients receiving palliative care (i.e., those with advanced, incurable disease) demonstrated acceptable internal consistency for the Existential Well-Being scale (alpha = .79; Cohen et al., 1997). Data from principal-components factor analysis supported the construct validity of the measure. Interestingly, among the various scales included in the instrument (i.e., Physical Symptoms, Psychological Symptoms, Support, Existential Well-Being), the Existential scale was one of the strongest predictors of global quality of life. However, little information is available concerning the association of this scale with other measures of existential or spiritual well-being, life satisfaction, or positive or negative affect (convergent validity). Nor has information been presented concerning its relationships with other measures of general religiousness or existential meaning.

Spiritual Well-Being Scale (SWBS)

The SWBS (Ellison, 1983) is a 20-item instrument with two subscales: (1) Religious Well-Being (e.g., "My relationship with God helps me not to feel lonely") and (2) Existential Well-Being (e.g., "I feel very fulfilled and satisfied with my life"). This measure has been popular, particularly in nursing research. It displayed good internal consistency and test–retest reliability for the total score and subscales in multiple samples, mostly involving religious participants (Bufford, Paloutzian, & Ellison, 1991). Acceptable internal consistency also has been demonstrated among breast cancer patients (Mickley & Soeken, 1993; Mickley, Soeken, & Belcher, 1992) and family caregivers of hospice patients (Kirschling & Pittman, 1989). In medically healthy samples, construct validity was supported by significant associations with meaning and purpose in life, emotional adjustment, marital adjustment, life satisfaction, self-concept, and physical health (Bufford et al., 1991). Studies with breast cancer patients have demonstrated significant associations between Spiritual Well-Being scores and intrinsic religiosity (Mickley & Soeken, 1993; Mickley et al., 1992). In some samples, scores were influenced by age and gender (Bufford et al., 1991). A limitation of this instrument is a ceiling effect, so it is not useful for assessing highly religious individuals (Bufford et al., 1991; Ledbetter, Smith, Vosler-Hunter, & Fischer, 1991). There has also been some question about its factor structure.

Each of these measures offers useful information about spiritual well-being. Both the FACIT Spiritual Well-Being scale (Fitchett, Peterman, & Cella, 1996) and Ellison's (1983) Spiritual Well-Being Scale allow for interesting distinctions between religious and existential well-being through provision of separate subscales. These measures have helped call attention to an important aspect of quality of life that traditionally has been neglected in health research. However, because the items on these scales (particularly the existential or meaning subscales) seem to overlap with mood and psychological well-being, these measures may not be useful in predicting psychosocial outcomes with which they are confounded.

RELATED MEASURES

Recently, a wave of measures has been developed to assess concepts that are related to religiousness, such as forgiveness, God locus of control, and altruism. As yet, only a few of them have been validated in health settings. In this section we note several of the instruments whose value for health research has been established or seems promising.

Forgiveness

Several measures of forgiveness have emerged in the past few years. Many of these focus on forgiveness in response to specific situations or transgressions. In contrast, the Trait Forgivingness Scale (Berry, Worthington, O'Connor, Parrott, & Wade, 2000) assesses the disposition to forgive across different circumstances, or "forgivingness" (Roberts, 1995; see also Worthington, Berry, & Parrott, Chapter 5, this volume). In a series of studies with healthy undergraduate students (Berry et al., in review), this 10-item instrument demonstrated acceptable internal consistency (alpha = .79) and test–retest reliability ($r = .78$). Construct validity was supported by significant correlations between self and other ratings on the scale, associations with other measures of forgiveness, and correlations with related constructs such as empathy, agreeableness, and anger. Another brief instrument is the Transgression-Related Interpersonal Motivations Inventory (TRIM; McCullough et al., 1998). This 12-item questionnaire focuses on motivations thought to underlie forgiving. It generates separate scores for transgression-related Avoidance (e.g., "I cut off the relationship with him/her") and Revenge (e.g. "I'm going to get even"). Evidence for internal consistency, test–retest reliability, and construct validity was obtained in studies with college students (McCullough et al., 1998). Advantages of the TRIM and the Trait Forgivingness Scale include their brevity compared with similar instruments and their focus on dimensions of forgiveness that are theoretically important. As yet, however, neither has been validated in medical or psychiatric populations.

God Locus of Control

Adjustment to difficult circumstances, including illness, is influenced by personal beliefs about the controllability of those events. The Multidimensional

Health Locus of Control (MHLC) scales, Form C, include four scales that assess the extent to which respondents believe their illness is due to (1) their own behavior, (2) the behavior of doctors, (3) the behavior of others (excluding doctors), and (4) chance or fate (Wallston, Stein, & Smith, 1994). Recently, a fifth scale was developed to evaluate beliefs that one's condition is controlled by God (e.g., "Whatever happens to my condition is God's will"; Wallston et al., 1999). Among patients with rheumatoid arthritis and systemic sclerosis, the six-item God Locus of Health Control (GLHC) scale demonstrated high internal consistency (alphas = .87–.94), significant associations with general religiousness and religious coping, and meaningful correlations with emotional adjustment. God locus of control was not strongly associated with the other locus of control scales, indicating that this scale provides distinct information. Perceptions that God influences one's health can take different forms (Pargament et al., 1988; see also the previous section of this chapter on religious problem solving). The wording of items on the GHLC scale and its pattern of associations with distress suggest that this scale primarily reflects a passive "deferring" style, in which primary responsibility is attributed to God as opposed to a "self-directing" style or a "collaborative" style of relating to God.

OTHER ASSESSMENT MODALITIES

Brief questionnaires such as those described in the preceding sections have distinct advantages in health research. They are easy to administer and score, are usually well accepted by patients, and are readily incorporated within the larger assessment batteries typically used by health investigators. Nevertheless, the limitations of conventional self-report questionnaires are well recognized. They reflect only a restricted range of experience, and are open to bias by defensiveness, impression management, limited memory, contextual demands, and so forth. There has been a growing call to incorporate richer, more creative approaches to assessing religious life, such as structured interviews, observer ratings, computer-coded written narratives, and momentary ecological ratings. Though our focus in this chapter has been on concise, pragmatic instruments, a few examples of more varied approaches to religious and spiritual assessment are noted below. (Qualitative assessment is discussed by Chirban in Chapter 11, this volume.)

Spiritual Strivings

Goal measures offer a promising avenue for exploring religious involvement. Using open-ended questions and self-ratings, methodologies have been developed to assess how motivational variables, variously construed as personal strivings (Emmons, 1999), life tasks (Cantor, 1990), or personal projects (Little, 1989), are expressed in everyday life. More recently, this approach to assessing personal goals has been used to explore spiritual or existential strivings (e.g., attempts to "deepen my relationship with God," "be more forgiving"; Emmons, 1999). This methodology provides both idiographic and nomothetic data. If ways can be found to minimize patient burden associated with some of the more elaborate rating systems, this approach may yield rich information about how spiritual goals are pursued in everyday life among medical and psychiatric patients, complementing the data from more global trait measures of religiousness.

Structured Interviews

The Royal Free Interview for Religious and Spiritual Beliefs (King, Speck, & Thomas, 1995) is a structured interview that provides quantitative data concerning medical patients' religious beliefs and their perceptions about their illness. The interview differentiates among respondents who express (1) a "religious" world view (i.e., affiliation with a faith tradition), (2) a "spiritual" world view (i.e., belief in a power beyond oneself, in the absence of a specific religion), and (3) a "philosophical" view (i.e., a search for existential meaning without reference to a power beyond oneself). Separate scales provide scores for Spiritual Beliefs and for Philosophical Beliefs; in addition, individual items assess participants' beliefs about the cause and meaning of their illness. Research with hospital staff and patients from a general medical practice suggested good internal consistency for the Spiritual scale (alpha = .81) but poor reliability for the Philosophical scale (alpha = .60; King et al., 1995; Seybold, 1999). Test–retest reliability, assessed among hospital staff, was good for both scales and for each of the individual items. A group of highly religious respondents (e.g., chaplains, ministers) obtained higher scores on the spiritual scales than did staff and patients. There is no additional information about validity.

Projective Assessment

The Spiritual Themes and Religious Responses Test (STARR; Saur & Saur, 1993; Brokaw, 1999) illustrates the adaptation of projective techniques for assessment of spirituality. The test includes 11 stimulus cards modeled on the Thematic Apperception Test (TAT). Respondents are invited to tell a story about the people depicted in the black and white photographs; alternately, a number of other instructions and inquiries can be used. Several scoring systems have been developed. Interrater reliability ranged from .46 to .88 for the 12 scoring dimensions developed by Misner (1995, cited in Brokaw, 1999), who also reported evidence of concurrent validity. Of course, use of this measure requires expertise in projective testing, in addition to training in this specific instrument. We are not aware of its use in health settings.

CONCLUSIONS

In sum, there has been significant progress in developing or adapting measures of religiousness for use in health settings. Investigators and clinicians have a growing array of options. Clearly, none of these instruments is without shortcomings. Except for the spiritual well-being scales, most measures focus on religiousness rather than spirituality (i.e., a concern with the sacred or transcendent that is not necessarily rooted in an established faith tradition). As far as we are aware, very few sound measures of spirituality or illness-specific spiritual coping (as distinct from spiritual well-being) have been developed. (Thoughtful consumers will appreciate that the label on a package does not always reflect its contents.) And although measures of spiritual well-being have opened new avenues of research, as noted, these instruments appear to be confounded with psychological well-being, so care should be taken in how they are interpreted. Other shortcomings for some instruments include limited information about temporal stability and convergent validity, potential ceiling effects, and lack of data about social desirability bias. In addition, most items on these questionnaires are framed in monotheistic language, so it is unclear how well they would be received by nontheistic respondents.

Nevertheless, there are now a number of brief, practical measures available to assess important dimensions of religiosity or spirituality in health settings. The recent work of the Fetzer Institute/National Institute on Aging (1999), which represents a collaborative effort to refine instruments, will contribute to further advances in this area. Ideally, scale development should focus on brief, practical measures that are grounded in theory, that avoid mixing together different dimensions of religiousness or spirituality, and that are appropriate for members of different religious and cultural traditions (including nontheistic respondents).

REFERENCES

Allport, G. W. (1950). *The individual and his religion*. New York: Macmillan.

Allport, G. W., & Ross, J. M. (1967). Personal religious orientation and prejudice. *Journal of Personality and Social Psychology, 5*, 432–443.

Almanza, J., Bimbela, A., Monroy, M., Cesarco, R., Iusin, S., Puig, M. E., Campillay, M., Torres, P., Ordenes, R., & Holland, J. (1999). Cross cultural adaptation of the Systems of Belief Inventory (SBI-15) in three Latin American Countries [Abstract]. *Psycho-Oncology*, 8(Suppl.), 172.

Altemeyer, B. (1988). *Enemies of freedom: Understanding right-wing authoritarianism*. San Francisco: Jossey-Bass.

Baider, L., Russak, S. M., Perry, S., Kash, K., Gronert, M., Fox, B., Holland, J., & Kaplan-Denour, A. (1999). The role of religious and spiritual beliefs in coping with malignant melanoma: An Israeli sample. *Psycho-Oncology*, 8, 27–35.

Batson, C. D. (1976). Religion as prosocial: Agent or double-agent? *Journal for the Scientific Study of Religion*, 15, 29–45.

Batson, C. D., & Schoenrade, P. (1991a). Measuring religion as quest: 1. Validity concerns. *Journal for the Scientific Study of Religion*, 30, 416–429.

Batson, C. D., & Schoenrade, P. (1991b). Measuring religion as quest: 2. Reliability concerns. *Journal for the Scientific Study of Religion*, 30, 430–447.

Batson, C. D., Schoenrade, P., & Ventis, W. L. (1993). *Religion and the individual: A social-psychological perspective*. New York: Oxford University Press.

Berry, J. W., Worthington, E. L., Jr., O'Connor, L. E., Parrott, L., & Wade, N. G. (2000). *The measurement of trait forgivingness*. Manuscript submitted for publication.

Boudreaux, E., Catz, S., Ryan, L., Amaral-Melendez, M., Brantley, P. J. (1995). The Ways of Religious Coping Scale: Reliability, validity, and scale development. *Assessment*, 2, 233–244.

Brady, M. J., Peterman, A. H., Fitchett, G., Mo, M., & Cella, D. (1999). A case for including spirituality in quality of life measurement in oncology. *Psycho-Oncology*, 8, 417–428.

Brokaw, B. F. (1999). Spiritual Themes and Religious Responses Test [Review]. In P. C. Hill & R. W. Hood, Jr. (Eds.), *Measures of religiosity* (pp. 371–374). Birmingham, AL: Religious Education Press.

Bufford, R. K., Paloutzian, R. F., & Ellison, C. W. (1991). Norms for the Spiritual Well-Being Scale. *Journal of Psychology and Theology*, 19, 56–70.

Burris, C. T. (1999a). Religious Orientation Scale [Review]. In P. C. Hill & R. W. Hood, Jr. (Eds.), *Measures of religiosity* (pp. 144–154). Birmingham, AL: Religious Education Press.

Burris, C. T. (1999b). Quest Scale [Review]. In P. C. Hill & R. W. Hood, Jr. (Eds.), *Measures of religiosity* (pp. 138–141). Birmingham, AL: Religious Education Press.

Burris, C. T. (1999c). The Mysticism Scale: Research Form D [Review]. In P. C. Hill & R. W. Hood, Jr. (Eds.), *Measures of Religiosity* (pp. 363–367). Birmingham, AL: Religious Education Press.

Burris, C. T., Jackson, L. M., Tarpley, W. R., & Smith, G. (1996). Religion as quest: The self-directed pursuit of meaning. *Personality and Social Psychology Bulletin*, 22, 1068–1076.

Cantor, N. (1990). From thought to behavior: "Having" and "doing" in the study of personality and cognition. *American Psychologist*, 45, 735–750.

Carver, C. S., Pozo, C., Harris, S. D., Noriega, V., Scheier, M. F., Robinson, D. S., Ketcham, A. S., Moffat, F. L., Jr., & Clark, K. C. (1993). How coping mediates the effect of optimism on distress: A study of women with early stage breast cancer. *Journal of Personality and Social Psychology*, 65, 375–390.

Carver, C. S., Scheier, M. F., & Weintraub, J. K. (1989). Assessing coping strategies: A theoretically based approach. *Journal of Personality and Social Psychology, 56*, 267–283.

Cella, D. F. (1997). *Functional Assessment of Chronic Illness Therapy Manual, version 4.* Evanston, IL: Evanston Northwestern Healthcare, Center on Outcomes, Research and Education.

Chatters, L. M., Levin, J. S., & Taylor, R. J. (1992). Antecedents and dimensions of religious involvement among older black adults. *Journal of Gerontology, 47,* S269–S278.

Cohen, S. R., Mount, B. M., Bruera, E., Provost, M., Rowe, J., & Tong, K. (1997). Validity of the McGill Quality of Life Questionnaire in the palliative care setting: A multi-centre Canadian study demonstrating the importance of the existential domain. *Palliative Medicine, 11,* 3–20.

Cohen, S. R., Mount, B. M., Strobel, M. G., & Bui, F. (1995). The McGill Quality of Life Questionnaire: A measure of quality of life appropriate for people with advanced disease: A preliminary study of validity and acceptability. *Palliative Medicine, 9,* 207–219.

Cotton, S. P., Levine, E. G., Fitzpatrick, C. M., Dold, K. H., & Tang, E. (1999). Exploring the relationships among spiritual well-being, quality of life, and psychological adjustment in women with breast cancer. *Psycho-Oncology, 8,* 429–438.

Crumbaugh, J. C., & Maholick, L. T. (1968). An experimental study in existentialism: The psychometric approach to Frankl's noogenic neurosis. *Journal of Clinical Psychology, 20,* 200–207.

David, J. P. (1999). Structure of Prayer Scale [Review]. In P. C. Hill & R. W. Hood, Jr. (Eds.), *Measures of religiosity* (pp. 70–72). Birmingham, AL: Religious Education Press.

Dudley, R. L., & Cruise, R. J. (1990). Measuring religious maturity: A proposed scale. *Review of Religious Research, 32,* 97–109.

Edwards, K. J. (1976). Sex-role behavior and religious experience. In W. J. Donaldson, Jr. (Ed.), *Research in mental health and religious behavior: An introduction to research in the integration of Christianity and the behavioral sciences* (pp. 224–238). Atlanta, GA: Psychological Studies Institute.

Ellison, C. G. (1983). Spiritual well-being: Conceptualization and measurement. *Journal of Psychology and Theology, 11,* 330–340.

Ellison, C. G., & Levin, J. S. (1998). The religion–health connection: Evidence, theory, and future directions. *Health Education and Behavior, 25,* 700–720.

Emmons, R. A. (1999). *The psychology of ultimate concerns: Motivation and spirituality in personality.* New York: Guilford Press.

Fawzy, F. I., Cousins, N., Fawzy, N. W., Kemeny, M. E., Elashoff, R., & Morton, D. (1990). A structured psychiatric intervention for cancer patients. I. Changes over time in methods of coping and affective disturbance. *Archives of General Psychiatry, 47,* 720–725.

Fehring, R. J., Miller, J. F., & Shaw, C. (1997). Spiritual well-being, religiosity, hope, depression, and other mood states in elderly people coping with cancer. *Oncology Nursing Forum, 24,* 663–671.

Fetzer Institute/National Institute on Aging. (1999). *Multidimensional measurement of religiousness/spirituality for use in health research.* Kalamazoo, MI: John E. Fetzer Institute.

Fitchett, G., Peterman, A. H., & Cella, D. F. (1996, November). *Spiritual beliefs and quality of life in cancer and HIV patients.* Paper presented at the meeting of the Society for the Scientific Study of Religion, Nashville, TN.

Folkman, S., & Lazarus, R. S. (1988). *Manual for the Ways of Coping Questionnaire.* Palo Alto, CA: Consulting Psychologists Press.

Friedel, L. A., & Pargament, K. I. (1995, August). *Religion and coping with crises in the work environment.* Paper presented at the annual convention of the American Psychological Association, New York.

Gorsuch, R. L., & McPherson, S. E. (1989). Intrinsic/Extrinsic measurement: I/E-Revised and single-item scales. *Journal of the Scientific Study of Religion, 28,* 348–354.

Gorsuch, R. L., & Miller, W. R. (1999). Assessing spirituality. In W. R. Miller (Ed.), *Integrating spirituality into treatment: Resources for practitioners* (pp. 47–64). Washington, DC: American Psychological Association.

Gorsuch, R. L., & Venable, G. D. (1983). Development of an "Age Universal" I-E scale. *Journal of the Scientific Study of Religion, 22,* 181–187.

Hall, M. E. L. (1999). Religious Experience Questionnaire [Review]. In P. C. Hill & R. W. Hood, Jr. (Eds.), *Measures of religiosity* (pp. 218–220). Birmingham, AL: Religious Education Press.

Harris, N. A., & Spilka, B. (1990). *The sense of control and coping with alcoholism: A multidimensional approach.* Paper presented at the meeting of the Rocky Mountain Psychological Association, Tucson, AZ.

Hill, P. C., & Hood, R. W., Jr. (Eds.). (1999). *Measures of religiosity.* Birmingham, AL: Religious Education Press.

Hoge, D. R. (1972). A validated intrinsic religious motivation scale. *Journal for the Scientific Study of Religion, 11,* 369–376.

Holland, J. C., Kash, K. M., Passik, S., Gronert, M. K., Sison, A., Lederberg, M., Russak, S. M., Baider, L., & Fox, B. (1998). A brief spiritual beliefs inventory for use in quality of life research in life-threatening illness. *Psycho-Oncology, 7,* 460–469.

Holland, J. C., Passik, S., Kash, K. M., Russak, S. M., Gronert, M. K., Sison, A., Lederberg, M., Fox, B., & Baider, L. (1999). The role of religious and spiritual beliefs in coping with malignant melanoma. *Psycho-Oncology, 8,* 14–26.

Hood, R. W., Jr. (1975). The construction and preliminary validation of a measure of reported mystical experience. *Journal for the Scientific Study of Religion, 14,* 29–41.

Kass, J. D., Friedman, R., Leserman, J., Zuttermeister, P. C., & Benson, H. (1991). Health outcomes and a new index of spiritual experience. *Journal of the Scientific Study of Religion, 30,* 203–211.

King, M., Speck, P., & Thomas, A. (1995). The Royal Free Interview for Religious and Spiritual Beliefs: Development and standardization. *Psychological Medicine, 25,* 1125–1134.

Kirkpatrick, L. A. (1989). A psychometric analysis of the Allport–Ross and Feagin measures of intrinsic–extrinsic religious orientation. In M. Lynn & D. Moberg (Eds.), *Research in the social scientific study of religion* (Vol. 1, pp. 1–30). Greenwich, CT: JAI Press.

Kirkpatrick, L. A., & Hood, R. W., Jr. (1990). Intrinsic–extrinsic religious orientation: The boon or bane of contemporary psychology of religion? *Journal for the Scientific Study of Religion, 29,* 442–462.

Kirschling, J. M., & Pittman, J. F. (1989). Measurement of spiritual well-being: A hospice caregiver sample. *Hospice Journal, 5,* 1–11.

Koenig, H. G., Meador, K., & Parkerson, G. (1997). Religion Index for Psychiatric Research: A 5-item measure for use in health outcomes studies [Letter to the editor]. *American Journal of Psychiatry, 154,* 885–886.

Koenig, H. G., Moberg, D. O., & Kvale, J. N. (1988). Religious activities and attitudes of older adults in a geriatric assessment clinic. *Journal of the American Geriatrics Society, 36,* 362–374.

Ledbetter, M. F., Smith, L. A., Vosler-Hunter, W. L., & Fischer, J. D. (1991). An evaluation of the research and clinical usefulness of the Spiritual Well-being Scale. *Journal of Psychology and Theology, 19,* 49–55.

Lederberg, M. S., & Fitchett, G. (1999). Can you measure a sunbeam with a ruler? *Psycho-Oncology, 8,* 375–377.

Little, B. R. (1989). Personal projects analysis: Trivial pursuits, magnificent obsessions, and the search for coherence. In D. M. Buss & N. Cantor (Eds.), *Personality psychology: Recent trends and emerging directions* (pp. 15–31). New York: Springer-Verlag.

Luckow, A., McIntosh, D. N., Spilka, B., & Ladd, K. (2000, February). *The multidimensionality of prayer.* Poster presented at the annual meeting of the Society for Personality and Social Psychology, Nashville, TN.

McBride, J. L., Arthur, G., Brooks, R., & Pilkington, L. (1998). The relationship between a patient's spirituality and health experiences. *Family Medicine, 30,* 122–126.

McCullough, M. E., Rachal, K. C,, Sandage, S. J., Worthington, E. L., Jr., Brown, S. W., & Hight, T. L. (1998). Interpersonal forgiving in close relationships: II. Theoretical elaboration and measurement. *Journal of Personality and Social Psychology, 75,* 1586–1603.

Mickley, J. R., & Soeken, K. (1993). Religiousness and hope in Hispanic- and Anglo-American women with breast cancer. *Oncology Nursing Forum, 20,* 1171–1177.

Mickley, J. R., Soeken, K., & Belcher, A. (1992). Spiritual well-being, religiousness and hope among women with breast cancer. *Image: Journal of Nursing Scholarship, 24,* 267–272.

Moos, R. H. (1993). *Coping Responses Inventory: CRI Adult Form, Professional Manual.* Odessa, FL: Psychological Assessment Resources.

O'Hea, E. L., Boudreaux, E. D., Martin, P. D., Catz, S. L., Scarinci, I. C., & Brantley, P. J. (2000, April). *The Ways of Religious Coping Scale: Norms and demographic predictors across several low-income medical samples.* Poster presented at the annual meeting of the Society of Behavioral Medicine, Nashville, TN.

Pardini, D., Plante, T. G., & Sherman, A. (2000). Strength of religious faith and its association with mental health outcomes among recovering alcoholics and addicts. *Journal of Substance Abuse Treatment, 19,* 1–8.

Pargament, K. I. (1997). *The psychology of religion and coping: Theory, research, practice.* New York: Guilford Press.

Pargament, K. I., Cole, B., VandeCreek, L., Belavich, T., Brant, C., & Perez, L.

(1999). The vigil: Religion and the search for control in the hospital waiting room. *Journal of Health Psychology, 4,* 327–341.

Pargament, K. I., Kennell, J., Hathaway, W., Grevengoed, N., Newman, J., & Jones, W. (1988). Religion and the problem-solving process: Three styles of coping. *Journal for the Scientific Study of Religion, 27,* 90–104.

Pargament, K. I., Koenig, H. G., & Perez, L. M. (2000). The many methods of religious coping: Development and initial validation of the RCOPE. *Journal of Clinical Psychology, 56,* 519–543.

Pargament, K. I., Smith, B. W., Koenig, H. G., & Perez, L. (1998). Patterns of positive and negative religious coping with major life stressors. *Journal of Scientific Study of Religion, 37,* 711–725.

Peterman, A. H. (2000, March). *Spirituality and quality of life among cancer and HIV/AIDS patients: The role of ethnicity.* Paper presented at the annual meeting of the American Psychosomatic Society, Savannah, GA.

Peterman, A. H., Fitchett, G., Brady, M. J., & Cella, D. (2000). *Psychometric validation of the FACIT Spiritual Well-being Scale.* Manuscript in preparation.

Plante, T. G., & Boccaccini, M. T. (1997a). Reliability and validity of the Santa Clara Strength of Religious Faith Questionnaire. *Pastoral Psychology, 45,* 429–437.

Plante, T. G., & Boccaccini, M. T. (1997b). The Santa Clara Strength of Religious Faith Questionnaire. *Pastoral Psychology, 45,* 375–387.

Plante, T. G., Yancey, S., Sherman, A. C., Guertin, M., & Pardini, D. (1999) Further validation for the Santa Clara Strength of Religious Faith Questionnaire. *Pastoral Psychology, 48,* 11–21.

Roberts, R. C. (1995). Forgivingness. *American Philosophical Quarterly, 32,* 289–306.

Saur, M. S., & Saur, W. G. (1993). *Spiritual Themes and Religious Responses Test (STARR): Preliminary manual.* Chapel Hill, NC: Author.

Schaefer, C. A., & Gorsuch, R. L. (1991). Psychological adjustment and religiousness: The multivariate belief–motivation theory of religiousness. *Journal for the Scientific Study of Religion, 30,* 448–461.

Seybold, K. S. (1999). The Royal Free Interview for Religious and Spiritual Beliefs [Review]. In P. C. Hill & R. W. Hood, Jr. (Eds.), *Measures of religiosity* (pp. 351–357). Birmingham, AL: Religious Education Press.

Sherman, A. C., Plante, T. G., Simonton, S., Adams, D. C., Burris, S. K., & Harbison, C. (1999). Assessing religious involvement in medical patients: Cross-validation of the Santa Clara Strength of Religious Faith Questionnaire. *Pastoral Psychology, 48,* 129–142.

Sherman, A. C., Plante, T. G., Simonton, S., Adams, D. C., Harbison, C., & Burris, S. K. (2000). A multidimensional measure of religious involvement for cancer patients: The Duke Religious Index. *Journal of Supportive Care in Cancer, 8,* 102–109.

Sherman, A. C., Plante, T. G., Simonton, S., Moody, V., & Wells, P. (2001). Patterns of religious coping among multiple myeloma patients: Associations with adjustment and quality of life [Abstract]. *Psychosomatic Medicine, 63,* 124.

Sherman A. C., Simonton, S., Adams, D. C., Latif, U., Plante, T. G., Burris, S. K., & Poling, T. (in press). Measuring religious faith in cancer patients: Reliability and construct validity of the Santa Clara Strength of Religious Faith Questionnaire. *Psycho-Oncology.*

Sherman, A. C., Simonton, S., Adams, D. C., Vural, E., & Hanna, E. (2000). Coping with head and neck cancer during different phases of treatment. *Head and Neck, 22,* 787–793.

Smith, C. A., Wallston, K. A., Dwyer, K. A., & Dowdy, S. W. (1997). Beyond good and bad coping: A multidimensional examination of coping with pain in persons with rheumatoid arthritis. *Annals of Behavioral Medicine, 19,* 11–21.

Stace, W. T. (1960). *Mysticism and philosophy.* Philadelphia: Lippincott.

VandeCreek, L., Ayres, S., & Bassham, M. (1995). Using the INSPIRIT to conduct spiritual assessments. *Journal of Pastoral Care, 49,* 83–89.

Vitaliano, P. P. (1991). *Revised Ways of Coping Checklist (RWCCL) and Appraisal Dimensions Scale (ADS) manual.* Seattle: University of Washington.

Wallston, K. A., Malcarne, V. L., Flores, L., Hansdottir, I., Smith, C. A., Stein, M. J., Weisman, M. H., & Clements, P. J. (1999). Does God determine your health? The God Locus of Health Control Scale. *Cognitive Therapy and Research, 23,* 131–142.

Wallston, K. A., Stein, M. J., & Smith, C. A. (1994). Form C of the MHLC scales: A condition-specific measure of locus of control. *Journal of Personality Assessment, 63,* 534–553.

Wulff, D. (1999). Humanistic Morality/Liberal Belief Scale [Review]. In P. C. Hill & R. W. Hood, Jr. (Eds.), *Measures of religiosity* (pp. 19–22). Birmingham, AL: Religious Education Press.

PART II

◄○►

FAITH AND HEALTH
IN SPECIAL
POPULATIONS

7

◄❍►

RELIGIOUS INVOLVEMENT AMONG CANCER PATIENTS
Associations with Adjustment and Quality of Life

ALLEN C. SHERMAN
STEPHANIE SIMONTON

Cancer is a jarring, life-altering experience for most patients and their families. Taxing treatments, disrupted functioning, and uncertainty about survival are among the burdens they face. For many, religion and spirituality play an important role in how they adapt to this crisis (Feher & Maly, 1999). Across studies of patients with diverse types of cancer, the great majority of participants reported that religion was important to them or helped them cope with their illness (Brandt, 1987; Fredette, 1995; Johnson & Spilka, 1991; Norum, Risberg, & Solberg, 2000; Ringdal, 1996; Silberfarb et al., 1991; Sodestrom & Martinson, 1987; Tebbi, Mallon, Richards, & Bigler, 1987; Yates, Chalmer, St. James, Follansbee, & McKegney, 1981). Indeed, religious activities usually rank among the most frequent coping responses reported by cancer patients (Carver et al., 1993; Fredette, 1995; Halstead & Fernsler, 1994; Sherman, Simonton, Adams, Vural, & Hanna, 2000; Sodestrom & Martinson, 1987). Clearly, religious beliefs and practices are a common resource in times of medical crisis. Aside from its potential impact on adjustment to illness, religion may also have relevance for cancer screening and early detection, health practices, treatment adherence, and perhaps even survival, though these areas are only beginning to be seriously explored.

In this chapter we review recent findings concerning religious involvement among cancer patients. We begin with a brief discussion of some of the practical and conceptual difficulties involved in trying to explore religiousness or spirituality in an oncology setting. Elusive phenomena in the best of circumstances, religiousness and spirituality are particularly difficult to evaluate in medical settings. Next we review recent findings concerning relationships between religious or spiritual involvement and quality-of-life outcomes. Are there reliable associations between faith and various aspects of well-being, such as distress, life satisfaction, physical symptoms, or relationship functioning? If so, which dimensions of religious involvement seem most salient? Then we consider how religious or spiritual concerns may change in response to the crisis of cancer. If faith sometimes influences the experience of cancer, does cancer in turn alter one's faith? Next we review the role of religion in cancer screening and early detection. We conclude with thoughts about future research in this area.

CHALLENGES IN EXPLORING RELIGIOUS AND SPIRITUAL INVOLVEMENT AMONG CANCER PATIENTS

As we discussed more fully in Chapter 6 (this volume), one of the challenges in investigating links between faith and health outcomes involves finding appropriate measures. What tools are available to help guide the search? Although a host of religious measures has been constructed, few are well suited for oncology patients (Sherman et al., 1999). Despite their convenience, single-item indices commonly used in epidemiological research (e.g., frequency of church attendance) have limited value in clinical studies because they provide little information and have questionable reliability (Park & Cohen, 1992). Conversely, questionnaires used by scholars of religion are sometimes long and complex, and this presents a significant burden for patients with severe illness. Some instruments are intended only for religious individuals or members of a particular faith, which further limits their applicability.

An additional problem in oncology research is the conceptual confusion that often characterizes explorations of religion (Sherman, Plante, et al., 2000). Important distinctions are sometimes blurred. For example, *general religious orientation*, an individual's typical involvement in religion, is sometimes confused with *cancer-specific religious coping*, that is, how an individual draws on religion to help him or her deal specifically with the crisis of cancer. Moreover, religion or spirituality as a *resource* variable (e.g., a source of strength or comfort) is sometimes confused with religion or spirituality as an *outcome* (e.g., as a reaction to illness or an aspect of quality of life). In particular, many religious measures include items that reflect general psychological adjustment or well-being. These instruments may offer valuable information, but they may not be appropriate for use in predicting other aspects of quality of life with which they are confounded (e.g., emotional adjustment, life satisfaction). Thus it is important to be clear about what aspects of religiousness or spirituality are being addressed. Fortunately, there has been significant progress in development of measures suitable for use with medical patients. We review a number of instruments that may be helpful in oncology settings in Chapter 6 (this volume)

ASSOCIATIONS BETWEEN RELIGIOUSNESS OR SPIRITUALITY AND QUALITY OF LIFE

Given the complexities involved in assessing such an ineffable area of human experience, what has been learned about relationships between faith and health among cancer patients? What dimensions of religiousness or spirituality have been associated with what aspects of illness and recovery? In the following sections we examine the correlates of (1) general religious or spiritual orientation, (2) cancer-specific religious coping, and (3) spiritual well-being.

Cancer encompasses a diverse array of illnesses. The particular difficulties that patients face vary with the site of illness (e.g., breast vs. lung cancer) and severity of disease (e.g., early stage vs. metastatic; Sherman & Simonton, 1999; Simonton & Sherman, 1998). Patients' experiences are also strongly colored by phase of treatment; the challenges associated with initial diagnosis, for example, are quite different from those evoked by active medical treatment or long-term survival. These characteristics of the illness may have an important bearing on the ties between faith and adjustment to cancer.

General Religious Orientation and Quality-of-Life Outcomes

A number of studies have focused on cancer patients' general involvement in religion or spirituality—their level of commitment to religion, depth of faith, private spiritual practices, or congregational activity. Many of these investigations have uncovered intriguing relationships between religious expression and adjustment to cancer, though the magnitude and breadth of these relationships and the methodological adequacy of the studies vary widely. These investigations have begun to chart the experience of individuals with various types of cancer.

Until recently, most investigations involved patients with advanced or terminal disease (e.g., Gibbs & Achterberg-Lawis, 1978; Ita, 1995–1996; Smith, Nehemkis, & Charter, 1983–1984; Swensen, Fuller, & Clements, 1993; Yates et al., 1981). Despite their methodological limitations, these pioneering studies generally suggest that, as they approach the end of life, religious individuals experience greater well-being, life satisfaction, and positive affect and more comforting attitudes toward death compared with their less religious peers. In contrast, religiousness appears to be less consistently tied to whether or not these patients experience emotional distress or functional impairment.

More recent investigations have broadened the focus to include individuals with more favorable prognoses. For example, an Israeli study examined the experience of patients with early-stage malignant melanoma—a type of skin cancer (Baider et al., 1999). Those participants who were more religious or spiritual, as assessed by a validated instrument (System of Beliefs Inventory—54; Holland et al., 1998), reported significantly lower levels of emotional distress on a number of measures relative to less religious patients. In addition, religious involvement was associated with an active–cognitive coping style. The ties between religiousness and greater active–cognitive coping and reduced emotional distress remained significant after accounting for demographic and disease variables. Religious involvement was not related to the other psychosocial outcomes assessed, including health-related quality of life, cancer-related intrusive or avoidance symptoms, or social support.

More limited findings emerged from a parallel study by this team of investigators, who used a similar research design and measures to assess American melanoma patients (Holland et al., 1999). Relative to the Israeli study, the American sample included patients with more extensive disease and those who had been ill for somewhat longer periods of time. Once again, more religious individuals displayed higher levels of active–cognitive coping than less religious patients, after controlling for demographic variables and tumor stage. These results challenge traditional assumptions that a religious orientation promotes a passive, regressive response to life crises (see also Pargament & Park, 1995). Religious participants in these studies appeared to acknowledge the reality of their illness and to search for positive meaning. On the other hand, the fact that religiousness was tied to lower emotional distress among Israeli patients but not among Americans suggests that religious and cultural context, in conjunction with medical factors, may be an important part of the picture.

Other investigations have focused attention on patients at different phases of medical treatment. For example, a Norwegian study explored the importance of faith among patients who had been hospitalized for treatment of various types of cancer (Ringdal, 1996). For these patients in the midst of active treatment, religiousness was associated with increased life satisfaction and reduced hopelessness, after controlling for demographic background and medical prognosis. Religiousness was not connected with emotional distress or quality-of-life scores. However, there is no information about the validity of the religious measure. On the other end of the spectrum, interesting findings emerged from a study of women who had successfully completed treatment and were well along in their recovery (Kurtz, Wyatt, & Kurtz, 1995). Among these cancer survivors, women who reported a stronger philosophical/spiritual view were more likely to have good health habits (e.g., exercise, healthful diet) than those with less philosophical/spiritual attitudes. These women were also more likely to report providing support to other cancer patients. A philosophical/spiritual view was not related to the other outcomes measured in this study, including emotional, sexual, or physical functioning. However, functioning was relatively well preserved among these long-term survivors. Findings may have been influenced by selection bias (55% participation rate).

Other studies have focused on patients at different phases of the life cycle. Fehring, Miller, and Shaw (1997) examined intrinsic religiousness—internalized values that guide one's daily life—among elderly hospitalized cancer patients with diverse sites and stages of disease. Among these older patients, those with higher levels of intrinsic religiousness reported significantly higher levels of hope and spiritual well-being, and lower levels of depression and emotional distress, relative to less intrinsically religious patients, after controlling for severity of physical symptoms. Such results are consistent with earlier investigations among middle-aged cancer patients that found modest evidence for associations between religiousness and increased hope and reduced distress (Acklin, Brown, & Mauger, 1983; Brandt, 1987; Herth, 1989; Mickley, Soeken, & Belcher, 1992).

In contrast, Tebbi and colleagues (1987) examined patients at a much earlier phase of life. In a study of adolescents with various types of cancer, most participants reported that religion offered security in the face of death and a sense of understanding regarding situations beyond their control. Religiosity scores were not significantly associated with locus of control.

Of course, not all investigations have yielded positive results. Negative findings were reported in a study of recently diagnosed multiple myeloma patients drawn from a large clinical trial (Silberfarb et al., 1991). Upon entrance into the study, most participants (90%) reported that religion was moderately or highly important to them. However, this self-rating was not associated with physicians' ratings of impaired functioning (e.g., employment limitations, social life restrictions, emotional instability). Findings may have been affected by reliance on physician ratings, which are generally regarded as a less sensitive index of quality of life than patient self-reports. The investigators also obtained standardized self-report measures of mood, but unfortunately associations with the religious item were not reported. Results also may have been influenced by selection bias (less than one-half of eligible patients participated in the psychosocial phase of the study), though there were no differences between participants and nonparticipants on the demographic and disease variables assessed.

Thus investigations have begun to explore religious resources among individuals from different age groups with diverse types of cancer at different phases of illness. Complementing these quantitative investigations, a growing number of qualitative studies also have highlighted connections between spiritual or religious engagement and well-being among cancer patients. These studies point to the potential value of religion in managing pain (Ferrell, Taylor, Grant, Fowler, & Corbisiero, 1993) and maintaining a sense of hope (Post-White et al., 1996).

Overall, despite broad differences in disease characteristics and measures used, most of the studies noted here hint at a modest but meaningful connection between religious or existential resources and adjustment to illness. For the most part, stronger religious or existential orientation is associated with more favorable outcomes. Because the great majority of these investigations used cross-sectional research designs (assessing religiousness and quality of life at the same point in time), no conclusions can be drawn about causal relationships. Moreover, much of the research is compromised by small samples and use of unvalidated measures of religiousness. Most studies report positive results for some outcomes but null findings for others. Which specific aspects of religiousness or spirituality are tied to which specific types of health outcomes are not yet clear. Some studies point to enhanced well-being and life satisfaction, while others highlight reduced emotional distress or functional impairment. Most investigations do not address the potential impact of patients' demographic background or disease characteristics. In particular, many studies mix together individuals with different sites and stages of disease and those at different phases of treatment, obscuring potentially important differences. If we are to better understand the ties between faith and adjustment to the crisis of cancer, there is a need for additional research that uses established measures to examine patients with particular types of disease as they transition through specific phases of illness.

In our own work, we also have found interesting ties between religiousness and quality of life, though results have varied with the type of cancer and personal background of the participants. In contrast to much of the previous research, in these studies we have tried to examine several dimensions of religious involvement among individuals with a particular type of disease at a particular phase of treatment. One ongoing study (Sherman, Plante, Simonton, Wells, & Moody, 2001) involves patients with multiple myeloma, a type of hematological cancer associated with high mortality. Patients were assessed prior to receiving an autologous bone marrow transplant, which is an aggressive, debilitating treatment. Bone marrow transplantation involves treatment with high-dose chemotherapy, which destroys tumor cells but also severely damages the immune system. Intensive chemotherapy is followed by autologous stem cell transplantation, in which patients receive back their own healthy stem cells that were harvested and stored prior to the high-dose chemotherapy. The stem cells regenerate the immune system and other blood products. Arkansas Cancer Research Center is a leading center for treatment of multiple myeloma, and patients come from all over the world seeking care. As might be expected, then, most participants came from middle- to upper-income families (see Table 7.1). Most were Protestant.

In this study, we examined participants' organizational religious behavior, nonorganizational religious behavior, and intrinsic religiosity, using the Duke Religious Index (DUREL; Koenig, Meador, & Parkerson, 1997). We

TABLE 7.1. Sample Characteristics for Multiple Myeloma Patients Assessed during Stem Cell Collection Prior to Bone Marrow Transplantation

Characteristic	Number (%)
Sex	
Female	26 (37.14)
Male	44 (62.86)
Ethnicity	
American Indian	1 (1.43)
African American	1 (1.34)
White	65 (92.86)
Other	3 (4.29)
Marital status	
Single	1 (1.43)
Married	63 (90.00)
Divorced/separated	4 (5.71)
Widowed	2 (2.86)
Family income	
$0–39,999	20 (28.57)
$40,000–99,999	26 (37.14)
$100,000 and over	22 (31.43)
Unknown	2 (2.86)
Religious affiliation	
Catholic	13 (18.57)
Protestant	46 (65.71)
Muslim	7 (10.00)
Jewish	3 (4.29)
None	1 (1.43)
Recurrent disease	
Nonrecurrent	59 (84.29)
Recurrent	11 (15.71)

Characteristic	Mean (SD)
Age	56.57 (8.46)
Months since initial diagnosis	14.16 (19.01)

also obtained measures of existential meaning (using the Meaning scale from the Sense of Coherence Scale; Antonovsky, 1993) and religious coping (see the following section). Outcome measures included emotional distress (a composite of Anxiety and Depression scales from the Brief Symptom Inventory, BSI; Derogatis, 1993), cancer-specific stress (Impact of Events Scale, IES; Horowitz, Wilner, & Alvarez, 1979), life satisfaction (Satisfaction with Life Scale; Diener, Emmons, Larsen, & Griffen, 1985), and health-related quality of life (FACIT; Cella, 1997). As anticipated, preliminary analyses with 70 participants indicated fairly high levels of distress. Overall, however, patients' general religious orientation had little to do with their adjustment to cancer. None of the indicators of religiousness was associated with health outcomes. On the other hand, individuals who perceived greater existential meaning experienced reliably better functioning across a broad range of outcomes relative to those with less sense of meaning in life (see Table 7.2). In particular, after controlling for relevant demographic and medical factors, we found that participants who regarded life as meaningful reported significantly better emotional well-being, greater life satisfaction, fewer cancer-related stress symptoms, and marginally less emotional distress. They also

TABLE 7.2. Associations between Existential Meaning and Quality-of-Life Outcomes among Multiple Myeloma Patients Prior to Bone Marrow Transplantation

Outcome	Control measures	Existential meaning	
		Zero-order correlation	Partial correlation
General distress (BSI Anxiety and Depression)	Income	$-.24^\dagger$	$-.23^\dagger$
Cancer-specific stress (IES)	Sex	$-.28^*$	$-.28^*$
Life satisfaction (SWLS)	Age	$.29^*$	$.31^*$
Physical well-being (FACIT-P)	—	$.29^*$	—
Functional well-being (FACIT-F)	Age, time since diagnosis	$.37^{**}$	$.38^{**}$
Emotional well-being (FACIT-E)	Age, income	$.29^*$	$.29^*$
Social well-being (FACIT-S)	Age, religious affiliation, time since diagnosis	$.19$	$.20$
Site-specific concerns (FACIT-BMT)	—	$.31^{**}$	—

Note. Partial correlations were used to control for medical or demographic variables that were significantly or marginally associated with outcomes. BSI, Brief Symptom Inventory; IES, Impact of Events Scale; SWLS, Satisfaction with Life Scale; FACIT, Functional Assessment of Chronic Illness Therapy. Higher scores reflect greater well-being on the FACIT scales.
$^\dagger p < .10$; $^* p < .05$; $^{**} p < .01$.

reported better physical well-being and functional well-being and fewer concerns about bone marrow transplantation.

These results imply that for middle- to upper-class myeloma patients facing aggressive treatment with bone marrow transplantation, existential resources—a perception that life is meaningful—may be more important for quality of life than religious resources. Of course, causal relationships cannot be determined from these data. A longitudinal study in progress may further clarify these relationships.

On the other hand, a rather different picture emerges from preliminary data from a study of patients with a different type of cancer, receiving a different type of treatment (Sherman, Simonton et al., 2001). This ongoing project involves women with newly diagnosed gynecological cancer, who are enrolled within 3 months of initial diagnosis. Though the sample is diverse, most of these women are poor and have limited education, in contrast to the myeloma patients discussed previously. Moreover, drawn from central Arkansas in the heart of the Bible Belt, most participants are from conservative Protestant denominations. Strength of religious faith is assessed with the Santa Clara Strength of Religious Faith questionnaire (SCSORF; Plante & Boccaccini, 1997), and organizational and nonorganizational religious practices are assessed with the DUREL (Koenig et al., 1997). The outcomes we are tracking among these women include their patterns of emotional distress (Hospital Anxiety and Depression Scale, HADS; Zigmond & Snaith, 1983), cancer-specific stress (IES; Horowitz et al., 1979), and health-related quality of life (Functional Assessment of Cancer Therapy, FACT; Cella, 1994). A substantial proportion of women enrolled in this project report high levels of distress and cancer-related stress symptoms.

Preliminary analyses from this ongoing study suggest that religious involvement is significantly correlated with a number of important health outcomes. Patients who scored higher in religious faith reported less distress and more favorable emotional well-being compared with less religious women, after accounting for relevant demographic and disease variables. A similar pattern emerged for organizational religious practices (e.g., attendance at religious services). Those with stronger organizational religiousness reported less distress, fewer cancer-related stress symptoms, better emotional well-being, and fewer concerns specific to this type of cancer (e.g., urinary incontinence, sexual difficulties). In contrast, private or nonorganizational religiousness (e.g., private prayer) did not play a significant role.

Once again, these results suggest that different dimensions of religious or spiritual involvement are differentially associated with adjustment to cancer. In particular, strength of faith and organizational religious practices were modestly tied to better adjustment, whereas private religious expression was not. Religiousness appears to be more strongly connected to psychosocial functioning than to physical functioning. These women are being followed longitudinally to examine whether religious involvement predicts outcomes over the course of the first year after diagnosis.

Religious Coping and Quality-of-Life Outcomes

Shifting the focus from general religious orientation to cancer-specific coping takes us from the resources a patient brings to this frightening illness to the particulars of how he or she makes use of those resources. A recent review of the stress and coping literature suggests that the effects of religious coping are distinct from those of nonreligious coping (Pargament, 1997). Moreover, adjustment to stressful circumstances appears to be more strongly predicted by religious coping than by general religiousness. As Pargament (1997) argues:

> It is not enough to find that general measures of religious faith or practice relate to general measures of adjustment or well-being. The central question remains: How does religion come to life in the immediate situation? . . . When we turn our attention to coping, we can see people moving from the generalities of their faith to the specifics of religious action in difficult moments. (p. 166)

Interest in religious or spiritual coping among cancer patients has generated growing interest, but research in this area is just beginning. Among the few investigations that have been completed, ethnicity and cultural context assume an important role. For example, in a study of 238 women with early-stage breast cancer, African American and Hispanic women reported relying on religious coping (measured by the COPE; Carver, Scheier, & Weintraub, 1989) significantly more frequently than non-Hispanic White women (Culver, Alferi, Carver, Kilbourn, & Antoni, 1999). Among Hispanic patients, greater religious coping was associated with less distress.

In another study of lower income Hispanic women with early-stage breast cancer, different patterns emerged for Catholic as opposed to evangelical patients (Alferi, Culver, Carver, Arena, & Antoni, 1999). Evangelical women reported significantly higher levels of general religiosity and cancer-related religious coping than Catholics. Interestingly, religiosity and religious coping tended to be associated with reduced distress during the course of the year for evangelical patients but with increased distress for Catholic patients. Though few of these associations were statistically reliable in this small sample of women ($N = 49$), turning to church members for support predicted significantly reduced distress at one of the follow-up periods for evangelical women. In contrast, for Catholic participants, getting support from church members and participating in religious gatherings predicted subsequent *increased* distress. These findings appear consistent with research in other clinical and nonclinical settings, which similarly suggested that religious coping may buffer distress for Protestants confronted by an uncontrollable stressor but may be less helpful for Catholics (Park, Cohen, & Herb, 1990; Tix & Frazier, 1998). These early observations hardly suggest that Catholics should be dissuaded from drawing on their faith to cope with the burdens of illness; however, they do indicate that religious affiliation is important to consider as we explore the complex ties between faith and health.

In contrast to the provocative findings obtained with Hispanic and African American cancer patients, research with white participants has generated much more limited results. A longitudinal study of predominantly European American women with newly diagnosed early-stage breast cancer found no effects for religious coping (Carver et al., 1993). Religious coping was among the most frequently reported coping strategies at multiple intervals throughout the course of the first year after diagnosis. However, this coping response was not associated with either optimism or distress, concurrently or prospectively.

We found a similar pattern of results in our own work with a predominantly European American sample of head and neck cancer patients (Sherman, Simonton, et al., 2000). Participants in this cross-sectional study included 120 patients with advanced head and neck cancer assessed at various phases of illness: (1) prior to treatment, (2) during active treatment, (3) within 6 months of completing treatment, or (4) more than 6 months posttreatment. Religious coping was one of the most commonly cited coping strategies for participants at each phase of illness. Older patients and women were especially likely to turn to their faith to manage the demands of illness. Nonetheless, religious coping was not significantly tied to emotional distress or cancer-related stress symptoms, echoing the earlier findings of Carver et al. (1993) with breast cancer patients. And similar results were reported in other cross-sectional (Ell, Mantell, Hamovitch, & Nishimoto, 1989) and longitudinal (Filipp, Klauer, Freudenberg, & Ferring, 1990) investigations involving patients with mixed sites and stages of disease.

Interestingly, a more complex picture emerges when we consider religious coping among family members of cancer patients. Abernethy, Chang, Duberstein, Seidlitz, and Evinger (1999) found a curvilinear relationship between religious coping and depression among predominantly White spouses of lung cancer patients. The investigators examined clinician ratings of depression, as well as self-reports of depression. Spouses who reported moderate levels of religious coping (assessed by the Religious Coping Interview; Koenig et al., 1992) were rated by clinicians as significantly less depressed than those who reported either no religious coping on the one hand or high levels of religious coping on the other. Findings were significant after accounting for the effects of neuroticism, social support, mastery, and optimism. The complex, presumably reciprocal relationships between religious coping and distress are difficult to interpret in cross-sectional studies such as these. Conceivably, spouses who turned to religion to cope with the crisis of illness in the family may have been buffered from depression. Those who did not use this coping strategy may have been more vulnerable, whereas those faced with high levels of distress may have turned more intensively to religious coping. In other words, heightened distress may have mobilized religious coping as a response, a finding consistent with research among family members of heart surgery patients (Pargament et al., 1999). Clearly, however, other interpretations are possible.

In part, whether religious coping is tied to favorable or unfavorable outcomes or is unrelated to health outcomes may depend on the type of coping efforts involved. In the face of tragedy, religious coping may be comforting and sustaining, but it may also embody conflict and struggle. Life-threatening illness may prompt a disconcerting reevaluation of one's spiritual beliefs and practices. Most of the research to date has used very basic measures of religious coping, which offer little information about the different ways that people might turn to their faith during crises. However, a recent qualitative study offers an intriguing glimpse of some of the religious struggles and ambiguities that may arise for patients coping with cancer (Taylor, Outlaw, Bernardo, & Roy, 1999). Participants were individuals with various types of malignancies, all of whom reported using prayer. Among the poignant religious challenges that participants encountered were questions about the fairness or capriciousness of God, doubts about personal and spiritual adequacy, and conflict about retaining a sense of personal control versus relinquishing control to God. Patients also struggled with uncertainty about the appropriateness of petitionary prayers (e.g., praying for oneself or praying for a cure) and the meaning of unanswered prayers. The experience of these patients reminds us that religious coping may sometimes encompass painful doubts rather than comforting convictions.

Struggles with religion in response to cancer also have emerged in our own research on religious coping. In the study introduced earlier concerning multiple myeloma patients facing aggressive treatment with bone marrow transplantation (Sherman, Simonton, Plante, et al., 2001), we found interesting connections between religious coping and quality of life. The most intriguing findings concerned patients who struggled with their faith in response to their illness. An adapted version of the Brief RCOPE (Pargament, Smith, Koenig, & Perez, 1998) was used to assess two broad patterns of religious coping: (1) "positive religious coping"—movement toward religion in response to cancer, and (2) "negative religious coping"— questioning, challenging, or turning away from religion. For these patients, negative religious coping was associated with a broad range of adverse outcomes (see Table 7.3). After controlling for relevant demographic and dis-

TABLE 7.3. Multiple Regression Analyses Predicting Quality-of-Life Outcomes from Negative Religious Coping, among Bone Marrow Transplant Patients

Outcome	Predictor	Standardized beta	Incremental R^2	
Distress	Low income[a]	$-.26^{\dagger}$	.01	Overall $F(3, 62)$ =
	High income[a]	$-.32^*$	.07	3.20, p = 03; R^2 = .13;
	Negative religious coping[b]	$.24^*$	.06	adjusted R^2 = .09
Cancer-related stress	Sex	$.24^*$	.04	Overall $F(2, 66)$ =
	Negative religious coping	$.32^{**}$	.10	5.72, p = .005; R^2 = .15; adjusted R^2 = .12
Life satisfaction	Age	$.26^*$	.07	Overall $F(2, 66)$ =
	Negative religious coping	$-.26^*$	.07	5.19, p = .008; R^2 = .14, adjusted R^2 = .11
Emotional well-being	Age	$.21^{\dagger}$	.04	Overall $F(4, 62)$ =
	Low income	$.34^*$	.06	3.66, p = .01; R^2 = .19; adjusted R^2 = .14
	High income	$.22^{\dagger}$	.03	
	Negative religious coping	$-.25^*$	.06	
Social/family well-being	Age	$.27^*$	.10	Overall $F(5,63)$ = 5.31,
	Religious affiliation1[c]	.20	.00	p =.0004; R^2 = .30; adjusted R^2 = .24
	Religious affiliation2[c]	$.26^{\dagger}$	.06	
	Time since diagnosis	$-.20^{\dagger}$	.07	
	Negative religious coping	$-.26^*$	.07	

[a]Low income was coded 1 for < $40,000, 0 for the higher two tertiles; high income was coded 1 for > $100,000, 0 for the lower two tertiles.
[b]Negative religious coping was coded 0 for low, 1 for high, using a median split due to its non-normal distribution.
[c]Religious affiliation1 was coded 1 for Catholic, 0 for others; religious affiliation2 was coded 1 for Protestant, 0 for others.
$^{\dagger}p < .10$; $^*p < .05$.

ease variables, we found that patients who relied on negative religious coping reported moderately but significantly increased distress and cancer-related stress symptoms. They also reported diminished life satisfaction, emotional well-being, and social and family well-being. There was no association with physical symptoms. Curiously, positive religious coping was not strongly tied to any of these psychosocial or physical outcomes (though there was a nonsignificant trend toward greater cancer-related stress).

Thus, in this study, how well patients adjusted to their illness was more strongly tied to religious coping, especially a questioning or turning away from religion, than to their general religious orientation. Of course, these results portray only a snapshot in time. The process of struggling with one's religion during a life-threatening crisis may be associated with very different outcomes in the long run than in the short term, as some individuals eventually find deeper faith, others arrive at a more comfortable detachment, and others continue to struggle actively with religious ambivalence.

In sum, research on religious coping among cancer patients is of more recent vintage and is generally stronger methodologically than research on general religiousness. Some investigations have found reliable associations with quality of life, whereas others yielded no significant relationships. Findings have been influenced by differences in the cultural and demographic background of the participants and by the way that coping is assessed. In particular, these relationships appear to be most salient among ethnic minority groups (e.g., Hispanics and African Americans versus non-Hispanic Whites). Moreover, it is possible that negative religious coping is more strongly tied to quality-of-life outcomes than is positive religious coping, a finding that, if confirmed, would parallel the differential effects of negative versus positive social support among cancer patients (Lepore, 1997; Lepore & Helgeson, 1998). As noted, most of the research completed thus far has used relatively simple tools to measure religious coping. With the recent arrival of more sophisticated instruments (e.g., RCOPE, Pargament, Koenig, & Perez, 2000; Brief RCOPE, Pargament et al., 1998; Ways of Religious Coping Scale, Boudreaux, Catz, Ryan, Amaral-Melendez, & Brantley, 1995; see also Sherman & Simonton, Chapter 6, this volume, for a review), we may be in a better position to learn about the myriad ways in which individuals draw on their faith to manage the demands of illness, how these coping efforts change over time, and how they influence quality of life.

Spiritual Well-Being and Quality-of-Life Outcomes

In the final part of this section, our attention shifts from the spiritual resources or coping efforts that individuals bring to their illness to the spiritual outcomes they experience. How does cancer affect patients' spiritual well-being—their sense of peacefulness, comfort, or meaning—and is spiritual well-being connected to other areas of functioning?

A number of investigations have found that spiritual well-being is tied to other important aspects of quality of life. Arguably, connections with emotional functioning may have limited meaning, given the fact that measures of spiritual well-being contain items that overlap with emotional well-being (e.g., comfort, unhappiness, satisfaction). Thus perhaps it is not surprising that individuals with greater spiritual well-being usually demonstrate more favorable psychological adjustment to cancer than those with lower spiritual well-being, despite differences in the particular measures that are used (Cohen et al., 1997; Cotton, Levine, Fitzpatrick, Dold, & Targ, 1999; Fitchett, Peterman, & Cella, 1996). For example, among patients with breast cancer (Mickley et al., 1992; Mickley & Soeken, 1993) or diverse types of malignancies (Kaczorowski, 1989), those with greater spiritual well-being reported higher levels of hope and lower state and trait anxiety compared with individuals with low spiritual well-being.

More interesting and less confounded are the associations between spiritual well-being and *physical* dimensions of quality of life. We can find initial hints about these connections by examining "global quality of life" or patient ratings of contentment, which usually reflect physical, as well as psychosocial, functioning. Global quality of life has been tied to spiritual or existential well-being in a number of studies (Cohen et al., 1997; Cotton et al., 1999; Fitchett et al., 1996), including some that controlled for demographic and medical factors, mood, and social desirability (Brady, Peterman, Fitchett, Mo, & Cella, 1999). When the focus turns more exclusively to physical symptoms, findings are less consistent (Cohen et al., 1997; Fitchett et al., 1996). In a sample of palliative care patients, Cohen and colleagues (1997) did not find any ties between existential well-being and various measures of physical functioning or activities of daily living. In contrast, in a broader study of patients with cancer or HIV disease who were assessed using different measures, Fitchett and colleagues (1996) reported significant associations between spiritual well-being and physical and functional well-being. This team of investigators then took a closer look at subgroups of patients who were burdened by high levels of pain or fatigue (Brady et al., 1999). In both groups of highly symptomatic patients, individuals with greater spiritual well-being were more likely to report continued enjoyment of life, despite their ailments, relative to those who scored low on spiritual well-being. Thus, a sense of existential or religious well-being appears to be tied to overall health-related quality of life among cancer patients. Relationships with physical functioning are less clear, but individuals with a more positive spiritual outlook may be better able to bear debilitating medical symptoms and still enjoy life.

CHANGES IN RELIGIOUSNESS OR SPIRITUALITY IN RESPONSE TO CANCER

Thus far much of our discussion has focused on how religious faith might influence the experience of cancer. Another intriguing question, hinted at in the previous section, concerns how an experience with cancer might alter one's religious faith. Does religious or spiritual involvement change in response to cancer? (Here we are not concerned with its impact on spiritual well-being but rather with its effects on more fundamental spiritual beliefs and commitments.) Which individuals seem most likely to experience these changes, and which dimensions of religious expression are most altered? How do these changes unfold over time, and are they enduring or ephemeral?

In part, finding changes in religiousness or spirituality may depend on where we look. Clinical experience and a newly emerging research literature offer many accounts of individuals who experience a shift in their spiritual or existential concerns in the aftermath of a cancer diagnosis (Andrykowski, Brady, & Hunt, 1993; Belec, 1992; Collins, Taylor, & Skokan, 1990; Curbow, Somerfield, Baker, Wingard, & Legro, 1993). They may report feeling closer to God, more attuned to the present moment, more apprecia-tive of the preciousness of life, more connected with forces beyond them-selves, or more imbued with a sense of mission (Sherman & Simonton, 2001). Cancer patients undergoing screening for bone marrow transplan-tation, for example, reported greater increases in religious satisfaction and meaning in life than did a comparison group of healthy individuals (Andrykowski et al., 1993). The majority of cancer patients reported feeling more satisfied with their religion since their diagnosis. Changes in spiritual or existential perspectives following personal crises are a core aspect of many theoretical models, ranging from Kierkegaard (1974) through Frankl (1963) and Tedeschi, Park, and Calhoun (1998).

Whether formal religious beliefs and rituals (as opposed to a personal sense of meaning or appreciation for life) change is less clear. Research with individuals confronted by other types of traumatic experiences suggests that, for most people, basic religious beliefs and practices are relatively stable (Croog & Levine, 1972; Pargament, 1997). Few studies have systematically explored this question among cancer patients. Findings are mixed (e.g., Curbow et al., 1993; Feher & Maly, 1999; Tebbi et al., 1987; Yates et al., 1981). In a qualitative cross-sectional study of older women with recently diagnosed breast cancer, half of the participants reported a strengthening of religious faith (Feher & Maly, 1999). Similar findings emerged in a cross-sectional study of patients receiving active treatment for various types of cancer (Moschella, Pressman, Pressman, & Weissman, 1997). Most reported increased religious involvement, with 67% reporting increased prayer and 51% expressing increased faith. As might be expected among medically ill individuals, increases in church attendance were less common (16%). A study of bone marrow transplant survivors suggested that a substantial pro-portion (40%) had experienced positive changes in their religious beliefs fol-lowing their difficult treatment experience (Curbow et al., 1993).

In contrast, in a longitudinal study of terminal cancer patients, who might be expected to report increased religiousness, there was little change over time in religious beliefs (Yates et al., 1981). Among those who died dur-ing the course of the study, there was a trend toward decreased or stable reli-gious beliefs rather than an increase. Changes in personal values, spiritual experiences, or day-to-day religious priorities may not be readily apparent in traditional measures of general religiousness, particularly those that lump together beliefs, attitudes, and practices. In his conceptual model of religious coping, Pargament (1997) distinguishes between two broad types of reli-gious changes. The first concerns changes in the "means" or pathways to significance—such as switching membership from one congregation to another, repenting, or reframing tragedy as part of God's plan. The second concerns changes in the "ends" or destinations of significance—such as developing new spiritual values and priorities or experiencing spiritual conversion. To capture specific changes such as these, investigators may need to move beyond sole reliance on global measures of religious traits or beliefs and focus on more fine-grained analyses, including religious coping (Pargament, 1997), spiritual striving (Emmons, 1999), religious doubts (Altemeyer, 1988; Krause, Ingersoll-Dayton, Ellison, & Wulff, 1999), forgiveness (Berry, Worthington, Parrott, O'Connor, & Wade, in press), volunteerism (Oman, Thoresen, & McMahon, 1999), mystical experiences (Hood, 1975), posttraumatic growth (Park, Cohen, & Murch, 1996; Tedeschi & Calhoun, 1996), or qualitative changes that patients themselves define as important (Taylor et al., 1999).

This work is only beginning. Preliminary studies of religious coping suggest little change or small decrements over time among patients with treatable disease (Alferi et al., 1999; Carver et al., 1993; Filipp et al., 1990; Sherman, Simonton, et al., 2000), but increased religious coping in patients with incurable illness (Hershberger, Pacheco, & Markert, 2000). These findings imply that a higher level of threat may mobilize greater religious coping or religious strivings. This notion—that greater threats elicit stronger religious expression (i.e., "there are no atheists in foxholes")—has been the subject of considerable interest (Pargament, 1997). In their model of posttraumatic growth, Calhoun and Tedeschi (1998) speculate that growth in the aftermath of crisis requires that individuals experience a relatively "seismic" level of threat or suffering, so that the experience disrupts their habitual assumptions about the world and sets in motion a process of cognitive reorganization (see also Carver, 1998; Kelly, 1955). Consistent with this expectation, a recent investigation of cancer patients found that individuals with Stage II (i.e., more advanced) disease reported greater posttraumatic growth than those with Stage I disease (Lechner & Zakowski, 2000). On the other hand, patients with the most extensive disease (Stage IV) reported less posttraumatic growth than those with regional disease (Stage III). Perhaps under some circumstances the level of threat is too overwhelming to sustain a serious reevaluation of one's basic world view. Whether spiritual changes are more likely to occur within certain thresholds of disease severity or subjective distress is an intriguing area for further study.

RELIGION AND CANCER SCREENING

Most research in oncology has focused on connections between faith and adjustment to illness. The potential impact of religiousness or spirituality on other important aspects of illness—such as treatment adherence, communication about symptoms, immunosuppression, or decisions about terminal care—has yet to be explored. However, one area in which religion is drawing growing attention concerns cancer screening and early detection. Some of the highest rates of cancer morbidity and mortality are found among rural elderly and minority populations. Cancer screening practices, such as mammograms, Pap smears, and colorectal screening, are alarmingly low in these groups (McCarthy et al., 1998). While access to health care services, health insurance, and health education are serious problems for these groups (Mickey, Durski, Worden, & Danigelis, 1995), traditional interventions targeting these needs have met with limited success. Given the central role of the church in the social fabric of these communities, some investigations have explored whether religion might have a meaningful role to play, either in facilitating or impeding health practices.

Some researchers have wondered whether religious involvement might have a negative impact on early detection of cancer, by encouraging counterproductive health beliefs. Do some religious communities contribute to avoidance of health care by fostering fatalistic expectations (e.g., "Cancer is a death sentence—this is God's will and there's nothing to be done"), or perceptions that healing is exclusively in the hands of God and not conventional health providers (e.g., "God is my doctor")? A study of elderly, poor, rural, predominantly African American individuals suggested that, although fatalistic attitudes about cancer were common, these assumptions did not seem to be linked to religious involvement (Powe, 1997). Participants with stronger spiritual beliefs and practices were no more likely to harbor these dire expectations about cancer than were their less religious counterparts. Similarly, a study of lower income, predominantly African American women indicated that religious beliefs about health did not have much impact on cancer screening practices (i.e., mammography and Pap smears; Paskett, Case, Tatum, Velez, & Wilson, 1999). Most women agreed that it was God's will for individuals to have cancer and that God was their doctor, but these beliefs were tempered by perceptions that God gives doctors wisdom and skill to heal and that God wants people to help themselves. Thus these studies suggest that religious involvement does not contribute to the low cancer screening rates characteristic of these underserved populations.

A more exciting possibility is the role local churches might play in encouraging cancer screening. Long used to promote education about heart disease and other health concerns in African American communities (Hatch & Lovelace, 1980; Paskett et al., 1999), local churches recently have become partners in efforts to increase cancer education and screening (Boehm et al., 1995; Weinrich et al., 1998). The Witness Project at Arkansas Cancer Research Center, for example, has enrolled African American cancer survivors to share their stories ("witness") in rural churches, where they serve as credible messengers and role models of successful survivorship (Erwin,

Spatz, Stotts, & Hollenberg, 1999; Erwin, Spatz, & Turtorro, 1992). The presentations include a strong spiritual component (e.g., hymns, statements of faith), consistent with participants' deep convictions about the ties between religion and healing. This program has been sufficiently successful in increasing screening and health education in medically underserved high-risk communities that it is currently being replicated on a national level. Innovative, church-based services such as these illustrate the potential practical benefits of cultivating links between religious faith and health. Other creative programs within the African American community have been designed to reduce smoking (Schorling et al., 1997), increase fruit and vegetable consumption (Campbell et al., 1999), bolster education about prostate cancer (Boehm et al., 1995) or provide services to geriatric cancer patients (Brown-Hunter & Price, 1998). These interventions do not place physicians in the ethically awkward position of advocating religious activity among their patients (Sloan, Bagiella, & Powell, 1999). Instead, they forge partnerships with a strongly valued indigenous community resource to promote health. These programs offer a promising approach in the battle against cancer.

CONCLUSIONS AND FUTURE DIRECTIONS

The work reviewed here suggests that faith is an important resource for many patients with cancer. General religious orientation and cancer-related religious coping have both been modestly associated with various dimensions of quality of life, including emotional distress, life satisfaction, social functioning, and sometimes physical symptoms. Spiritual well-being has also been tied to several important aspects of quality of life. The relationships between religion and cancer appear to be complex, however. On balance, stronger religious or spiritual involvement usually has been associated with more favorable quality of life outcomes, but negative outcomes sometimes have been noted as well, as have null findings.

Current results are provocative, but systematic research in this area is in its infancy, and considerable work has yet to be done. To borrow a phrase from musician Stephen Stills, "There's something happening here, what it is ain't exactly clear." Many studies have used idiosyncratic, unvalidated, or very narrow measures of religious involvement. Although this is understandable for a field in its early stages, it means that the reliability of results from these investigations is open to question and that comparability across studies is difficult. Different dimensions of religious involvement have sometimes been confused (e.g., general religious commitment, cancer-specific coping, and religious/spiritual well-being). Fortunately, there has been meaningful progress in the development or refinement of measures for use in medical settings (see Chapter 6, this volume). The growing availability of brief, psychometrically sound instruments means that health researchers have better tools to work with as they explore different facets of religious or spiritual involvement. Additional research is needed to clarify which dimensions of faith are most strongly tied to which health outcomes. Aside from examinations of emotional, social, or functional aspects of quality of life, a wide array of other important endpoints merits investigation. For example, the potential impact of faith on prevention behaviors, cancer screening, treatment adherence, and lifestyle changes are areas ripe for study. Moreover, the potential effects on biological endpoints, such as treatment toxicities, chemotherapy-induced immune suppression, or recurrence rates, would be fascinating avenues for exploration.

Relative to religiousness, spirituality remains a concept that is vaguely understood and poorly operationalized by health researchers. Advances have been made in studying spiritual outcomes (e.g., spiritual or existential well-being), but efforts to explore spirituality as a *predictor* or *resource* variable are stymied by conceptual and psychometric difficulties. Measures of spirituality tend to be confounded by psychological well-being. Although spirituality is a notoriously difficult construct to operationalize, we suspect that definitions that emphasize concepts such as comfort, inner peacefulness, harmony, or hope may be less a theoretical necessity than a conceptual and methodological drawback (see Chapter 1, this volume). Perhaps a more compelling theoretical case should be made for the centrality of these concepts as defining features of spirituality, or instruments should be developed with greater divergent validity.

Among other methodological limitations of the literature, most studies are characterized by small samples, which limits statistical power and the prospects for uncovering meaningful relationships. In addition, most investigations have used cross-sectional designs (i.e., religiousness and health outcomes are assessed at a single point in time). There is a pressing need for longitudinal studies, particularly because faith has sometimes been associated with negative, as well as favorable, outcomes. Do higher levels of adversity and distress prompt increased reliance on religion, does religious coping sometimes lead to negative outcomes, or are these associations influenced by other, as yet unidentified, factors? If religious faith does enhance adaptation to illness for some individuals, when does it foster recovery to premorbid levels of functioning (i.e., "resilience") and when does it facilitate *higher* functioning or growth (i.e., "thriving") (Carver, 1998)? Longitudinal studies would help shed light on these fundamental questions.

In addition, longitudinal studies (both qualitative and quantitative) might help clarify changes in religiousness or spirituality over time in response to the crisis of cancer. If life-threatening illness sometimes leads to painful doubts or conflicts concerning spiritual values, under what circumstances does this process of reevaluation lead eventually to stronger faith, when does it lead to a transformation or conversion to a different kind of faith, and when does it lead to more enduring withdrawal from spiritual pursuits? Do such changes in spirituality have relevance for health outcomes? If so, is the level of integration and personal comfort with these spiritual changes more important than the direction of the changes (i.e., toward or away from spiritual involvement)?

For which individuals are relationships between faith and health most important? The current oncology literature provides few clues. In general, levels of religious commitment and religious coping are higher among members of ethnic minority groups, the elderly, women, and individuals with less education and fewer economic resources (Gallup, 1990; Pargament, 1997). In studies of cancer patients, links between faith and health appear to be stronger among minority groups (e.g., Culver et al., 1999; Feher & Maly, 1999). We know less about the potential influence of other characteristics, such as disease severity and phase of treatment.

Another area that has received little attention is the social or family context of religious coping. Only a few studies have examined the relationship between religiousness and quality of life for family members of cancer patients (Abernethy et al., 1999; Rabins, Fitting, Eastham, & Zabora, 1990). Which dimensions of faith might be helpful to family members coping with disruptive changes in family life, and how does religious coping within the family change over the trajectory of the disease? What impact does the family, in turn, have on the patient's religious coping efforts? Are health outcomes influenced by social support for or undermining of a patient's religious coping efforts?

Finally, we have little information about the mediating pathways that might help explain the relationships between faith and health among cancer patients. Among other benefits, religious or spiritual involvement is thought to offer a framework for creating meaning (Andrykowski et al., 1993; Geertz, 1966), a sense of control and coherence (Koenig, 1997; Pargament et al., 1999), a forum for social support (Durkheim, 1915/1965; Feher & Maly, 1999), a reservoir of hope and comfort (Koenig, 1997; Pargament, 1997), and a mandate for constructive health behaviors and coping strategies (Kurtz et al., 1995; Van Ness, 1999). Each of these factors has been associated with health outcomes. As yet, however, we know little about the differential importance of these mechanisms, alone or in interaction, for explaining how faith might be tied to various health outcomes. A recent qualitative study suggested that religious faith provided emotional comfort, social support, and a sense of meaning for older women with newly diagnosed breast cancer (Feher & Maly, 1999). Similarly, a pioneering study by Moschella and colleagues (1997) hinted at the role of faith in providing a sense of meaning to explain suffering (i.e., theodicy). In our work with gynecological cancer patients, there are preliminary indications that optimism mediates the relationships between general religious orientation and psychological adjustment (Sherman, Simonton, et al., 2000); social support did not seem to play a comparable role. Additional studies may help us better understand these important pathways.

A life-threatening illness such as cancer represents a nodal, transformative experience for most individuals. Heightened spiritual concerns, embodying a search for comforting resources or a struggle with disconcerting ambiguities, are a natural response to the crisis of illness. There are indications that spirituality and religiousness are tied to important health outcomes for cancer patients, but we have only begun to trace these connections. Within the next few years, the burgeoning research activity in this area should do much to deepen our understanding and sharpen our questions.

REFERENCES

Abernethy, A. D., Chang, H. T., Duberstein, P. R., Seidlitz, L., & Evinger, J. S. (1999). Religious coping and depression in spouses of lung cancer patients [Abstract]. *Annals of Behavioral Medicine, 21*(Suppl.), S124.

Acklin, M. W., Brown, E. C., & Mauger, P. A. (1983). The role of religious values in coping with cancer. *Journal of Religion and Health, 22*, 322–333.

Alferi, S. M., Culver, J. L., Carver, C. S., Arena, P. L., & Antoni, M. H. (1999). Religiosity, religious coping, and distress: A prospective study of Catholic and Evangelical women in treatment for early-stage breast cancer. *Journal of Health Psychology, 4*, 343–356.

Andrykowski, M. A., Brady, M. J., & Hunt, J. W. (1993). Positive psychosocial adjustment in potential bone marrow transplant recipients: Cancer as a psychosocial transition. *Psycho-Oncology, 2*, 261–276.

Altemeyer, B. (1988). *Enemies of freedom: Understanding right-wing authoritarianism.* San Francisco: Jossey-Bass.

Antonovski, A. (1993). The structure and properties of the Sense of Coherence Scale. *Social Science and Medicine, 36*, 725–733.

Baider, L., Russak, S. M., Perry, S., Kash, K., Gronert, M., Fox, B., Holland, J., & Kaplan-Denour, A. (1999). The role of religious and spiritual beliefs in coping with malignant melanoma: An Israeli sample. *Psycho-Oncology, 8*, 27–35.

Belec, R. H. (1992). Quality of life: Perceptions of long-term survivors of bone marrow transplantation. *Oncology Nursing Forum, 19*, 31–37.

Berry, J. W., Worthington, E. L., Jr., Parrott, L., III, O'Connor, L. E., & Wade, N. G. (in press). Dispositional forgiveness: Development and construct validity of the Transgression Narrative Test of Forgivingness (TNTF). *Personality and Social Psychology Bulletin.*

Boehm, S., Coleman-Burns, P., Schlenk, E. A., Funnell, M. M., Parzuchowski, J., & Powell, I. J. (1995). Prostate cancer in African American men: Increasing knowledge and self-efficacy. *Journal of Community Health Nursing, 12*, 161–169.

Boudreaux, E., Catz, S., Ryan, L., Amaral-Melendez, M., & Brantley, P. J. (1995). The Ways of Religious Coping Scale: Reliability, validity, and scale development. *Assessment, 2*, 233–244.

Brady, M. J., Peterman, A. H., Fitchett, G., Mo, M., & Cella, D. (1999). A case for including spirituality in quality of life measurement in oncology. *Psycho-Oncology, 8*, 417–428.

Brandt, B. T. (1987). The relationship between hopelessness and selected variables in women receiving chemotherapy for breast cancer. *Oncology Nursing Forum, 14*, 35–39.

Brown-Hunter, M., & Price, L. K. (1998). The Good Neighbor Project: Volunteerism and the elderly African-American patient with cancer. *Geriatric Nursing, 19*, 139–141.

Calhoun, L. G., & Tedeschi, R. G. (1998). Posttraumatic growth: Future directions. In R. G. Tedeschi, C. L. Park, & L. G. Calhoun (Eds.), *Posttraumatic growth: Positive changes in the aftermath of crisis* (pp. 215–238). Mahwah, NJ: Erlbaum.

Campbell, M. K., Demark-Wahnefried, W., Symons, M., Kalsbeek, W. D., Dodds, J., Cowan, A., Jackson, B., Motsinger, B., Hoben, K., Lashley, J., Demissie, S., & McClelland, J. W. (1999). Fruit and vegetable consumption and prevention of cancer: The Black Churches United for Better Health Project. *American Journal of Public Health, 89*, 1390–1396.

Carver, C. S. (1998). Resilience and thriving: Issues, models, and linkages. *Journal of Social Issues, 54*(2), 245–266.

Carver, C. S., Pozo, C., Harris, S. D., Noriega, V., Scheier, M. F., Robinson, D. S., Ketcham, A. S., Moffat, F. L., Jr., & Clark, K. C. (1993). How coping mediates the effect of optimism on distress: A study of women with early stage breast cancer. *Journal of Personality and Social Psychology, 65*, 375–390.

Carver, C. S., Scheier, M. F., & Weintraub, J. K. (1989). Assessing coping strategies: A theoretically based approach. *Journal of Personality and Social Psychology, 56*, 267–283.

Cella, D. F. (1994). *Functional Assessment of Cancer Therapy Manual.* Chicago, IL: Rush-Presbyterian-St. Luke's Medical Center.

Cella, D. F. (1997). *Functional Assessment of Chronic Illness Therapy Manual, version 4.* Evanston, IL: Evanston Northwestern Healthcare, Center on Outcomes, Research and Education.

Cohen, S. R., Mount, B. M., Bruera, E., Provost, M., Rowe, J., & Tong, K. (1997). Validity of the McGill Quality of Life Questionnaire in the palliative care setting: A multi-centre Canadian study demonstrating the importance of the existential domain. *Palliative Medicine, 11*, 3–20.

Collins, R. L., Taylor, S. E., & Skokan, L. A. (1990). A better world or a shattered vision? Changes in life perspectives following victimization. *Social Cognition, 8*, 263–285.

Cotton, S. P., Levine, E. G., Fitzpatrick, C. M., Dold, K. H., & Targ, E. (1999). Exploring the relationships among spiritual well-being, quality of life, and psychological adjustment in women with breast cancer. *Psycho-Oncology, 8*, 429–438.

Croog, S. H., & Levine, S. (1972). Religious identity and response to serious illness: A report on heart patients. *Social Science and Medicine, 6,* 17–32.

Culver, J. L., Alferi, S. M., Carver, C. S., Kilbourn, K. M., & Antoni, M. H. (1999). Ethnic differences in coping strategies among early-stage breast cancer patients [Abstract]. *Annals of Behavioral Medicine, 21*(Suppl.), S230.

Curbow, B., Somerfield, R., Baker, F., Wingard, J. R., & Legro, M. W. (1993). Personal changes, dispositional optimism, and psychological adjustment to bone marrow transplantation. *Journal of Behavioral Medicine, 16,* 423–443.

Derogatis, L. R. (1993). *Brief Symptom Inventory: Administration, scoring, and procedures manual.* Minneapolis, MN: National Computer Systems.

Diener, E., Emmons, R., Larsen, R., & Griffen, S. (1985). The Satisfaction with Life Scale. *Journal of Personality Assessment, 49,* 71–75.

Durkheim, E. (1965). *The elementary forms of the religious life.* New York: Free Press. (Original work published 1915)

Ell, K. O., Mantell, J. E., Hamovitch, M. B., & Nishimoto, R. H. (1989). Social support, sense of control, and coping among patients with breast, lung, or colorectal cancer. *Journal of Psychosocial Oncology, 7,* 63–89.

Emmons, R. A. (1999). *The psychology of ultimate concerns: Motivation and spirituality in personality.* New York: Guilford Press.

Erwin, D. O., Spatz, T. S., Stotts, R. C., & Hollenberg, J. A. (1999). Increasing mammography practice by African American women *Cancer Practice, 7,* 78–85.

Erwin, D. O., Spatz, T. S., & Turtorro, C. L. (1992). Development of an African-American role model intervention to increase breast self-examination and mammography. *Journal of Cancer Education, 7,* 311–319.

Feher, S., & Maly, R. C. (1999). Coping with breast cancer in later life: The role of religious faith. *Psycho-Oncology, 8,* 408–416.

Fehring, R. J., Miller, J. F., & Shaw, C. (1997). Spiritual well-being, religiosity, hope, depression, and other mood states in elderly people coping with cancer. *Oncology Nursing Forum, 24,* 663–671.

Ferrell, B. R., Taylor, E. J., Grant, M., Fowler, M., & Corbisiero, R. M. (1993). Pain management at home: Struggle, comfort, and mission. *Cancer Nursing, 16,* 169–178.

Filipp, S.-H., Klauer, T., Freudenberg, E., & Ferring, D. (1990). The regulation of subjective well-being in cancer patients: An analysis of coping effectiveness. *Psychology and Health, 4,* 305–317.

Fitchett, G., Peterman, A. H., & Cella, D. F. (1996, November). *Spiritual beliefs and quality of life in cancer and HIV patients.* Paper presented at the meeting of the Society for the Scientific Study of Religion, Nashville, TN.

Frankl, V. (1963). *Man's search for meaning: An introduction to logotherapy* (I. Lasch, Trans.). New York: Pocket Books.

Fredette, S. L. (1995). Breast cancer survivors: Concerns and coping. *Cancer Nursing, 18,* 35–46.

Gallup, G., Jr. (1990). *Religion in America: 1990.* Princeton, NJ: Princeton Religious Research Center.

Geertz, C. (1966). Religion as a cultural system. In M. Banton (Ed.), *Anthropological approaches to the study of religion* (pp. 1–46). London: Tavistock.

Gibbs, H. W., & Achterberg-Lawlis, J. (1978). Spiritual values and death anxiety: Implications for counseling with terminal cancer patients. *Journal of Counseling Psychology, 25,* 563–569.

Halstead, M. T., & Fernsler, J. I. (1994). Coping strategies of long-term cancer survivors. *Cancer Nursing, 17,* 94–100.

Hatch, J., & Lovelace, K. (1980). Involving the southern rural church and students of health professions in health education. *Public Health Reports, 595,* 23–25.

Hershberger, P. J., Pacheco, J., & Markert, R. J. (2000, April). *Stability of attitudes toward physician-assisted suicide and euthanasia among patients with non-curable malignancy.* Paper presented at the annual meeting of the Society of Behavioral Medicine, Nashville, TN.

Herth, K. A. (1989). The relationship between level of hope and level of coping response and other variables in patients with cancer. *Oncology Nursing Forum, 16,* 67–72.

Holland, J. C., Kash, K. M., Passik, S., Gronert, M. K., Sison, A., Lederberg, M., Russak, S. M., Baider, L., & Fox, B. (1998). A brief spiritual beliefs inventory for use in quality of life research in life-threatening illness. *Psycho-Oncology, 7,* 460–469.

Holland, J. C., Passik, S., Kash, K. M., Russak, S. M., Gronert, M. K., Sison, A., Lederberg, M., Fox, B., & Baider, L. (1999). The role of religious and spiritual beliefs in coping with malignant melanoma. *Psycho-Oncology, 8,* 14–26.

Hood, R. W., Jr. (1975). The construction and preliminary validation of a measure of reported mystical experience. *Journal for the Scientific Study of Religion, 14,* 29–41.

Horowitz, M. H., Wilner, N., & Alvarez, W. (1979). Impact of Events Scale: A measure of subjective stress. *Psychosomatic Medicine, 41,* 209–218.

Ita, D. J. (1995–1996). Testing of a causal model: Acceptance of death in hospice patients. *Omega, 32,* 81–92.

Johnson, S. C., & Spilka, B. (1991). Coping with breast cancer: The roles of clergy and faith. *Journal of Religion and Health, 30,* 21–33.

Kaczorowski, J. M. (1989). Spiritual well-being and anxiety in adults diagnosed with cancer. *Hospice Journal, 5,* 105–116.

Kelly, G. A. (1955). *The psychology of personal constructs.* New York: Norton.

Kierkegaard, S. (1974). *Fear and trembling* (Lowrie, Trans.). Princeton, NJ: Princeton University Press. (Original work published 1984)

Koenig, H. G. (1997). Use of religion by patients with severe medical illness. *Mind/Body Medicine, 2,* 31–36.

Koenig, H. G., Cohen, H. J., Blazer, D. G., Pieper, C., Meador, K. G., Shelp, F., Goli, V., & DiPasquale, B. (1992). Religious coping and depression among elderly, hospitalized medically ill men. *American Journal of Psychiatry, 149,* 1693–1700.

Koenig, H. G., Meador, K., & Parkerson, G. (1997). Religion Index for Psychiatric Research: A 5-item measure for use in health outcome studies [Letter to the editor]. *American Journal of Psychiatry, 154,* 885–886.

Krause, N., Ingersoll-Dayton, B., Ellison, C. G., & Wulff, K. M. (1999). Aging, religious doubt, and psychological well-being. *Gerontologist, 39,* 525–533.

Kurtz, M. E., Wyatt, G., & Kurtz, J. C. (1995). Psychological and sexual well-being, philosophical/spiritual views, and health habits of long-term cancer survivors. *Health Care for Women International, 16,* 253–262.

Lechner, S., & Zakowski, S. (2000, April). *Disease severity influences found meaning in cancer.* Paper presented at the annual meeting of the Society of Behavioral Medicine, Nashville, TN.

Lepore, S. J. (1997, April). *Social constraints, intrusive thoughts, and negative affect in women with cancer.* Paper presented at the annual meeting of the Society of Behavioral Medicine, San Francisco, CA.

Lepore, S. J., & Helgeson, V. S. (1998). Social constraints, intrusive thoughts, and mental health after prostate surgery. *Journal of Social and Clinical Psychology, 17,* 89–106.

McCarthy, E. P., Burns, R. B., Coughlin, S. S., Freund, K. M., Rice, J., Marwill, S. L., Ash, A., Shwartz, M., & Moskowitz, M. A. (1998). Mammography use helps to explain differences in breast cancer stage at diagnosis between older black and white women. *Annals of Internal Medicine, 128,* 729–736.

Mickey, R. M., Durski, J., Worden, J. K., & Danigelis, N. L. (1995). Breast cancer screening and associated factors for low-income African American women. *Preventive Medicine, 24,* 467–476.

Mickley, J. R., & Soeken, K. (1993). Religiousness and hope in Hispanic- and Anglo-American women with breast cancer. *Oncology Nursing Forum, 20,* 1171–1177.

Mickley, J. R., Soeken, K., & Belcher, A. (1992). Spiritual well-being, religiousness and hope among women with breast cancer. *Image: Journal of Nursing Scholarship, 24,* 267–272.

Moschella, V. D., Pressman, K. R., Pressman, P., & Weissman, D. E. (1997). The problem of theodicy and religious response to cancer. *Journal of Religion and Health, 36,* 17–20.

Norum, J., Risberg, T., & Solberg, E. (2000). Faith among patients with advanced cancer: A pilot study on patients offered "no more than" palliation. *Journal of Supportive Care in Cancer, 8,* 110–114.

Oman, D., Thoresen, C. E., & McMahon, K. (1999). Volunteerism and mortality. *Journal of Health Psychology, 4,* 301–316.

Pargament, K. I. (1997). *The psychology of religion and coping: Theory, research, practice.* New York: Guilford Press.

Pargament, K. I., Cole, B., VandeCreek, L., Belavich, T., Brant, C., & Perez, L. (1999). The vigil: Religion and the search for control in the hospital waiting room. *Journal of Health Psychology, 4,* 327–341.

Pargament, K. I., Koenig, H. G., & Perez, L. M. (2000). The many methods of religious coping: Development and initial validation of the RCOPE. *Journal of Clinical Psychology, 56,* 519–543.

Pargament, K. I., & Park, C. L. (1995). Merely a defense? The variety of religious means and ends. *Journal of Social Issues, 51,* 13–32.

Pargament, K. I., Smith, B. W., Koenig, H. G., & Perez, L. (1998). Patterns of positive and negative religious coping with major life stressors. *Journal of Scientific Study of Religion, 37,* 711–725.

Park, C., & Cohen, L. H. (1992). Religious beliefs and practices and the coping process. In B. M. Carpenter (Ed.), *Personal coping: Theory, research, and application* (pp. 185–198). Westport, CT: Praeger.

Park, C., Cohen, L. H., & Herb, L. (1990). Intrinsic religiousness and religious coping as life stress moderators for Catholics versus Protestants. *Journal of Personality and Social Psychology, 59,* 562–574.

Park, C. L., Cohen, L. H., & Murch, R. (1996). Assessment and prediction of stress-related growth. *Journal of Personality, 64,* 71–105.

Paskett, E. D., Case, D., Tatum, C., Velez, R., & Wilson, A. (1999). Religiosity and cancer screening. *Journal of Religion and Health, 38,* 39–51.

Plante, T. G., & Boccaccini, M. T. (1997). Reliability and validity of the Santa Clara Strength of Religious Faith Questionnaire. *Pastoral Psychology, 45,* 429–437.

Post-White, J., Ceronsky, C., Kreitzer, M. J., Nickelson, K., Drew, D., Mackey, K. W., Koopmeiners, L., & Gutknecht, S. (1996). Hope, spirituality, sense of coherence, and quality of life in patients with cancer. *Oncology Nursing Forum, 23,* 1571–1579.

Powe, B. D. (1997). Cancer fatalism: Spiritual perspectives. *Journal of Religion and Health, 36,* 135–144.

Rabins, P. V., Fitting, M. D., Eastham, J., & Zabora, J. (1990). Emotional adaptation over time in care-givers for chronically ill elderly people. *Age and Ageing, 19,* 185–190.

Ringdal, G. I. (1996). Religiosity, quality of life, and survival in cancer patients. *Social Indicators Research, 38,* 193–211.

Schorling, J. B., Roach, J., Siegel, M., Baturka, N., Hunt, D. E., Guterbock, M., & Stewart, H. L. (1997). The trial of church-based smoking cessation interventions for rural African Americans. *Preventive Medicine, 26,* 92–101.

Sherman, A. C., Plante, T. G., Simonton, S., Adams, D. C., Burris, S. K., & Harbison, C. (1999). Assessing religious involvement in medical patients: Cross-validation of the Santa Clara Strength of Religious Faith Questionnaire. *Pastoral Psychology, 48,* 129–142.

Sherman, A. C., Plante, T. G., Simonton, S., Adams, D. C., Harbison, C., & Burris, S. K. (2000). A multidimensional measure of religious involvement for cancer patients: The Duke Religious Index. *Journal of Supportive Care in Cancer, 8,* 102–109.

Sherman, A. C., Plante, T. G., Simonton, S., Wells, P., & Moody, V. R. (2001). Associations between religious/existential resources and quality of life outcomes for multiple myeloma patients [Abstract]. *Psychosomatic Medicine, 63,* 128.

Sherman, A. C., & Simonton, S. (1999). Family therapy for cancer patients: Clinical issues and interventions. *Family Journal, 7,* 38–49.

Sherman, A. C., & Simonton, S. (2001). Coping with cancer in the family. *Family Journal, 9,* 193–200.

Sherman, A. C., Simonton, S., Adams, D. C., Vural, E., & Hanna, E. (2000). Coping with head and neck cancer during different phases of treatment. *Head and Neck, 22,* 787–793.

Sherman, A. C., Simonton, S., Latif, U., Eaves, A., France, M., & Parham, G. (2001). *Religiousness and quality of life among newly-diagnosed gynecological cancer patients.* Manuscript in preparation.

Sherman, A. C., Simonton, S., Plante, T. G., Moody, V. R., & Wells, P. (2001). Patterns of religious coping among multiple myeloma patients: Associations with adjustment and quality of life [Abstract]. *Psychosomatic Medicine, 63,* 124.

Silberfarb, P. M., Anderson, K. M., Rundle, A. C., Holland, J. C., Cooper, M. R., & McIntyre, O. R. (1991). Mood and clinical status in patients with multiple myeloma. *Journal of Clinical Oncology, 9,* 2219–2224.

Simonton, S., & Sherman, A. C. (1998). Psychosocial dimensions of mind/body medicine: Promises and pitfalls from research with cancer patients. *Alternative Therapies in Health and Medicine, 4,* 50–67.

Sloan, R. P., Bagiella, E., & Powell, T. (1999). Religion, spirituality, and medicine. *Lancet, 353,* 664–667.

Smith, D. K., Nehemkis, A. M., & Charter, R. A. (1983–1984). Fear of death, death attitudes, and religious conviction in the terminally ill. *International Journal of Psychiatry in Medicine, 13,* 221–232.

Sodestrom, K. E., & Martinson, I. M. (1987). Patients' spiritual coping strategies: A study of nurse and patient perspectives. *Oncology Nursing Forum, 14,* 41–46.

Swensen, C. H., Fuller, S., & Clements, R. (1993). Stage of religious faith and reactions to terminal cancer. *Journal of Psychology and Theology, 21,* 238–245.

Taylor, E. J., Outlaw, F. H., Bernardo, T. R., & Roy, A. (1999). Spiritual conflicts associated with praying about cancer. *Psycho-Oncology, 8,* 386–394.

Tebbi, C. K., Mallon, J. C., Richards, M. E., & Bigler, L. R. (1987). Religiosity and locus of control of adolescent cancer patients. *Psychological Reports, 61,* 683–696.

Tedeschi, R., & Calhoun, L. (1996). The Post-Traumatic Growth Inventory: Measuring the positive legacy of trauma. *Journal of Traumatic Stress, 9,* 455–471.

Tedeschi, R. G., Park, C. L., & Calhoun, L. G. (1998). *Posttraumatic growth: Positive changes in the aftermath of crisis.* Mahwah, NJ: Lawrence Erlbaum.

Tix, A. P., & Frazier, P. A. (1998). The use of religious coping during stressful life events: Main effects, moderation, and mediation. *Journal of Consulting and Clinical Psychology, 66,* 411–422.

Van Ness, P. H. (1999). Religion and public health. *Journal of Religion and Health, 38,* 15–26.

Weinrich, S., Holdford, D., Boyd, M., Creanga, D., Cover, K., Johnson, A., Frank-Stromborg, M., & Weinrich, M. (1998). Prostate cancer education in African American churches. *Public Health Nursing, 15,* 188–195.

Yates, J. W., Chalmer, B. J., St. James, P., Follansbee, M., & McKegney, F. P. (1981). Religion in patients with advanced cancer. *Medical and Pediatric Oncology, 9,* 121–128.

Zigmond, A. S., & Snaith, R. P. (1983). The Hospital Anxiety and Depression Scale. *Acta Psychiatrica Scandinavica, 67,* 361–370.

8

―◄O►―

RELIGION AND HEALTH
IN HIV/AIDS COMMUNITIES

R. COREY REMLE
HAROLD G. KOENIG

In this chapter, we review research that explores religiousness or spirituality as a means of reducing stress and enhancing psychological well-being in the lives of people who are infected with the human immunodeficiency virus (HIV) or have acquired immune deficiency syndrome (AIDS). We also note clinical applications and discuss avenues for future research.

The growing focus on the relationship between religion, spirituality, and health among individuals with HIV/AIDS is a timely one. When faced with a chronic physical condition or terminal illness, people have turned to religion for many reasons; researchers have a growing interest in exploring correlations among religiousness, spirituality, physical health and mental health and understanding the possible mechanisms that might explain these relationships (Ellison & Levin, 1998). Notwithstanding impressive treatment advances, HIV infection and AIDS disease progression have characteristics of both a chronic physical condition and a terminal illness; moreover, this illness has profound effects on both physical and mental health. HIV/AIDS provides a unique, albeit complex, opportunity to study how religion and/or spirituality influences individual and community responses to an epidemic. In this chapter we focus on five aspects of this role: (1) the use of religion or spirituality as a source of comfort, (2) the potential mental health and social benefits of religion/spirituality, (3) the possible physical health benefits of religion/spirituality, (4) the negative effects that religion/

spirituality can have on persons with HIV/AIDS, and (5) the types of interventions health and religious professionals can use to enhance the quality of life of people with HIV/AIDS. Before proceeding with our research review, however, we offer some background information to place this disease and its relationships with religion and spirituality in perspective.

BACKGROUND: THE AIDS EPIDEMIC

According to the UNAIDS Committee of the World Health Organization, by the end of 2000 an estimated 21.8 million men, women, and children around the world had died due to AIDS illnesses (UNAIDS/WHO, 2001). Another 36.1 million had become infected with HIV—many of whom have suffered AIDS-defining illnesses. Within the United States, the history of the Centers for Disease Control and Prevention's (CDC) surveillance of what came to be known as HIV/AIDS has been well documented (Shilts, 1987; Ward & Drotman, 1996). Twenty years ago, the rise of rare illnesses such as lymphodenopathy, pneumocystis corinii pneumonia (PCP), and Kaposi's sarcoma appearing in patients with severe unexplained immunosuppression signified the beginning of the AIDS epidemic (Centers for Disease Control [CDC], 1981; Oppenheimer, 1992). The case definition of AIDS was expanded in 1987 to include laboratory results indicating infection with HIV and/or the presence of one or more of a longer list of opportunistic infections (including cryptosporidiosis, toxoplasmotic encephalitis, persistent herpes simplex virus, wasting syndrome, dementia, and oral candidiasis). The list of AIDS-related illnesses was expanded again in 1993 to include pulmonary tuberculosis, recurrent pneumonia, and cervical cancer (CDC, 1992a, 1992b; Osmond, 1999).

CD4+ cell counts (also known as helper T-cells) were an early measurement of the severity of disease progression. Low CD4+ counts reflect a diminished capacity of the immune system to combat infection. After the 1993 case definition revision, a person could be diagnosed with AIDS if they had a CD4+ cell count below 200/mL. Subsequently, researchers and clinicians also focused on a significant measure called "viral load," the amount of HIV RNA copies in the bloodstream. By 1987, zidovudine, commonly known as AZT, was the recommended treatment for individuals with HIV; in order to reduce the amount of virus in the bloodstreams, combination antiretroviral therapies were subsequently developed that appear quite promising, though they require patients to take many medications per day with complex scheduling requirements (Chesney, Morin, & Sherr, 2000). Prior to the development of AZT and for years afterward, however, many AIDS sufferers were desperately looking for answers to this devastating illness. Anecdotal reports from friends, loved ones, and fellow sufferers about any treatment that offered hope were pursued by many AIDS patients. Some such treatments included meditation, affirmations, spiritual soul cleansings, support groups, and herbal medicine (Shilts, 1987; Gavzer, 1988; Hay, 1988). Thus many individuals pursued spiritually oriented interventions not only to enhance quality of life and find meaning in illness but also as part of treatment.

Time Course of the Disease

AIDS incidence cases and mortality have decreased in yearly statistics since 1996. The HIV clinical latency period is now estimated to last 7 to 10 years or longer, but scientists know that HIV begins attacking the immune system right away through rapid replication and destruction of CD4+ immune cells. A major goal for current treatments of HIV infection is to increase the clinical latency period before infection progresses to AIDS-related illnesses. The issues of latency period and AIDS-related illness diagnoses underscore an important point: An AIDS diagnosis represents a different disease state from HIV infection. Current clinical explanations of HIV infection see it as a progressive illness moving from an acute syndrome experienced within the first 3 weeks of seroconversion to clinical latency through middle and advanced stages of HIV disease to AIDS. As the disease progresses, the clinical manifestations include various combinations of the illnesses described previously, as well as pain, dementia, bacterial infections, and certain cancers.

Populations Affected

In the first 10 years of the AIDS crisis, gay and bisexual men were the most affected cultural population in the United States. By the end of 1991, 55% of all reported AIDS cases were attributed to men who had sex with men (CDC, 1992b). However, from July 1999 to June 2000 (the year for which the most recent statistics are available), 44% of new AIDS cases were designated to the same exposure category, demonstrating a marked decline (CDC, 2000).

Injecting drug users (IDU) are the second largest group to receive the attention of scientists and epidemiologists tracking AIDS prevalence. Since the beginning of the AIDS crisis, approximately 26% of cumulative U.S. AIDS cases among adults and adolescents have been attributed to exposures through injecting drug use (CDC, 2000). Unfortunately, through the past 20 years, IDU has remained at steady levels as an exposure category despite HIV prevention and education efforts.

Before 1992, women represented approximately 10% of all documented AIDS cases in the United States (CDC, 1992a). Gradual increases in AIDS cases have been seen among women of all ages, regardless of exposure category; the potential for infection among 13- to 24-year-old women has caused particular concern for health safety experts. Young women account for nearly half of the annual HIV infection rates over recent years (CDC, 2000).

Racial and ethnic minority groups bear a disproportionate burden of the AIDS epidemic (Washington, 1996). In particular, of overall female AIDS cases, African Americans represent nearly 57% of the cumulative total, whereas Hispanics represent 20%, and Caucasians represent 22% (CDC, 2000).

Given the profound threats and demands associated with HIV infection and AIDS, what role does religiousness or spirituality play in adjustment to the illness?

RELIGION/SPIRITUALITY AS A SOURCE OF COMFORT

In recent years, research has began to explore some of the ways in which HIV/AIDS patients turn to religious or spiritual resources in the wake of their illness (Hall, 1998; Jenkins, 1995; Schwartzberg, 1996). A life-threatening disease often intensifies spiritual or religious concerns. However, many individuals with HIV feel alienated or estranged from formal religious institutions, which often have been antagonistic toward their lifestyle or their illness (Bell, 1991; Worth, 1990). Still, religious organizations have varied widely in their response to patients afflicted with the AIDS epidemic, from bitter reproach to staunch advocacy (Crawford, Allison, Robinson, Hughes, & Samaryk, 1992; Jenkins, 1995), and individuals with HIV vary greatly in their faith. What role do religion and spirituality play for those whose lives have been disrupted by this disease?

Perreault and Perreault (1996) compared several dimensions of spirituality among 48 HIV-positive and 47 HIV-negative men. They found a significant difference between the two groups on eight of nine dimensions of the Elkins Spiritual Orientation Inventory. Those with HIV disease scored higher on transcendence, fruits of spirituality, altruism, mission in life, sacredness of life, meaning in life, awareness, and idealism. There was no difference on the ninth dimension, materialism. Although these results don't demonstrate causal relationships, they suggest that HIV disease may prompt stronger spiritual involvement, offering a sense of meaning, purpose, and existential support after infection.

Jenkins (1995) examined patterns of religious involvement and religious coping among HIV-positive U.S. military personnel. Most of the 422 participants were male (93%) and were on duty or employed; only a minority had CD4+ counts below 200/ml and qualified for a definition of AIDS. In other words, the majority faced HIV disease as a chronic illness but were not in the terminal stage of AIDS. As might be expected, relative to the general population, participants were less likely to be members of a particular religious denomination or to attend services regularly and more likely to profess personal spiritual beliefs. Nonetheless, some participants held personal spiritual beliefs while they continued their involvement in organized religious institutions.

Jenkins examined three broad styles of religious coping: a style of self-directed coping without God's help and two styles based on collaboration between self and God—collaborative/self, which emphasized the role of self in coping, and collaborative/deferral, which emphasized the role of God. Forty-one percent of participants reported using a self-directing style of coping, whereas 41.5% used a collaborative/deferral style, and 18% used a collaborative/self approach. African Americans were much more likely than Caucasians to cope using the collaborative/deferral style and much less likely to use the self-directed coping style. Moreover, the collaborative/deferral coping style was more common among participants with advanced as opposed to early-stage disease.

In addition to exploring broad styles of religious coping, Jenkins also examined more specific religious coping strategies (e.g., performance of good deeds, turning to clergy or the congregation for emotional support, pleading for a miracle, etc.). Most of these religious coping strategies were used more frequently by African Americans and by women (exceptions included pleading and expressing discontent with God). Disease stage did not seem to affect use of these coping patterns. In fact, patterns of increased reliance on religious coping among women and African Americans with HIV is consistent with other research. Overall, these findings begin to shed light on the different types of religious coping employed by HIV-infected individuals and highlight the influence of ethnicity, gender, and disease severity. Spiritual beliefs and practices were relatively common, and although many participants were ambivalent or disenchanted with organized religion, others maintained stronger ties.

PSYCHOLOGICAL AND SOCIAL BENEFITS OF RELIGION/SPIRITUALITY

Benefits for the Patient

Research has begun to examine how patients with HIV/AIDS make use of religion/spirituality to cope with the emotional stress, social isolation, and physical symptoms of their illness. Are these religious or spiritual beliefs and activities associated with better mental health, greater well-being, or greater social support?

In the investigation of HIV-positive military personnel noted above, Jenkins (1995) examined connections between religious coping strategies and psychosocial adjustment. Participants whose coping was marked by religious discontent, involving anger or alienation from God, were significantly more likely to report depressive symptoms and loneliness on standardized questionnaires.

A study by Coleman and Holzemer (1999) examined spiritual well-being among 117 predominantly lower income African Americans with HIV/AIDS. Twenty-six percent of the participants had received an AIDS diagnosis, but all participants reported substantial HIV symptoms. Psychological well-being was measured by a composite of depression, anxiety, and hope. In multivariate analyses, existential well-being—a sense of life satisfaction and purpose—was significantly associated with psychological well-being. In contrast, religious well-being, which reflects satisfaction with one's relationship with God, was not significantly related to psychological well-being. Interestingly, although 84% of participants retrospectively reported that religion was important to them before their HIV infection, many fewer (61%) indicated that religion was important after infection. The authors were unable to identify reasons for this change except to suggest that it may be due to shifting life priorities after learning of HIV infection. One wonders whether a sense of stigmatization or shame also played some role in the decreased salience of religion after infection.

Schwartzberg (1996) suggests that HIV-positive gay men with a "transformation" coping style have greater overall psychological well-being. Through extensive interviews with 19 HIV-infected men, Schwartzberg explored issues such as changes in personal sense of meaning and purpose, in self-image, and in emotional acceptance after learning of their HIV infection. The author suggested that the coping styles of these men clustered into four categories, including a "transformation" category. Several of the participants in this category referred to spiritual or religious viewpoints as helpful in coping with the disease through the creation of a new sense of purpose in their lives. One in particular, a former minister, best exemplified transformational coping through spirituality. Despite the small participant pool for this study, the findings illustrate the potential value of spirituality for creating meaning in adversity and enhancing adjustment.

Long-term survivors of AIDS (those who have had an AIDS diagnosis for more than 3 years, according to the CDC) are of particular interest to clinicians; anecdotes from these survivors suggest that hardiness, a psychological construct composed of the personality dimensions of commitment, challenge, and control, may be correlated with better health over time. Thus several studies have focused on hardiness among individuals with HIV or AIDS (e.g., Blaney et al., 1991; Carson, 1993; Farber, Schwartz, Schaper, Moonen, & McDaniel, 2000; Zich & Temoshok, 1987).

In one study, 100 HIV-positive participants completed a survey regarding spiritual activities, health practices, AIDS-related activities, and hardiness (Carson, 1993). Fifty-five percent of the participants had been diagnosed with HIV infection over the previous 2 years. The investigator wished to determine if hardiness was related to involvement in spiritual or religious activities such as prayer, meditation, visualization or imagery, reading religious literature, or attendance at congregational services or spiritual retreats. Hardiness was significantly correlated with a composite measure of all spiritual activities combined; greater hardiness was tied to more spiritual involvement. When these spiritual activities were examined independently, only prayer and meditation were positively related to hardiness. These activities, along with visualization and imagery, were used much more frequently by participants compared with the other spiritual activities.

Hardiness has received further attention from other investigators. Farber and colleagues (2000) examined the dimensions of commitment, challenge, and control as resilience factors in adaptation among 200 predominantly African American (68%) patients with symptomatic HIV disease and AIDS. The investigators found that high hardiness was significantly related to lower psychological distress levels, higher perceived quality of life, and more positive personal beliefs regarding the benevolence of the world and randomness of life events. Among the three dimensions of hardiness, commitment (a sense of meaning and purpose in life) was most consistently associated with favorable adjustment. Although religious or spiritual beliefs were not specifically examined, one would expect that they might play an important role in promoting a sense of meaning and a positive, optimistic world view.

Benefits for the Caregiver

Not only do individuals with HIV/AIDS experience great distress from their disease, but also the persons who care for them are confronted by a profound emotional burden during caregiving activities and after the death of their loved one (Schwartzberg, 1992; Folkman, Chesney, Cooke, Boccellari, & Collette, 1994; Folkman, 1997; Richards, Acree, & Folkman, 1999). These burdens are compounded if the caregivers also have HIV disease themselves. In a longitudinal project at University of California in San Francisco, Susan Folkman and her colleagues examined stress, coping, and bereavement among male partners caring for men with HIV/AIDS (Folkman et al., 1994). The project included in-depth interviews regarding the spiritual aspects of bereavement for these caregivers both at the time of loss and after 3 or 4 years had passed (Folkman, 1997; Richards & Folkman, 1997; Richards et al., 1999). The qualitative and quantitative data collected during the course of illness and after bereavement offer valuable insights into the role of spirituality in coping with this terminal illness over time.

As the project began, Folkman et al. (1994) assessed religious/spiritual beliefs and activities among 305 men involved in homosexual relationships directly affected by HIV/AIDS. The participants included two groups of caregivers of AIDS patients; one group (N = 82) included caregivers who were HIV-infected themselves, and the second group (N = 162) was composed of HIV-negative caregivers. In addition, a comparison group of 61 HIV-positive men whose partners did not have HIV infection was included. The HIV-positive caregiving group, who were confronted by their own illness, as well as that of their partners, had significantly poorer immune status, more illness symptoms, lower income, and more depression. Interestingly, they also reported higher religiosity/spirituality than the HIV-negative caregivers. Perhaps they drew on spiritual resources to help them manage their daunting circumstances. (The average score of the HIV-positive participants with healthy partners fell in between those of the other two groups.) A regression analysis was used to explore the factors that contribute to caregiving burden. As might be expected, the needs of the ill partner, the quality of the couple's relationship, and other stressful events each contributed to caregiver burden. In addition, however, HIV-positive participants who had stronger religiosity/spirituality reported less burden. This relationship was not significant for HIV-negative caregivers. Thus for those participants who faced the greatest challenges (caregivers who were HIV-positive), spirituality seemed to help lessen the burden.

As the project continued, quantitative assessments and qualitative in-depth interviews were conducted with the participants every 2 months. By the 2-year follow-up, a substantial proportion of caregivers had lost their partners to AIDS. In open-ended interviews at the time of bereavement, Richards and Folkman (1997) found that many caregivers (54%) spontaneously mentioned spiritual phenomena even though such accounts were not solicited. Several themes emerged from the interviews in which spirituality was discussed. Although not present in each interview, these themes included: easing the passage of the dying person's spirit, beliefs in spiritualism (the dying person's spirit leaves the body at death and goes on), beliefs in and/or experiences of a higher order (God's plan or an intelligence permeating life), belief that the relationship between the two men persists in some way, and use of rituals to mark the death or to celebrate life.

Qualitative analyses of the interviews were supplemented by quantitative data from questionnaires. Caregivers who referred to spirituality during their interviews turned to a number of coping strategies more frequently than those who did not mention spirituality: They made more use of positive reappraisal, planful problem solving, and confrontive coping—strategies that generally reflect adaptive engagement rather than avoidance of adverse circumstances. On the other hand, caregivers who referred to spirituality also had significantly higher depressive symptoms, higher anxiety, less positive states of mind, and more physical symptoms. The caregivers' own HIV status was not associated with discussion of spirituality. Overall, these findings hint that greater distress and a decline in the caregivers' own health may have mobilized stronger reliance on spirituality and adaptive coping, though of course the cross-sectional research design leaves questions about causality unresolved. Pointing to similar research among bereaved parents, the authors suggest that spiritual involvement may be associated with heightened distress at the time of bereavement but reduced distress in the longer term.

Seventy members of the same cohort were evaluated again 3 to 4 years later (Richards et al., 1999). Interestingly, the proportion of bereaved caregivers who spontaneously discussed spirituality during the open-ended interviews (77%) was substantially greater than it had been at the time of bereavement (54%). At this point, participants' discussions focused less on spirituality as a means of coping with the loss of their partners, and more on spirituality as an internalized sense of purpose, growth, and direction. Affiliation with a religion had little impact on whether participants discussed spiritual issues during their interviews. Forty-three percent reported no religious affiliation, yet 77% mentioned spirituality.

Once again, in quantitative analyses those who mentioned spirituality during their interviews scored more highly on coping through positive reappraisal relative to those who did not mention spiritual issues. There were no significant differences on any of the other measures in this small sample, though moderate effect sizes hinted at increased planful problem solving, decreased behavioral escape/avoidance, increased optimism, decreased anxiety, and increased physical symptoms among more spiritual individuals.

When reviewed in combination, this series of studies, stemming from one longitudinal research program, suggests that spirituality is concurrently associated with adaptive coping and reduced burden for caregivers, particularly those who are also ill. Participants also reported that spiritual involvement provided a sense of comfort and meaning in dealing with bereavement. Unfortunately, no prospective analyses were reported (in which spirituality at one point is used to predict outcomes at another), and the data do not demonstrate that spiritual involvement leads to reduced distress or illness symptoms over time. These relationships are complex. Whether spirituality is associated with long-term changes in illness-related distress for some individuals awaits further investigation.

PHYSICAL HEALTH BENEFITS
OF RELIGION/SPIRITUALITY

If there are psychosocial benefits associated with religious or spiritual faith for some patients with HIV, do these translate into better physical health, slowed disease progression, or increased survival? There is growing evidence that psychological stress, social isolation, and depression are associated with neuroendocrine and immunological changes (Rabin, 1999) that, at least theoretically, could affect the course of HIV/AIDS, given the enormous role that the immune system plays in this disease.

Some studies suggest that factors that reduce psychological stress and increase social support may affect the course of HIV infection through immunological mechanisms. Ironson and colleagues (1990) conducted a prospective study of HIV-positive and HIV-negative men, examining psychological functioning and immune responses. As anticipated, men testing positive reported significantly more acute anxiety and traumatic stress; more provocatively, there was also a significant inverse correlation between self-reported anxiety and natural killer (NK) cell activity. Evans et al. (1997) examined 93 HIV-positive homosexual men, all without clinical symptoms at study entry. Physical examinations and comprehensive interviews were conducted at 6-month intervals for 42 months; these evaluations included assessment of stressful life events that had occurred between examinations (omitting HIV-related stresses). Those with high life stress ($N = 38$) had a significantly greater risk of early HIV disease progression compared with those with low life stress ($N = 55$, $RR = 2.0$). In other words, the risk of disease progression doubled for each stressful life event per 6-month study interval. Interestingly, depression was unrelated to disease progression.

Religious or spiritual activities may affect the course of HIV disease through similar mechanisms, although this area is only beginning to be explored. For example, Woods, Antoni, Ironson, and Kling (1999) surveyed 106 HIV-positive gay men to determine if religiosity (measured as either religious activities or religious coping) is associated with less depression or better immune function in this population. Religious activities, such as prayer, religious attendance, spiritual discussions, and reading religious/spiritual literature, were associated with significantly higher CD4+ counts and CD4+ percentages (T-helper-inducer cells). The investigators were careful to ensure that this association was *not* due to participants becoming unable to participate in religious activity as their disease worsened and immune function decreased. Religious coping (putting trust in God, seeking God's help, increasing prayer, etc.) was related to lower Beck Depression Inventory scores and lower Spielberger Trait Anxiety Inventory scores, but not to specific immune markers. One possible explanation for the latter finding might be that participants with more severe disease turned to religion for comfort, disguising any cross-sectional association between religious coping and better immune function. Additional research would help clarify whether spiritual or religious involvement influences immune status or disease progression among individuals with different levels of disease severity.

PRAYER, MEDITATION,
AND OTHER SPIRITUAL ACTIVITIES

As indicated previously, many early sufferers of AIDS searched far and wide for treatments, cures, and coping mechanisms to deal with the physical and emotional onslaughts associated with immunological impairment, especially in the absence of any standard treatment before the FDA's 1987 approval of zidovudine (also known as AZT) (Shilts, 1987; Abrams, 1996). The holistic and alternative health care that AIDS patients could receive outside the United States gained considerable attention from rumors and stories about Rock Hudson after information about his condition was released to the public (Shilts, 1987). Some patients continue to turn to spiritual tools such as prayer, meditation, or affirmation to enhance their overall health (Hay, 1988; Carson, 1993).

Very few investigations have examined the potential impact of these activities on disease endpoints. Recently, one intervention study suggested a possible effect of spiritual practices on health outcomes. Researchers reported a randomized, double-blind study of the effects of distant healing on the health outcomes of 40 patients with advanced AIDS (Sicher, Targ, Moore, & Smith, 1998). Distant healing, defined as "a conscious, dedicated act of mentation attempting to benefit another person's physical or emotional well-being," includes prayer and forms of psychic healing on behalf of the patient (Sicher et al., 1998, p. 356). Participants were unaware of whether or not they had been randomized to the group that was being prayed for. The investigators documented significant improvement among patients who received the distant healing intervention compared with control patients. At 6 months after treatment, the treated group had a lower number of outpatient visits, fewer hospitalizations, fewer AIDS-defining illnesses acquired, and less illness severity. Not surprisingly, this line of investigation is controversial, and further research is needed to substantiate these findings. However, the results seem particularly interesting in light of the mixed, sometimes negative, response to the AIDS epidemic among some religious/spiritual communities.

NEGATIVE PERCEPTIONS OR EXPERIENCES
OF RELIGION/SPIRITUALITY

In contrast to the idea that religion or spirituality may help those with HIV/ AIDS, some believe that divine retribution, for homosexuality in particular, *caused* the AIDS crisis in the United States (Chilton, 1987). Because gay men and intravenous drug users were the first populations to enter societal awareness as AIDS sufferers, this disease has never escaped the moral judgments made by some about its origins or its sufferers. Researchers have reported that many patients encounter stigmatizing experiences among religious congregations because of such attitudes (Fortunato, 1987; Schwartzberg, 1996; Shilts, 1987).

There are numerous ways in which religious/spiritual beliefs and actions can have a negative impact on people with HIV/AIDS. Some experiences are based on self-induced fears and expectations, and others involve stigmatizing interactions with people who use a judgmental religious framework or show fear of the person with HIV/AIDS. Such fears or stigmatizing experiences can lead to higher levels of anxiety, depression, or isolation through two possible emotional responses: (1) an increased sense of alienation and/or (2) an increased sense of guilt or punishment.

Increased Alienation

HIV-positive individuals may feel alienated from public worship as a result of expressed, or even expected, moral condemnation from others. Some have experienced moral judgment pronounced upon them by congregational leaders or members. Others have avoided organized religion due to fears of the judgment and derision they could face if they attended church (Schaefer & Coleman, 1992). Hall (1998) conducted in-depth, directed interviews with 10 people living with advanced HIV disease who discussed spiritual beliefs and experiences that helped them to cope with their illness. Her concluding statement aptly captures how stigmatization from religious organizations can block the potential benefits some receive through spirituality:

> For most of the participants, organized religion acted as a barrier to attaining spirituality until their anger was ameliorated, first by discernment that the beliefs of the religions that labeled and persecuted them were in themselves flawed by their absence of caring and authenticity, and second when they discovered what were for them more valid and cogent spiritual ideas. (Hall, 1998, p. 152)

An Increased Sense of Guilt or Punishment

Some patients view their disease as a punishment for their behaviors, whether visited upon them by divine will or as a result of "indulgences," leading to considerable guilt and self-condemnation (Hall, 1994, 1998; Schwartzberg, 1992, 1996). The diagnosis of HIV is often associated with embarrassment and shame. According to Barbee, Verlega, Sherburne, and Grimshaw (1999), how patients contract the virus greatly influences their perceptions of the types of support they receive from others. Negative self-perceptions and feared judgment about the route of transmission may influence whether an individual with HIV disease turns for help to religious leaders, members of the congregation, or even a transcendent Higher Power.

INTERVENTIONS BY HEALTH
AND RELIGIOUS PROFESSIONALS

Ultimately, the arenas of clinical care and spiritual services overlap as health providers, and AIDS social service agencies often must respond to the spiritual distress expressed by AIDS patients. Sometimes service providers offer referrals to spiritual or religious resources; on other occasions they provide much more (Belcher, Dettmore, & Holzemer, 1989). Nurses are often encouraged to listen to patients' spiritual or religious concerns and in some cases to advocate for nonstandard health care options (Sowell, Lowenstein, & Spicer, 1996). Some writers view this advocacy role as part of a holistic health care perspective that includes addressing spiritual as well as medical distress (Belcher et al., 1989). An obstacle to this type of spiritual support is the homophobia and fear of occupational HIV exposure that some health professionals harbor, which can create difficulties in developing positive clinician–patient relationships and compound the stigma and discrimination that AIDS patients encounter in the broader society (Mackareth, 1995).

Rather than addressing spiritual distress themselves, most social service agencies refer patients to a church, temple, or spiritual center to assist with the many psychospiritual issues surrounding a chronic or terminal illness. Aside from offering spiritual support, these resources may also provide social support, educational prevention programs, or other outreach services. Many churches offer compassionate ministry programs for individuals with HIV/AIDS, which may include financial assistance, visits from volunteers, support groups, and educational programs (Washington, 1996). These ministries have taken various forms, including:

- Regional AIDS Interfaith Networks that link area churches together to share resources, experiences, and opportunities for training volunteers
- Nonprofit organizations such as Balm in the Gilead, Inc., a national organization based in New York City that works through black churches to stop the spread of HIV and to support HIV-infected individuals and the African American community.
- Individual congregational ministries.
- Books and training manuals to help congregations create an AIDS ministry (including several published by the Balm in the Gilead's Black Church National HIV/AIDS Technical Assistance Center; Sunderland, 1987; Weatherford & Weatherford, 1999).

Some community efforts have integrated HIV prevention with Buddhist theological concepts in order to tailor the message to Southeast Asian communities in the United States; the temple is used as an educational forum for HIV prevention discussions (Loue, Lane, Lloyd, & Loh, 1991). Although there may be superb benefits from any of these programs and proposals, as yet most of them have not been researched to verify their efficacy.

SUMMARY AND CONCLUSIONS

Although interest in this area is growing, relationships between religion, spirituality, and health among individuals with HIV disease are complex and poorly understood. Seropositive individuals, family, friends, and caregivers search for meaning and purpose within, or as a result of, the suffering they experience. As Victor Frankl (1963) pointed out, this search for meaning is an important aspect of human growth and adaptation in response to adversity. Like those affected by other serious illnesses, some people afflicted by HIV/AIDS are drawn toward a spiritual or religious framework in which to make sense of the disease, their losses and expectations, and the meaning of their lives (Koenig, McCullough, & Larson, 2000; Pargament, 1997; Richards et al., 1999). Others may employ religious or spiritual forms of coping as a means of finding emotional comfort and alleviating the stresses of illness, discrimination, financial hardship, and inadequate support services.

It is among HIV/AIDS communities, in particular, that a division can appear between religion and spirituality. For years, many religious organizations shunned or ignored the plight of HIV-infected individuals or argued that this was a moral punishment for sexual or drug-use behaviors. In response to the moral stigma and alienation they experienced from families, friends, and fellow congregation members, many infected gay and bisexual men, for example, turned away from the religions of their childhood or from organizationally supported worship in general. Yet, as this chapter makes clear, spirituality remains quite important for many individuals with HIV disease, and some retain strong ties to organized religion. Research in this area has only begun to clarify the role of spirituality and religion in the lives of those with HIV or AIDS.

Avenues for Future Research

Most of the research reviewed here does not distinctly differentiate between religion and spirituality; nor does it always distinguish between those infected with HIV without presenting illnesses and those with "full-blown"

AIDS. However, relationships between faith and health among HIV-infected persons are bound to depend in part on differences in their disease status, social and cultural communities, relationships with religion, world views, and spiritual histories. For example, religious/spiritual beliefs and practices for African American or Hispanic women are bound to differ from those of gay or bisexual white men. Relationships between faith and health, and the mechanisms underlying these relationships, are apt to differ as well. It would be important for future research in this area to carefully account for these contextual and medical variables. An additional shortcoming in the literature is the limited number of longitudinal studies concerning relationships between religion and/or spirituality and health outcomes for AIDS patients. Additional longitudinal investigations are clearly needed. However, lack of standardized medical definitions and treatments over time make these studies difficult to conduct. For example, the AIDS-related complex referred to in early studies (e.g., Carson, 1993) is no longer a clinical term. The changing clinical vocabulary offers a challenge in reviewing literature from more than 5 years ago, and the recent introduction of new treatment regimens could alter possible conclusions from longitudinal data.

Thus there are many gaps in our current knowledge. We present a few important researchable questions:

- How do religious/spiritual activities and beliefs affect immune function?
- Among those for whom the current multidrug treatment regimens do not work, how does incorporation of religion or spirituality affect quality of life and survival?
- How do spiritual or religious resources affect quality of life or disease endpoints among individuals from different age groups and different cultures and genders?
- How do religious or spiritual concerns differ now from those of 10 to 15 years ago for HIV-infected individuals (e.g., does present knowledge about AIDS alter one's spiritual outlook compared with the days when comparatively little was known?)
- How does neurological impairment associated with AIDS limit the use of religious/spiritual activities as a cognitive coping strategy or source of meaning? Do other aspects of spiritual involvement (e.g., social support, emotional comfort) become more important?
- Does the experience of being a long-term survivor of AIDS lead to changes in an individual's religious or spiritual world view?

Exploring the connections between faith and health in the context of this disease offers exciting opportunities for further research.

ACKNOWLEDGMENT

Support for this chapter was provided by the John Templeton Foundation, Radnor, Pennsylvania.

REFERENCES

Abrams, D. I. (1996). Alternative therapies. In G. P. Wormser (Ed.), *A clinical guide to AIDS and HIV* (pp. 379–396). Philadelphia, PA: Lippincott-Raven.

Barbee, A. P., Verlega, V. J., Sherburne, S. P., & Grimshaw, A. (1999). Helpful and unhelpful forms of social support for HIV-positive individuals. In V. J. Verlega & A. P. Barbee (Eds.), *HIV and social interaction* (pp. 83–105). Thousand Oaks, CA: Sage.

Belcher, A. E., Dettmore, D., & Holzemer, S. P. (1989). Spirituality and sense of well-being in persons with AIDS. *Holistic Nursing Practice, 3*, 16–25.

Bell, N. K. (1991). Social/sexual norms and AIDS in the South. *AIDS Education and Prevention, 3*, 164–180.

Blaney, N. T., Goodkin, K., Morgan, R. O., Feaster, D., Millon, C., Szapocznik, J., & Eisdorfer, C. (1991). A stress-moderator model of distress in early HIV-1 infection: Concurrent analysis of life events, hardiness, and social support. *Journal of Psychosomatic Research, 35*, 297–305.

Carson, V. B. (1993). Prayer, meditation, exercise, and special diets: Behaviors of the hardy person with HIV/AIDS. *Journal of the Association of Nurses in AIDS Care, 4*,18–28.

Centers for Disease Control. (1981, July 4). Kaposi's sarcoma and *Pneumocystis carinii* pneumonia among homosexual men: New York City and California. *Mortality and Morbidity Weekly Report, 30*, 305–308.

Centers for Disease Control. (1992a, January 17). The second 100,000 cases of acquired immune deficiency syndrome: United States, 1981–December 1991. *Mortality and Morbidity Weekly Report, 41*, 28–29.

Centers for Disease Control. (1992b, January 17). 1993 revised classification for HIV infection and expanded surveillance case definition for AIDS among adolescents and adults. *Mortality and Morbidity Weekly Report, 41*, 1–19.

Centers for Disease Control and Prevention. (2000). *HIV/AIDS Surveillance Report: Mid-Year Edition, 12*(1), 1–41.

Chesney, M. A., Morin, M., & Sherr, L. (2000). Adherence to HIV combination therapy. *Social Sciences and Medicine, 50*, 1599–1605.

Chilton, D. (1987). *Power in the blood: A Christian response to AIDS*. Brentwood, TN: Wolgemuth & Hyatt.

Coleman, C. L., & Holzemer, W. L. (1999). Spirituality, psychological well-being, and HIV symptoms for African Americans living with HIV disease. *Journal for the Association of Nurses in AIDS Care, 10*, 42–50.

Crawford, I., Allison, K. W., Robinson, W. L., Hughes, D., & Samaryk, M. (1992). Attitudes of African-American Baptist ministers towards AIDS. *Journal of Community Psychology, 20*, 304–308.

Ellison, C. G., & Levin, J. S. (1998). The religion–health connection: Evidence, theory, and future directions. *Health Education and Behavior, 25,* 700–720.

Evans, D. L., Leserman, J., Perkins, D. O., Stern, R. A., Murphy, C., Zheng, B., Gettes, D., Longmate, J. A., Silva, S. G., van der Horst, C. M., Hall, C. D., Folds, J. D., Golden, R. N., & Petitto, J. M. (1997). Severe life stress as a predictor of early disease progression in HIV infection. *American Journal of Psychiatry, 154,* 630–634.

Farber, E. W., Schwartz, J. A. J., Schaper, P. E., Moonen, D. J., & McDaniel, J. S. (2000). Resilience factors associated with adaptation to HIV disease. *Psychosomatics, 41,* 140–146.

Folkman, S. (1997). Positive psychological states and coping with severe stress. *Social Science and Medicine, 45,* 1207–1221.

Folkman, S., Chesney, M. A., Cooke, M., Boccellari, A., & Collette, L. (1994). Caregiver burden in HIV-positive and HIV-negative partners of men with AIDS. *Journal of Consulting and Clinical Psychology, 62,* 746–756.

Fortunato, J. (1987). *AIDS: The spiritual dilemma.* San Francisco, CA: Harper & Row.

Frankl, V. (1962). *Man's search for meaning: An introduction to logotherapy* (I. Lasch, Trans.). New York: Simon & Schuster.

Gavzer, B. (1988, September 18). Why some people survive AIDS. *Parade,* 4–7.

Hall, B. A. (1994). Ways of maintaining hope in HIV disease. *Research in Nursing and Health,* 17, 283–293.

Hall, B. A. (1998). Patterns of spirituality in persons with advanced HIV disease. *Research in Nursing and Health, 21,* 143–153.

Hay, L. (1988). *The AIDS book: Creating a positive approach.* Santa Monica, CA: Hay House.

Ironson, G., LaPerrier, A., Antoni, M., O'Hearn, P., Schneiderman, N., Klimas, N., & Fletcher, M. A. (1990). Changes in immune and psychological measures as a function of anticipation and reaction to news of HIV-A antibody status. *Psychosomatic Medicine, 52,* 247–270.

Jenkins, R. (1995). Religion and HIV: Implications for research and intervention. *Journal of Social Issues, 51,* 131–144.

Koenig, H. G., McCullough, M. E., & Larson, D. B. (2000). *Religion and health: A century of research reviewed.* New York: Oxford University Press.

Loue, S., Lane, S. D., Lloyd, L. S., & Loh, L. (1999). Integrating Buddhism and HIV prevention in US Southeast Asian communities. *Journal of Health Care for the Poor and Underserved, 10,* 100–121.

Mackareth, P. A. (1995). HIV and homophobia: Nurses as advocates. *Journal of Advanced Nursing, 22,* 670–676.

Oppenheimer, G. M. (1992). Causes, cases, and cohorts: The role of epidemiology in the historical construction of AIDS. In E. Fee & D. M. Fox (Eds.), *AIDS: The making of a chronic disease* (pp. 49–83). Berkeley: University of California Press.

Osmond, D. H. (1999). Classification, staging, and surveillance of HIV. In P. T. Cohen, M. A. Sande, & P. A. Volberding (Eds.), *The AIDS knowledge base: A textbook on HIV disease from the University of California, San Francisco and San Francisco General Hospital* (3rd ed., pp. 3–12). Philadelphia, PA: Lippincott, Williams & Wilkins.

Pargament, K. I. (1997). *The psychology of religion and coping: Theory, research, practice.* New York: Guilford Press.

Perreault, L. T., & Perreault, M. (1996, July 7–12). A comparative study on the spirituality of men living with and without HIV/AIDS. *International Conference Abstracts on AIDS, 11*(1), 404.

Rabin, B. S. (1999). *Stress, immune function, and health: The connection.* New York: Wiley-Liss.

Richards, T. A., Acree, M., & Folkman, S. (1999). Spiritual aspects of loss among partners of men with AIDS: Post bereavement follow-up. *Death Studies, 23,* 105–127.

Richards, T. A., & Folkman, S. (1997). Spiritual aspects of loss at the time of a partner's death from AIDS. *Death Studies, 21,* 527–552.

Schaefer, S., & Coleman, E. (1992). Shifts in meaning, purpose, and values following a diagnosis of HIV infection among gay men. *Journal of Psychology and Human Sexuality, 5,* 13–29.

Schwartzberg, S. (1992). AIDS-related bereavement among gay men: The inadequacy of current theories of grief. *Psychotherapy, 29,* 422–429.

Schwartzberg, S. (1996). *A crisis of meaning: How gay men are making sense of AIDS.* New York: Oxford University Press.

Shilts, R. (1987). *And the band played on: Politics, people, and the AIDS epidemic.* New York: St. Martin's Press.

Sicher, F., Targ, E., Moore, D., & Smith, H. S. (1998). A randomized, double-blind study of the effect of distant healing in a population with advanced AIDS. *Western Journal of Medicine, 169,* 356–363.

Sowell, R. L., Lowenstein, A. J., & Spicer, T. (1996). Nursing perspectives in the care of patients with HIV infection. In G. P. Wormser (Ed.), *A clinical guide to AIDS and HIV* (pp. 379–396). Philadelphia: Lippincott-Raven.

Sunderland, R. (1987). *AIDS: A manual for pastoral care.* Philadelphia: Westminster Press.

UNAIDS/WHO. (2001). Global AIDS statistics. *AIDS Care, 13,* 263–272.

Ward, J. W., & Drotman, D. P. (1996). The epidemiology of HIV and AIDS. In G. P. Wormser (Ed.), *A clinical guide to AIDS and HIV* (pp. 1–19). Philadelphia: Lippincott-Raven.

Washington, H. (1996, Spring–Summer). HIV among African Americans. *Harvard AIDS Review* [On-line]. Available: http://www.hsph.harvard.edu/hai/publications/HAR_Archive/special96-2.html/

Weatherford, R. J., & Weatherford, C. B. (1999). *Somebody's knocking at your door: AIDS and the African-American Church.* New York: Haworth Press.

Woods, T. E., Antoni, M. H., Ironson, G. H., & Kling, D. W. (1999). Religiosity is associated with affective and immune status in symptomatic HIV-infected gay men. *Journal of Psychosomatic Research, 46,* 165–176.

Worth, D. (1990). Minority women and AIDS: Culture, race, and gender. In D. A. Feldman (Ed.), *Culture and AIDS* (pp. 111–135). New York: Praeger.

Zich, J., & Temoshok, L. (1987). Perceptions of social support in men with AIDS and ARC: Relationships with distress and hardiness. *Journal of Applied Social Psychology, 17,* 193–215.

9

◄○►

TOBACCO AND ALCOHOL USE AMONG YOUNG ADULTS

Exploring Religious Faith,
Locus of Health Control,
and Coping Strategies as Predictors

A. SANDRA WILLIS
KENNETH A. WALLSTON
KAMAU R. S. JOHNSON

Discovering the predictors of tobacco and alcohol use is an important stage in understanding, preventing, and modifying health-compromising behavior of adolescents and young adults. The health attitudes and behaviors of college students, who are in transition between adolescence and adulthood, have enormous impact on later quality of life. Health promotion and prevention programs target this population to prevent the adoption of health-compromising behaviors that may lead to chronic disease later in life. The purpose of this chapter is to examine individual differences in religiosity, perceived control over health, and coping factors that place young adults at risk for initiating and regularly using tobacco and alcohol. In doing so, we may gain insight into psychosocial factors that may have protective value.

Prevalence statistics from the Monitoring the Future study (Johnston, 1996) showed that 39.3% of college students had smoked in the past year, 26.9% in the past month. Statistics are similar for young adults of the same age who do not attend college. Sixty-two million people in the United States

(29% of the population aged 12 and older) use tobacco. According to the National Center for Health Statistics (Centers for Disease Control and Prevention [CDC], 1998), 43% of men 18 and older and 33% of women above the age of 18 smoke. Although adult smoking has declined sharply over the last quarter century, especially among educated people, smoking has made a partial comeback (1990–1996) among high school seniors (Johnston, 1996). Sax (1997) found that the incidence of smoking among college freshmen nationwide increased over a 30-year period. In a Virginia college sample, white females with lower grade point averages and low life satisfaction have emerged as the most frequent users of tobacco among the different gender and ethnic groups (Schorling, Gutgesell, Klas & Smith, 1994). Cigarette smoking, compared with other types of substance use, showed the least decline from adolescent initiation to usage in young adulthood (Bachman, Wadsworth, O'Malley, Johnston, & Schulenberg, 1997).

Fifty-one percent of Americans aged 12 and above admitted to drinking alcohol in the previous month. Of these, 15% binged (five or more drinks in a short period of time) at least once in the previous month (CDC, 1998). Though several researchers (see Prendergast, 1994, for review) report a 9–12% decline in heavy drinking (use of more than one ounce of alcohol per day during the past 30 days) within adolescent and young adult populations between 1980 and 1992, some report that college students showed less than a 1% decline (Johnston, O'Malley, & Bachman, 1993) and that the percentage of heavy drinkers among college students remained constant at 20% (Engs & Hanson, 1988).

Although they have higher levels of education, usually associated with more readily adopting health-enhancing behaviors, college students show high levels of alcohol use. They do, however, show a lower prevalence of smoking behaviors, are less likely to be overweight, and more likely to use seat belts than young adults not enrolled in college. Social norms that support alcohol use on and in proximity to college campuses still exist (Wechsler & Issac, 1991). Concern associated with excessive alcohol use is based on problems with immediate consequences and development of long-term patterns of alcohol use. Globetti, Stem, Morasco, and Haworth-Hoeppner (1988) review studies of college students and report percentage ranges for the following alcohol-related problems: drinking and driving, 33–41%; destruction of property, 6–7%; loss of friends, 7–8%; academic problems, 17–23%; problems with authorities, 3–15%; and student judiciary problems, 20–60%. Kim, Larimer, Walker, and Marlatt (1997) discovered more frequent use of tobacco and other drugs and more frequent sexual activity among heavy drinkers in college as compared with students who were abstinent or light to moderate alcohol consumers; however, no associations were found for heavy drinking and psychological health.

This chapter considers the role of religious/spiritual beliefs, perceptions of control over health, and coping mechanisms that may confer protection to older adolescents and young adults faced with choices concerning smoking and drinking. We offer a brief review of past research on religiousness and substance use among adolescents and young adults in the first section. The second section of the chapter reviews research concerning health and perceived control and religious and nonreligious coping strategies. We discuss new questions relevant to previous research and propose a conceptual model to explain how the effects of religiosity on health may be mediated by various dimensions of health locus of control and coping. In an attempt to begin to answer the questions posed, the third section reports research from the Health Beliefs and Behaviors Study (HBBS; Willis et al., 1999; Willis, 1999, 2000) of tobacco and alcohol use behaviors in a religiously and geographically diverse sample of black and white college students between the ages of 16 and 23. Subsequent sections include a discussion of the HBBS findings, support for the proposed model, and resultant evidence for risk and protective factors. The chapter concludes by examining the application of religion/spirituality to health promotion and intervention programs designed for adolescents and young adults.

FACTORS INFLUENCING TOBACCO AND ALCOHOL USE IN YOUNG PEOPLE

Religiosity

The effects of religious beliefs and involvement on the physical and mental well-being and coping strategies of elderly adults have been relatively well researched (Koenig, George, & Siegler, 1988; Langer & Rodin, 1976; Levin, 1994). More recently, attention has been focused on the effects of religious factors in the lives of adolescents and their impact on decision-making processes involved in engaging in the potentially health-compromising behaviors of tobacco and alcohol use. In a review of research on religion and health-compromising behaviors, Wallace and Williams (1997) report that studies on adolescent health show inverse relationships between religion and both sexual involvement and drug use; however, most researchers have not included religiosity as a focal variable when exploring factors associated with risk and protection and have viewed it primarily as a form of social control against delinquency or deviance.

Recent studies have explored religiosity as a potential protective factor. Dryfoos (1990) and Hawkins, Catalano, and Miller (1992) identified lack of religiosity or low religiosity as a risk factor for adolescent problem behaviors. Yarnold (1998) reported that religion was unrelated to alcohol use, whereas other researchers (e.g., Kunz & Giesbrecht, 1999; Patlock-

Peckham, Hutchinson, Cheong, & Nagoshi, 1998; Perkins, 1987) have found significant associations. In the Patlock-Peckham et al. (1998) study, college students with no religious affiliation used alcohol more often and in greater quantity than did Protestants or Catholics. Two-thirds of a national sample of college students (Hanson & Engs, 1986) reported using alcohol, whereas 90% of those who deemed religion unimportant used alcohol. Foshee and Hollinger (1996) report that maternal religiosity and religious attendance (more so than religious importance) is negatively related to alcohol use in young adolescents (aged 12–14). Pullen, Modrcin-Talbott, West, and Muenchen (1999) examined church attendance and drug use in adolescents ranging from 12 to 19 years of age. Their findings indicated that as frequency of church attendance increased, alcohol and other substance use decreased. Similar results have also been found in a study of religious attitudes, belief in God, and church attendance among 1,500 students in the Netherlands (Mullen & Francis, 1995).

Social support, a salient part of religious involvement, also emerges as a protective factor in the form of connectedness to family and school community. Resnick et al. (1997) reported that parent–family connectedness, perceived school connectedness, and parental expectations of school achievement were associated with lower levels of risky behaviors. Additional research found an inverse relationship between health-compromising behaviors and protective factors such as stronger emotional well-being, higher self-esteem, school connectedness and achievement, family connectedness, and more conventional family structure, as well as religiosity (Neumark-Sztainer, Story, French, & Resnick, 1997). Hardesty and Kirby (1995) examined 475 students who had disciplinary problems and/or who had dropped out of high school and were presumed to be at higher risk for substance abuse. Students from actively religious families, who attended church services, prayed, and observed religious holidays, were less likely to use drugs and more likely to choose drug-abstinent friends. This positive relationship remained when controlling for the family climate (family cohesion, expressiveness, and conflict). The investigators contend that their results are encouraging given the strong influence that peer pressure may have on initiating and maintaining substance use in this age group. Gorsuch (1995) reported that nurturing and supportive religious experiences are associated with decreased substance use, whereas religiosity characterized by restrictiveness, harshness, and punishment may be associated with substance abuse.

Perceived Control of Health

Individuals' perceived control over their health has been examined extensively to discover the nature and extent of its relationship to health knowledge, health behavior, and health status. Given the influence of conformity to peer norms for substance use behavior among adolescents and young adults, perceived control over health status is a relevant factor to investigate. Wallston, Wallston, and DeVellis (1978) developed the Multidimensional Health Locus of Control (MHLC) scale to measure three loci of control over one's health: internal, chance, and powerful others. Internality refers to the belief that a person's own behaviors influence his or her health status. Powerful others, in this schema, refer to health professionals, such as physicians, nurses, or therapists, but also encompass friends, co-workers, and family members. Those with a chance health locus of control orientation do not see their health status as controllable; rather, they believe their health status is determined by random factors such as fate, luck, or chance (Wallston et al., 1978).

Many researchers have found correlations between the MHLC scales and health practices. Bennett, Norman, Moore, Murphy, and Tudor-Smith (1997), using a random sample of Welsh adults, found some support for the Wallstons' health locus of control model as related to smoking behavior: Smokers held higher internal, chance, and powerful others beliefs than those who never smoked, though chance locus alone emerged as a significant predictor of smoking frequency. Lemos-Giráldez and Fidalgo-Aliste (1997) found that the MHLC scale was not an adequate predictor of health-related behaviors and attitudes in college students. However, several other studies (Chassin, Presson, Pitts, & Sherman, 2000; Eiser, Eiser, Gammage, & Morgan, 1989) found a significant negative relationship between smoking and internal locus of control in adolescents.

In the past, the MHLC scales assessed only three loci of health control—internality, powerful others, and chance. Welton, Adkins, Ingle, and Dixon (1996) hypothesized that beliefs in God control constituted a fourth dimension. They developed scales to assess God control in general, as well as God control over health, and administered their measures to two samples of college students, along with a measure of health habits and lifestyles. Both the general internal and general God control scales predicted a composite of measures of health habits, but only in one of their two samples did they find that health control beliefs predicted health habits (Welton et al., 1996). Interestingly, it was the God control of health subscale that was predictive in that instance. Coincidentally, unaware of the work by Welton et al., Wallston and his colleagues (1999) had developed their own version of a God locus of health control scale and had been using it in a longitudinal study of persons with rheumatoid arthritis. Those participants were considerably older and less healthy than the college students studied by Welton et al. (1996). Later in this chapter, we present data relating the God control scale developed by Wallston to health behaviors of college students. It is possible that part of the reason for the inconsistent findings relating MHLC scores to health behaviors is that the path from health beliefs (such as those assessed by the MHLC) to health behaviors is mediated by a variety of coping strategies that the participants use when confronted with health-related stressors. Thus we turn now to a discussion of coping strategies and the role they may play in determining specific health behaviors.

Religious and Nonreligious Coping Strategies

A variety of coping strategies used by adolescents may influence their engagement in risky behavior. Individuals of all ages have long claimed that relief from stress is one of their motivations for smoking and drinking. Research on coping strategies has yielded two general categories of coping: problem-focused, used to alter the source of stress when an individual believes that a constructive solution exists, and emotion-focused, used to reduce distress associated with a problem that an individual believes will be enduring (Carver, Scheier, & Weintraub, 1989; Folkman & Lazarus, 1980). Carver et al. (1989; Carver, 1997) developed a tool called the COPE Inventory as an assessment for several distinctive aspects of both problem-focused and emotion-focused strategies.

In general, research evidence supports the idea that problem-focused coping tends to be more adaptive in the long run than emotion-focused coping (McCrae & Costa, 1986; Rippetoe & Rogers, 1987), though individual and situational differences should be taken into account (Lehman, Ellard, & Wortman, 1986). Problem-focused strategies attempt to remove or reduce the effects of a stressor. These mechanisms include active coping (executing direct action), planning (thinking of a plan for an active strategy after appraising the stressor), and seeking instrumental support (requesting information or assistance in solving the problem). Emotion-focused coping strategies include seeking emotional support (looking for emotional comfort and understanding), venting (releasing emotions related to the stressor), reframing (appraising the stressor in a more positive light), and humor (making jokes about the stressor). Acceptance (awareness of the reality of the stressor) and denial (refusing to accept the reality of the stressor) may represent two ends of the same coping dimension. Using self-blame, some individuals tend to criticize themselves as a response to stress. Behavioral disengagement (reducing efforts or giving up attempts to deal with the stressor), self-distraction (using cognitive tactics to mentally disengage from the stressor), and substance use are also considered to be less adaptive emotion-focused strategies (Carver et al., 1989).

Turning to religion for support is also categorized as an emotion-focused coping mechanism. One of the subscales of the COPE assesses this construct. To distinguish types of religious coping, Boudreaux, Catz, Ryan,

Amaral-Melendez, and Brantley (1995) designed a scale to measure external/social religious coping, focused on social support within the religious community, and internal/private religious coping, emphasizing coping through one's personal relationship with God.

Most research on religious coping strategies of adolescents and young adults has focused on the study of well-being, adjustment-related factors, and stress (Maton, 1989; Park, Cohen, & Herb, 1990). Maton (1989) found that spiritual support, defined as "the perceived, personally supportive components of an individual's relationship with God," was positively related to college adjustment in freshmen undergoing high stress but that spiritual support was not related to well-being in students encountering low levels of stress. Researchers have investigated the use of substances as a method of coping with stress (e.g., Cooper, Russell, Skinner, & Windle, 1992). McKee, Hinson, Wall, and Spriel (1998), as well as Williams and Clark (1998), have found substance use as a coping strategy to be predictive of frequency of alcohol use. Use of substances may sometimes function as an avoidant coping strategy, along with denial and behavioral disengagement. MacLean, Lecci, and Croteau (1999) report that substance use, denial, and "partying" were strongly predictive of alcohol-related problems.

Emotion-focused and avoidance coping strategies have been found to predict alcohol use (Karwacki & Bradley, 1996; McCreary & Sadava, 1998). In other studies (Evans & Dunn, 1995; Simpson & Arroyo, 1998; Windle & Windle, 1996), avoidance coping was associated with alcohol-related problems but not with quantity or frequency of alcohol consumption. Protective strategies include religious coping by females and males (MacLean et al., 1999), religious coping by females and suppression of competing activities by males (McKee et al., 1998), and problem-solving coping (McCreary & Sadava, 1998). However, several studies have failed to support any coping strategy as a predictor of not using substances (Evans & Dunn, 1995; Karwacki & Bradley, 1996; Williams & Clark, 1998).

WHY ARE RELIGIOUS/SPIRITUAL BELIEFS ASSOCIATED WITH REDUCED ALCOHOL AND TOBACCO USE?

Evidence from the majority of studies reviewed supports religiosity as conferring a salutary effect on adolescents and young adults. If religious faith and involvement are negatively related to adoption of tobacco and alcohol use, how can we explain these effects? Religiosity may act as a protective factor by offering contextual coping mechanisms, for example, positive reframing or seeking emotional and instrumental support. Do youth strong in faith use more adaptive coping mechanisms than nonreligious youth, for example, active, problem-solving strategies as opposed to venting, denial, and disengagement?

Religious/spiritual beliefs within an organized system may provide protection by offering contextual coping mechanisms, but it is likely that other mediating factors are operating as well. Is strong faith associated with the perception that God's omnipotence includes control over health? Are religious youth more likely to place the control of their health in God's hands? If so, how does this perception influence adolescents' and young adults' decision making regarding their health? If adolescents have a strong belief that God controls their health status, are they less likely to engage in potentially health-compromising behaviors? Conversely, might religious youth with strong beliefs that God controls their health feel protected to the point that they perceive themselves invulnerable to health risks, thus making them more likely to engage in tobacco and alcohol use? See Figure 9.1 for a representation of the conceptual framework guiding these questions.

THE HEALTH BELIEFS
AND BEHAVIORS STUDY (HBBS)

As a means of addressing the questions posed in the previous section, this study (Willis et al., 1999) examined several variables that might predict tobacco and alcohol use among currently healthy college students. We examined strength of religious faith, four health control loci (God, Internal, Powerful Others, and Chance), and use of religious and nonreligious coping strategies. Religious/spiritual factors, including strength of faith, God locus of health control beliefs, and religious coping strategies were hypothesized to operate as protective factors, such that high levels would be associated with healthier behaviors concerning tobacco and alcohol use—for example,

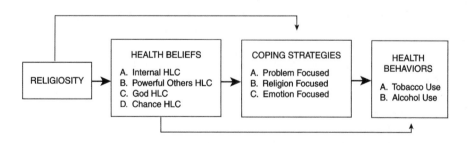

FIGURE 9.1. Coping–Control Model.

the avoidance of substance use, a lowered frequency of tobacco and alcohol use in regular users, attempts to stop using tobacco, and lower frequency of driving when drinking or riding with a drinking driver. It was also expected that college students high in internal locus of health control would be less likely to initiate smoking and more likely to stop tobacco use after beginning and less likely to use substances as a coping mechanism. It was further hypothesized that emotion-focused and avoidance-based coping strategies would be associated with increased college student drinking; therefore, the use of such coping strategies may be viewed as a risk factor.

Undergraduate students (N = 551; 69.5% female, 30.5% male) attending selected universities in north central Alabama, central Tennessee, Washington, DC, northern Iowa, and central coastal California were surveyed. The combined sample included students randomly selected across university majors and students recruited from introductory psychology courses. For results reported in this chapter, the age of the participants ranged from 16 to 23 years (M = 19.17, SD = 1.35). Participants' ethnic backgrounds were diverse: 52.3% white, 42.6% black, 2.0% Hispanic, 1.6% Asian, and 1.5% from other ethnic groups. Participants were asked to complete the HBBS battery of questionnaires as a mail-in survey or in a classroom setting in which they received extra credit points as incentive.

Predictor and Mediator Measures

Religiosity was operationalized by the Santa Clara Strength of Religious Faith Scale (SCSORF; Plante & Boccaccini, 1997). With these 10 items, participants used a 5-option response scale (ranging from 1 = *strongly disagree* to 5 = *strongly agree*) to indicate their level of agreement with statements designed to measure their strength of religious faith (e.g., "My religious faith is extremely important to me"). In the current sample, the alpha reliability of the SCSORF was .92.

Perceived control of health was measured by the three subscales—Powerful Others (PHLC), Internal (IHLC), and Chance (CHLC)—from Form A of the Multidimensional Health Locus of Control (MHLC) scale (Wallston et al., 1978). Interspersed throughout were items from the recently developed God Locus of Health Control (GLHC) subscale (Wallston et al., 1999). These 24 items (6 per subscale) have a 6-option response format (ranging from 1 = *strongly disagree* to 6 = *strongly agree*) to measure participants' beliefs in the loci of control of their health status. The GLHC contains items such as, "Whatever happens to my health is God's will," whereas a prototypical PHLC item states, "When I recover from an illness, it's usually because other people (for example, doctors, nurses, family friends) have taken good care of me." A typical IHLC item reads, "The main thing that affects my health is what I myself do"; a sample item from the CHLC subscale is, "My good health is largely a matter of good fortune." High scores on each of the MHLC/GLHC subscales signify agreement with that particular belief. The Cronbach alphas for the subscales were .93, .65, .68, and .59 respectively.

Both nonreligious and religious coping strategies were assessed in this study. The main instrument for assessing nonreligious coping was the Brief COPE (Carver, 1997). The shortened version of the COPE consists of two items for each of 14 strategies that people might use when they confront difficult or stressful events in their lives. These coping strategies range from Use of Humor (e.g., "I make fun of the situation") to Active Coping (e.g., "I try to come up with a strategy about what to do"). Other strategies such as planning, seeking instrumental support, seeking emotional support, venting emotions, reframing, acceptance, denial, self-blame, behavioral disengagement, self-distraction, and substance use were also assessed with the Brief COPE. Participants responded to each of the 28 items with a rating from 1 ("I usually *don't* do this *at all*") to 4 ("I usually do this *a lot*"). According to Carver (1997), Cronbach's alpha for the subscales ranges between .50 (Venting) and .90 (Substance Use).

The Brief COPE also contains a subscale assessing Turning to Religion (e.g., "I've been praying or meditating"). Because this subscale contained only two items, we also administered the 40-item Ways of Religious Coping Scale (WORCS; Boudreaux et al., 1995), to bolster our assessment of religious coping strategies. The WORCS was specifically designed to determine how participants used religion to cope with stressful events. The participants indicated how often they engaged in 40 religious behaviors by circling a number from 0 = *not used at all/does not apply* to 4 = *used always*. Two subscales are derived for the WORCS: one designed to measure external/social religious coping (e.g., "I talk to church/mosque/temple members") and one that measures internal/private religious coping (e.g., "I pray for strength").

To provide aggregate measures of coping strategies, a principal-components factor analysis with orthogonal rotation was conducted on the data from this sample using the 14 subscales from the Brief COPE and the two subscales from the WORCS. The best solution resulted in three factors: Problem-Focused Coping, consisting of Active Coping (loading = .72), Planning (.73), Behavioral Disengagement (-.60), and Positive Reframing (.53); Religious-Focused Coping, consisting of Internal/Private Religious Coping (.90); External/Social Religious Coping (.83), and Turning to Religion (.80); and Emotion-Focused Coping [consisting of Seeking Instrumental Support (.62), Seeking Emotional Support (.61), Venting Emotions (.57), Denial (.52), Self-Blame (.50), and Self-Distraction (.47). Three scales from the Brief COPE (Acceptance, Humor, and Substance Use) did not load on any of these three factors.

Measures of the Use of Tobacco and Alcohol

Six items adapted from questions on the Youth Risk Behavior Survey (Alabama State Department of Education, 1998; CDC, 1998) assessed tobacco use. The items included trying smoking, age at initiation of smoking, days of smoking each month, cigarettes smoked daily, and attempts to quit smoking. A smoking behavior index was also formed by multiplying the number of days the individual smoked in the past month by the average number of cigarettes smoked daily. The two components of this index correlated .70.

Alcohol-related behaviors were assessed with five items: age at first drink, number of days in which an alcoholic drink was consumed within the previous 30, number of days in which five or more alcoholic drinks were consumed over a short time period (i.e., "binge drinking") within the previous 30 days, frequency of drinking when driving, and frequency of riding with a drinking driver. The number of days out of the previous 30 that the student reported having at least one drink of alcohol and the number of times the student reported binging (i.e., having 5 or more drinks in a short period of time) were highly correlated ($r = .77$), so the two measures were standardized and combined into an index of drinking frequency. In this sample, the index of drinking frequency was positively correlated ($r = .26$; $p < .001$) with the index of smoking behavior, indicating that among college students the use of tobacco and alcohol go hand in hand.

Characteristics of HBBS Sample

Sixty-one percent of the sample had tried smoking; 12% of the sample had tried smoking before the age of 13. The mean age for smoking for the first time was 15.66 ($SD = 2.47$). Forty-one percent had smoked in the previous 30 days. For those who smoked on at least one day out of the previous 30, the number of cigarettes smoked daily was relatively low, averaging four per day. For respondents who had tried alcohol (approximately 80% of the sample), the mean age at drinking their first alcoholic beverage was 15.64 ($SD = 3.54$). Almost 10% had tried alcohol before the age of 13. Sixty-two percent of the sample had consumed alcohol within the previous 30 days ($M = 3.46$, $SD = 5.3$). Over half of this percentage (31.7%) reported that they had had five or more drinks in sequence on at least one occasion ($M = 1.41$; $SD = 3.3$) in the previous 30 days. Within the previous 30 days, 17% of the sample had driven a vehicle while drinking alcohol ($M = .49$ times, $SD = 2.08$) and 32% had ridden in a vehicle driven by someone who had been drinking ($M = 1.14$ times, $SD = 2.99$). Refer to Figures 9.2 and 9.3 for a comparison of alcohol and tobacco use between the Youth Risk Behavior Surveillance national sample (grades 9–12; CDC, 1997) and the Health Beliefs and Behaviors Survey sample (ages 16–23; Willis et al., 1999).

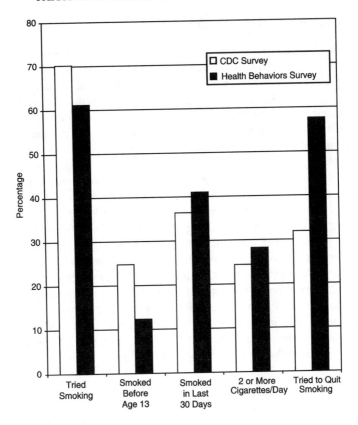

FIGURE 9.2. Comparison of smoking behaviors in CDC Youth Risk Behavior Survey (CDC, 1997) and HBBS (Willis et al., 1999) samples.

Multivariate analysis of variance revealed differences between races in rates of alcohol consumed monthly and in binge drinking, such that whites drank on more days in the previous 30 than blacks and that whites engaged in more binge drinking than blacks. There were race differences in God locus: blacks had a stronger God locus than whites. Chance locus was also perceived to a different extent: Whites had stronger beliefs in chance than blacks. The only sex difference was in God locus, such that women were lower in God locus. A single difference in coping strategies was noted between races in that blacks reported greater use of religion. Females were significantly more likely than males to use emotional support as a coping strategy.

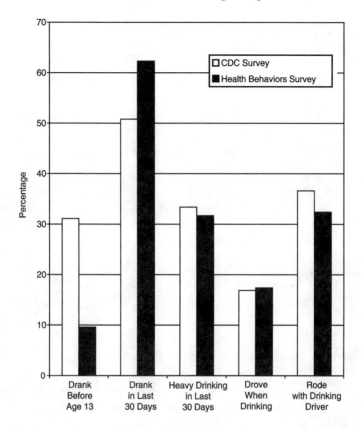

FIGURE 9.3. Comparison of drinking behaviors in CDC Youth Risk Behavior Survey (CDC, 1997) and HBBS (Willis et al., 1999) samples.

Tobacco Use Behaviors

Initiating Smoking

Table 9.1 contains Pearson product–moment correlations between various measures of tobacco use and all of the individual difference measures. Whether the student had ever tried smoking was negatively associated with strength of religious faith, God locus of health control beliefs, and the use of religion-focused coping strategies. Positive associations with having tried smoking were found for the use of emotion-focused coping and for the use of humor, substances, and self-blame as coping mechanisms.

TABLE 9.1. Pearson Correlations between Tobacco Use and Strength of Religious Faith, Multiple Dimensions of Health, Locus of Control, and Coping Strategies

	Ever tried smoking	Age at first try	Smoking frequency	Ever tried quitting
Strength of Faith	−.20**	.06	−.19**	.01
God LHC	−.14**	.03	−.13*	.08
Internal LHC	.03	.04	.02	.06
Powerful Others LHC	−.05	.02	.01	−.03
Chance LHC	.00	−.03	.21***	.01
Problem-Focused	−.05	−.05	−.28***	−.02
Religion-Focused	−.18***	.02	−.17**	.03
Emotion-Focused	.09*	.01	.11	.06
Active Coping	−.01	−.06	−.22***	−.02
Planning	−.07	−.08	−.13*	.04
Positive Reframing	−.05	.00	−.13*	.03
Acceptance	.06	−.06	−.13*	−.02
Humor	.13**	.01	.10*	−.05
Religion	−.18***	.03	−.21***	−.02
Emotional Support	.02	.04	−.01	−.01
Instrumental Support	−.03	−.03	−.05	.05
Self-Distraction	−.01	.13*	−.06	−.05
Denial	.00	−.02	.04	−.04
Venting	.03	.04	.06	.16*
Substance Use	.28***	−.03	.34***	.07
Behavioral Disengagement	.01	.02	.04	.04
Self-Blame	.08*	−.02	.07	.00
External WORC	−.15**	.08	−.18**	.07
Internal WORC	−.15**	.07	−.16**	.07

Note. Boldface is used to indicate aggregate coping strategies.
*$p < .05$; **$p < .01$; ***$p < .001$.

Extent of Smoking

The index of smoking frequency was negatively correlated with strength of religious faith, God locus of health control beliefs, and the use of both problem-focused and religion-focused coping strategies. Young adults who smoked more often had stronger beliefs in chance factors and were more likely to use substances in general as a way to cope. None of the individual difference measures were significantly associated with ever having attempted to quit smoking.

Alcohol Use and Exposure to Alcohol–Related Risks

Table 9.2 presents the Pearson product–moment correlations between the various measures of alcohol use (including exposure to alcohol-related risks) and the individual difference measures examined in these analyses of the

HBBS data. With the exception of ILHC, many of the individual difference measures were significantly related to the index of alcohol use. Those measures having a religious orientation (i.e., strength of faith, God locus, and the use of religion-focused coping strategies) had the strongest negative associations. Individuals who consumed less alcohol were also more likely to believe that powerful others controlled their health. Conversely, strong beliefs that random factors (CHLC) determined health status were related to increased drinking among students.

Several of the specific coping strategies assessed by the Brief COPE were differentially related to drinking in the previous 30 days and to binge drinking in the previous month. Behavioral disengagement and not realistically accepting the elements of a stressful situation were associated with increased binge drinking only. Being less likely to positively reframe a stressful situation was associated with drinking more but not with binge drinking.

TABLE 9.2. Pearson Correlations between Alcohol Use and Strength of Religious Faith, Multiple Dimensions of Health Locus of Control, and Coping Variables

	Age at first drink	Frequency of drinking/ 30 days	Frequency of binge drinking/ 30 days	Times/ 30 days drove drunk	Times/30 days rode with drunk driver
Strength of Faith	.05	−.26***	−.22***	−.04	−.08*
God LHC	.00	−.25***	−.22***	−.03	−.07
Internal LHC	−.02	.02	.01	.03	.04
Powerful Others LHC	.06	−.12**	−.12**	−.06	−.02
Chance LHC	−.01	.04	.05	.04	.05
Problem-Focused	.00	−.24***	−.13**	−.19**	−.21**
Religion-Focused	.04	−.27***	−.30***	−.03	−.04
Emotion-Focused	−.03	.11*	−.02	.03	.15**
Active Coping	.01	−.13**	−.13**	−.01	−.06
Planning	−.01	−.18***	−.16***	−.13**	−.12**
Positive Reframing	−.05	−.11**	−.08	−.06	−.04
Acceptance	.00	−.06	−.10*	−.10*	−.05
Humor	.00	.12**	.13**	.04	.07
Religion	.07	−.30***	−.29***	−.08	−.12**
Emotional Support	.01	−.05	−.07	−.04	−.04
Instrumental Support	.05	−.09*	−.09*	−.11*	−.07
Self-Distraction	.01	−.04	−.04	−.01	−.04
Denial	−.12*	.11**	.10*	.17***	.16***
Venting	−.03	−.02	−.07	−.05	.00
Substance Use	−.06	.44***	.43***	.28***	.38***
Behavioral Disengagement	.04	.05	.10*	.11*	.14**
Self-Blame	−.04	.13**	.13**	.05	.08
External WORC	.05	−.21***	−.21***	−.04	−.06
Internal WORC	.04	−.25***	−.26***	−.08	−.08

Note. Boldface is used to indicate aggregate coping strategies.
*$p < .05$; **$p < .01$; ***$p < .001$.

Driving Behaviors and Alcohol Use

Surprisingly, none of the locus of control or religion-oriented variables was related to driving choices (see Table 9.2). As expected, students who used problem-focused coping were less likely to drive after drinking or ride with a driver who had been drinking. Use of emotion-focused coping was associated with riding with a driver who had been drinking, but not with driving after drinking.

The number of times in the previous 30 days that the students reported riding with a driver who had been drinking was strongly correlated ($r = .71$; $p < .001$) with the number of times they admitted driving while drinking. Thus these two items were standardized and summed to create an index of alcohol-related risk exposure. Among the coping subscales from the Brief COPE, the strongest predictor of alcohol-related risk exposure was substance use, followed by denial, behavioral disengagement, and lack of planning.

Tests of the Coping–Control Model

The conceptual framework guiding these analyses suggests that college students' use of tobacco and alcohol is most proximately mediated by their use of coping strategies. These coping strategies are, in turn, partially mediated by the students' control beliefs. If this model is correct, the influence of religiosity, which appears to be associated with the use of tobacco and alcohol, will become insignificant once control beliefs and coping strategies are accounted for. To more fully test this conceptual model, a series of path analyses (using hierarchical regression analysis) was conducted. The dependent variables for these path analyses were the initiation of smoking, the two indices of smoking behavior and alcohol use already described, and alcohol-related driving behaviors. The three coping factors were entered on the first step of the analyses; the four health locus of control subscales were entered on the second step; and, finally, the third step contained the measure of religious faith.

For initiation of smoking, 4% of the variance was explained by religion-focused coping ($\beta = -.19$; $p < .001$); other factors did not contribute significantly. Approximately 9% of the variance in the index of smoking behavior (number of days smoked times number of cigarettes per day) was explained by the coping strategies that students typically utilized for handling stressors, with problem-focused coping ($\beta = -.23$; $p < .001$) contributing more weight than religious-focused coping ($\beta = -.14$; $p = .02$) and emotion-focused coping ($\beta = .14$; $p = .02$) in explaining the use of tobacco. Only one of the health locus of control scores, Chance ($\beta = .18$; $p = .005$), contributed significantly, explaining an additional 2.8% of the variance. Strength of faith made no further contribution to the explanation of the smoking behaviors.

When the dependent variable was the index of alcohol use (i.e., number of days drinking plus binging), the three coping strategy factors together explained about 13% of the variance. The standardized regression weights for problem-focused (ß = –.08, p = .06) and emotion-focused (ß = .04, p = ns) coping were not significant; however, the use of religion-focused coping strategies emerged as a striking predictor (ß = –.30, p < .0001) of alcohol use. Compared with frequency of tobacco use, a different pattern also emerged in Step 2 of the alcohol use analysis. Whereas the Chance health locus of control scores contributed to explanation of smoking frequency, Powerful Others (ß = –.11, p = .02) and God (ß = –.14, p = .009) loci contributed independently (an additional 2.6%, p < .01) to the explanation of the variance in alcohol consumption. Interestingly, the external locus of Powerful Others and God locus, typically considered external, accounted for drinking behavior over and above the variance explained by the coping measures, whereas the internal subscale (ß= .04; p = ns) did not add anything unique to the model. Coping strategies, however, remained the stronger mediators of both sets of substance use behaviors.

Thus there is support for the general conceptual model showing that the use of coping strategies, particularly those that are religion focused or problem focused, mediate the relationship between strength of religious faith and the health-compromising behaviors under consideration. There is also evidence that control beliefs contribute independently, though to a lesser degree and in different patterns, to the frequency of tobacco and alcohol use. In the case of alcohol-related driving behaviors, strength of belief in chance factors is the sole mediator. In sum, as predicted, having strong religious faith is, indeed, related to diminished smoking and drinking, but its effects upon these health behaviors are entirely explained by a combination of religious and nonreligious health beliefs and coping strategies.

THE COPING–CONTROL MODEL:
EVIDENCE FOR PROTECTIVE AND RISK FACTORS

Findings from the HBBS suggest that coping strategy and control belief profiles may be useful in predicting smoking and drinking risk in adolescents and young adults.

Risk Factors

Students who smoked more frequently had stronger beliefs in chance factors as determinants of health. However, coping strategies explained more of the variance in health-compromising behavior. Students who initiated smoking were more likely to use emotion-focused coping, humor, and self-blame as ways of handling stress. Humor and self-blame were associated with more frequent use of both tobacco and alcohol. The association between using humor to cope and using substances was unexpected. It was not, as one might presume, related to positive reframing in this sample. Humor may be functioning as an alternative form of self-distraction or disengagement. Self-blame is likely to be related to low self-efficacy and self-esteem. Adolescents may use substances to superficially enhance their image for the benefit of user-peers or may use substances to enhance mood.

Denial was revealed as an additional coping strategy associated with alcohol use and alcohol-related driving behaviors, but not with smoking. Lack of acceptance and behavioral disengagement were associated specifically with binge drinking. Youth who drink, and particularly drink heavily, apparently rely on emotion-focused, avoidance strategies for dealing with stress. More research is needed to determine whether youth under excessive stress are more likely to smoke and/or drink than those with less stressful lifestyles and to see if smoking and drinking are more frequent among adolescents with poor management skills. If so, substance use prevention programs should aim to inoculate young adults with problem-focused coping strategies and, when appropriate, religion-focused strategies as well.

Protective Factors

Young people who employed religion-focused coping were less likely to try smoking. Both religion-focused and problem-focused coping were associated with less frequent tobacco and alcohol use. Within these coping aggregates, active coping, planning, and positive reframing, in addition to religious coping, appeared to be most influential in mediating the protective effects of religious faith.

Individuals who believe that their health status is determined by parents and health practitioners, as well as by God, may be less likely to use alcohol. Use of alcohol, certainly no less risky than smoking in producing long-term ill effects, may be associated with stricter proscriptions from the religious community, schools, and parents due to the salience of alcohol's short-term effects on perceptual and motor skills.

Internal locus of control, hypothesized to be a protective factor, had less impact than God or powerful-others loci on substance use. Adolescents and young adults, as compared with older adults, may be developmentally unprepared to understand the potential long-term hazards of their current health-compromising behaviors. Perceptions of uniqueness or invulnerability, limited role commitments, and tendencies toward sensation-seeking may also account for these differences. People in this age group may be more responsive to immediate cues for substance use and react more impulsively. Conversely, these effects may be present as individual differences in smokers and drinkers regardless of age.

COMPONENTS OF RELIGIOSITY THAT CONTRIBUTE TO ITS PROTECTIVE VALUE

Why do certain coping strategies and perceived control over health mediate the salutary effects of religiosity on older adolescents' and young adults' use of tobacco and alcohol? Various aspects of religious context may be important.

Control Beliefs and Religious Proscriptions

Adolescents and young adults are concerned with issues of identity and impression management (Haden & Edmundson, 1991; Haworth-Hoeppner, Globetti, Stem, & Morasco, 1989). Engagement in risky behavior often follows the norms set by peers and/or family in which a risky behavior is part of a favorable image, making a young person more willing to engage in smoking and drinking (Gibbons, Gerrard, Blanton, & Russell, 1998). Religion, conceptualized as exercising control over members' behavior, especially that of youth, may provide specific proscriptions concerning inappropriate behavior. Strong religious beliefs and long-term participation in a religious community may create a prototypical model for a social image that is different from the one promoted by nonreligious peers, one that is accompanied by cognitions and behaviors that include engaging in healthy behaviors. The HBBS provides support for the God and powerful-others loci of health control dimensions within the coping–control model: Students who perceived that their health status was controlled by God and powerful others, which may include clergy and adult and peer members of a faith community, consumed less alcohol.

Adaptive Coping and Religion as a Source of Meaning and Support

The HBBS revealed religion-focused coping and problem-focused coping as protective factors associated with less frequent tobacco and alcohol use. Several contextual features of religious involvement may help to explain these relationships.

Religious affiliation and participation may offer a meaningful framework for the development of self-concept and purpose in life. Awareness of self as a loved, important person connected to a divine, omnipotent being and participation in religious endeavors, such as outreach missions and service to others, may enhance self-esteem and self-efficacy and may also promote the use of planning and active coping in one's own life. The variety of life situations encountered while providing services to others may provide a knowledge base for the adaptive use of positive reframing.

Spiritual support may influence well-being for those undergoing stressful life events in two ways: cognitive mediation and emotional support (Maton, 1989; Pargament, 1997; Pargament et al., 1990). Within the cognitive mediation model, spiritual support encourages positive appraisals of the meaning and implications of stressful life events, that is, the use of positive reframing. An atmosphere of emotional support may lead to general beliefs, such as enhanced self-esteem, and possibly to specific beliefs including those about God's and powerful others' control over health. In addition, religious involvement offers a support system that may enhance coping through the use of instrumental and emotional assistance, such as that provided by guidelines in Scripture or by support from congregation members and clergy.

Religion-Focused and Problem-Focused Coping Used in Tandem

Results from the HBBS revealed that religion-focused and problem-focused strategies were strongly related and, particularly in the case of smoking, are adaptive when used together. This finding supported our hypothesis that religious faith is not solely associated with emotion-based coping mechanisms aimed at reducing distress. In fact, coping associated with religiosity appears to be uniquely composed of adaptive strategies from both the problem-based and emotion-based coping aggregates, based on our factor analysis. Students with strong religious faith, in addition to using religious coping, were significantly more likely to engage in positive reframing, active coping, seeking instrumental support, seeking emotional support, and planning. Of these coping strategies, active coping, planning, and positive reframing (from the problem-focused component), in addition to religious coping, seem to be most influential in mediating the protective effects of religious faith on tobacco and alcohol use in older adolescents and young adults.

TOWARD INTERVENTION STRATEGIES

Integrating religiosity/spirituality into structured health promotion and intervention programs for adolescents and young adults has been of considerable interest (Kutter & McDermott, 1997; Pullen et al., 1999; Wallace & Forman, 1998). This interest has occurred in part due to the gradual acceptance by health professionals and the scientific community that spiritual factors may be salient in health and illness (McCullough, Hoyt, Larson, Koenig, & Thoreson, 2000). Pullen et al. (1999) suggest that the inclusion of spirituality in substance use programs may improve recovery and/or decrease relapse. Plante and Pardini (2000) found that strong religious faith was associated with greater resilience to stress and lower anxiety among recovering substance abusers; denomination affiliation appeared to moderate the beneficial effects.

Within traditional 12-step programs, such as Alcoholics Anonymous (AA), spiritual awareness and growth are considered essential in helping members maintain sobriety (Thoreson et al., 1998). Members provide emotional and instrumental support during group meetings in which emotional disclosure is encouraged. AA emphasizes developing or strengthening spirituality and, tacitly, God locus of control concerning all matters, including health (see Step 11, AA, 2000). During the past 2 decades, 12-step programs have been increasingly likely to serve younger substance abusers. Beck and Olivet (1988) provide an abbreviated version of the traditional 12 steps for adolescents, focusing on three components: admit, accept, and surrender. Vaughn and Long (1999) conducted a qualitative study to examine the process and outcomes of an adolescent AA program. Adolescents in the group were observed to gradually surrender to a higher power, forgive themselves and others, and begin to live in the moment. Self-reflective prayer, company of recovering peers, and nurturing adults provided them the support necessary to confront their addiction and enhance their progression through the program. In general, these programs are considered successful by many, although it remains difficult to determine effectiveness empirically (Thoreson et al., 1998).

The continuing concern about increasing substance use among young people has led laypeople, as well as researchers and practitioners, to propose that religion and spirituality may enhance traditional health promotion and treatment regimens. Community-based spiritual interventions are drawing more attention (Schorling et al., 1997; Swaddiwudhipong, Chaovakiratipong, Ngunttra, Khumklum, & Silarug, 1993). Church congregations may consider prevention and reduction of alcohol and tobacco use among their youth membership as a major priority and may implement peer education programs to supplement and enrich health education in community school curricula. In turn, successful programs may be adopted as part of the outreach mission of churches and implemented in the wider community. Youth and parents should be encouraged to recognize who may be at risk due to their perceptions of control, coping choices, self-efficacy levels, and tendencies toward sensation seeking. Programs that integrate the learning and practiced use of problem-based coping strategies and that offer opportunities for instrumental and emotional support from trusted peers and older adults should be more effective than programs based primarily on presentation of health information. In addition to abstinence-based programs, religious organizations might also consider pragmatic models such as Marlatt's harm reduction approach (Dimeff, Baer, Kivlahan, & Marlatt, 1999; Marlatt, 1998).

Have we reached a point at which we can confidently disseminate public health messages such as, "Just say no to drugs, yes to church and God"? Although many are eager to include spiritual factors in health promotion and prevention, using this adage would be premature. Empirical research to support the use of religion-infused programs is needed (Harris, Thoresen, McCullough, & Larson, 1999; Miller, 1999), and ethical issues require careful consideration (see Tan & Dong, Chapter 12, and Chirban, Chapter 11, this volume). There is a paucity of intervention studies that provide insight into effective integration of religion/spirituality into health promotion programs (for discussion of research suggestions and guidelines, see Airhihenbuwa, 1996; Harris et al., 1999; Worthington, Kurusu, McCullough, & Sandage, 1996). Hence, although research has consistently demonstrated that religion is related to decreased alcohol and tobacco use among adolescents and young adults, there is much to learn about how these findings may be effectively applied toward formulation of intervention strategies.

REFERENCES

Airhihenbuwa, C. O. (1996). The paradigm war, the future of education, and the paradox of health education as a casualty. *Journal of Health Education, 27,* 384–386.

Alabama State Department of Education. (1998). *The 1997 Alabama State Department of Education Youth Risk Behavior Survey Report.* Montgomery, AL: Author.

Alcoholics Anonymous. (2000). *The twelve steps of Alcoholics Anonymous* [Online]. Available: www.carburettor.co.nz/12Steps.htm.

Bachman, J. G., Wadsworth, K., O'Malley, P. M., Johnston, P., & Schulenberg, J. (1997). *Smoking, drinking, and drug use in young adulthood: The impacts of new freedoms and new responsibilities.* Hillsdale, NJ: Erlbaum.

Beck, S., & Olivet, D. C. (1988). Adapting the Alcoholics Anonymous model in adolescent alcohol treatment. *Holistic Nursing, 2*(4), 28–33.

Bennett, P., Norman, P., Moore, L., Murphy, S., & Tudor-Smith, C. (1997). Health locus of control and value for health in smokers and nonsmokers. *Health Psychology, 16*(2), 179–182.

Boudreaux, E., Catz, S., Ryan, L., Amaral-Melendez, M., & Brantley, P. J. (1995). The Ways of Religious Coping scale: Reliability, validity, and scale development. *Assessment, 2*(3), 233–244.

Carver, C. S. (1997). You want to measure coping but your protocol's too long? Consider the Brief COPE. *International Journal of Behavioral Medicine, 4*(1), 92–100.

Carver, C. S., Scheier, M. F., & Weintraub, J. K. (1989). Assessing coping strategies: A theoretically based approach. *Journal of Personality and Social Psychology, 56*(2), 267–283.

Centers for Disease Control and Prevention (1998). Youth Risk Behavior Surveillance—United States, 1997. *Morbidity and Mortality Weekly Report—Surveillance Summaries, 47*(SS-3), 1–89.

Chassin, L., Presson, C. C., Pitts, S. C., & Sherman, S. J. (2000). The natural history of cigarette smoking from adolescence to adulthood in a midwestern community sample: Multiple trajectories and their psychosocial correlates. *Health Psychology, 19*(3), 223–231.

Cooper, M. L., Russell, M., Skinner, J. B., & Windle, M. (1992). Development and validation of a three-dimensional measure of drinking motives. *Psychological Assessment, 4,* 123–132.

Dimeff, L. A., Baer, J. S., Kivlahan, D. R., & Marlatt, G. A. (1999). *Brief Alcohol Screening and Intervention for College Students (BASICS): A harm reduction approach.* New York: Guilford Press.

Dryfoos, J. G. (1990). *Adolescents at risk: Prevalence and prevention.* New York: Oxford University Press.

Eiser, J. R., Eiser, C., Gammage, P., & Morgan, M. (1989). Health locus of control and health beliefs in relation to adolescent smoking. *British Journal of Addiction, 84,* 1059–1065.

Engs, R. C., & Hanson, D. J. (1988). University students' drinking patterns and problems: Examining the effects of raising the purchasing age. *Public Health Reports, 103,* 667–673.

Evans, D. M., & Dunn, N. J. (1995). Alcohol expectancies, coping responses, and self-efficacy judgments: A replication and extension of Cooper et al.'s 1988 study in a college sample. *Journal of Studies on Alcohol, 56,* 186–193.

Folkman, S., & Lazarus, R. S. (1980). An analysis of coping in a middle-aged community sample. *Journal of Health and Social Behavior, 21,* 219–239.

Foshee, V. A., & Hollinger, B. R. (1996). Maternal religiosity, adolescent social bonding, and adolescent alcohol use. *Journal of Early Adolescence, 16,* 451–469.

Gibbons, F. X., Gerrard, M., Blanton, H., & Russell, D. W. (1998). Reasoned action and social action: Willingness and intention as independent predictors of health risk. *Journal of Personality and Social Psychology, 74*(5), 1164–1180.

Globetti, G., Stem, J. T., Morasco, F., & Haworth-Hoeppner, S. (1988). Student residence arrangements and alcohol use and abuse: A research note. *Journal of College and University Student Housing, 18*(1), 28–33.

Gorsuch, R. L. (1995). Religious aspects of substance abuse and recovery. *Journal of Social Issues, 51*(2), 65–83.

Haden, T. L., & Edmundson, E. W. (1991). Personal and social motivations as predictors of substance abuse among college students. *Journal of Drug Education, 21*(4), 303–312.

Hanson, D. J., & Engs, R. C. (1986). College students' drinking problems: 1982–1985. *Psychological Reports, 58*(1), 276–278.

Hardesty, P. H., & Kirby, K. M. (1995). Relation between family religiousness and drug use within adolescent peer groups. *Journal of Social Behavior and Personality, 10,* 421–430.

Harris, A. H. S., Thoresen, C. E., McCullough, M. E., & Larson, D. B. (1999). Spirituality and religiously oriented health interventions. *Journal of Health Psychology, 4,* 413–433.

Hawkins, J. D., Catalano, R. F., & Miller, J. Y. (1992). Risk and protective factors for alcohol and drug problems in adolescence and early adulthood: Implications for substance abuse prevention. *Psychological Bulletin, 112*(1), 64–105.

Haworth-Hoeppner, S., Globetti, G., Stem, J. T., & Morasco, F. (1989). Quantity and frequency of drinking among undergraduates at a southern university. *International Journal of Addictions, 24*(9), 829–857.

Johnston, L. D. (1996, December 19). *Monitoring the future study of drug use.* News and Information Services, University of Michigan, pp. 233, 236

Johnston, L. D., O'Malley, P. M., & Bachman, J. G. (1993). *National survey results on drug use from Monitoring the Future Study, 1975–1992: Vol. II. College students and young adults* (NIH Publication No. 93–3598). Rockville, MD: National Institute of Drug Abuse.

Karwacki, S. B., & Bradley, J. R. (1996). Coping, drinking motives, goal attainment expectancies and family models in relation to alcohol use among college students. *Journal of Drug Education, 26*(3), 243–255.

Kim, E. L., Larimer, M. E., Walker, D. D., & Marlatt, G. A. (1997). Relationship of alcohol use to other health behaviors among college students. *Psychology of Addictive Behaviors, 11*(3), 166–173.

Koenig, H. G., George, L. K., & Siegler, I. C. (1988). The use of religion and other emotion-regulating coping strategies among older adults. *Gerontologist, 28*(3), 303–310.

Kunz, J. L., & Giesbrecht, N. (1999). Gender, perceptions of harm, and other social predictors of alcohol use in a Punjabi community in the Toronto area. *Substance Use and Misuse, 34,* 403–419.

Kutter, C. J., & McDermott, D. S. (1997). The role of the church in adolescent drug education. *Journal of Drug Education, 27,* 293–305.

Langer, E. J., & Rodin, J. (1976). The effects of choice and enhanced personal responsibility for the aged: A field experiment in an institutional setting. *Journal of Personality and Social Psychology, 34,* 191–198.

Lehman, D. R., Ellard, J. H., & Wortman, C. B. (1986). Social support for the bereaved: Recipients' and providers' perspectives on what is helpful. *Journal of Consulting and Clinical Psychology, 54*(4), 438–446.

Lemos-Gir ldez, S., & Fidalgo-Aliste, A. M. (1997). Personality dispositions and health-related habits and attitudes: A cross-sectional study. *European Journal of Personality, 11*(3), 197–209.

Levin, J. S. (1994). Religion and health: Is there an association, is it valid, is it causal? *Social Science and Medicine, 38*(11), 1475–1482.

MacLean, M. G., Lecci, L., & Croteau, N. (1999, June). *Substance use coping, related coping strategies, and alcohol-related problems.* Poster presented at the annual convention of the American Psychological Society, Denver, CO.

Marlatt, G. A. (Ed.). (1998). *Harm reduction: Pragmatic strategies for managing high-risk behaviors.* New York: Guilford Press.

Maton, K. I. (1989). The stress-buffering role of spiritual support: Cross-sectional and prospective investigations. *Journal for the Scientific Study of Religion, 28*(3), 310–323.

McCrae, R. R., & Costa, P. T. (1986). Personality, coping and coping effectiveness in an adult sample. *Journal of Personality, 54*(2), 385–405.

McCreary, D. R., & Sadava, S. W. (1998). Stress, drinking, and the adverse consequences of drinking in two samples of young adults. *Psychology of Addictive Behaviors, 12*(4), 247–261.

McCullough, M. E., Hoyt, W. T., Larson, D. B., Koenig, H. G., & Thoreson, C. (2000). Religious involvement and mortality: A meta-analytic review. *Health Psychology, 19*(3), 211–222.

McKee, S. A., Hinson, R. E., Wall, A. M., & Spriel, P. (1998). Alcohol outcome expectancies and coping styles as predictors of alcohol use in young adults. *Addictive Behaviors, 23*(1), 17–22.

Miller, W. R. (Ed.). (1999). *Integrating spirituality into treatment: Resources for practitioners.* Washington, DC: American Psychological Association.

Mullen, K., & Francis, J. (1995). Religiosity and attitudes toward drug use among Dutch school children. *Journal of Alcohol and Drug Education, 41*(1), 16.

Neumark-Sztainer, D., Story, M., French, S. A., & Resnick, M. D. (1997). Psychosocial correlates of health compromising behaviors among adolescents. *Health Education Research: Theory and Practice, 12*(1), 37–52.

Pargament, K. I. (1997). *The psychology of religion and coping: Theory, research, practice.* New York: Guilford Press.

Pargament, K. I., Ensing, D. S., Falgout, K., Olsen, H., Reilly, B., Van Haitsma, K., & Warren, R. (1990). God help me: I. Religious coping efforts as predictors of the outcomes to significant negative life events. *American Journal of Community Psychology, 18*(6), 793–824.

Park, C., Cohen, L. H., & Herb, L. (1990). Intrinsic religiousness and religious coping as life stress moderators for Catholics versus Protestants. *Journal of Personality and Social Psychology, 59*(3), 562–574.

Patlock-Peckham, J. A., Hutchinson, G. T., Cheong, J., & Nagoshi, C. T. (1998). Effect of religion and religiosity on alcohol use in a college student sample. *Drug and Alcohol Dependence, 49*, 81–88.

Perkins, H. W. (1987). Parental religion and alcohol use problems as intergenerational predictors of problem drinking among college youth. *Journal for the Scientific Study of Religion, 26*(3), 340–357.

Plante, T. G., & Boccaccini, M. T. (1997). The Santa Clara Strength of Religious Faith Questionnaire. *Pastoral Psychology, 45*(5), 375–387.

Plante, T. G., & Pardini, D. A. (2000, August). Religious denomination affiliation and psychological health: Results from a substance abuse population. In A. S. Willis (Chair), *Health and religious denomination affiliation.* Symposium conducted at the annual convention of the American Psychological Association, Washington, D.C.

Prendergast, M. L. (1994). Substance use and abuse among college students: A review of recent literature. *Journal of American College Health, 43*(3), 99–114.

Pullen, L., Modrcin-Talbott, M. A., West, W. R., & Muenchen, R. (1999). Spiritual high vs high on spirits: Is religiosity related to adolescent alcohol and drug abuse? *Journal of Psychiatric and Mental Health Nursing, 6*, 3–8.

Resnick, M. D., Bearman, P. S., Blum, R. W., Bauman, K. E., Harris, K. M., Jones, J., Tabor, J., Beuhring, T., Sieving, R. E., Shew, M., Ireland, M., Bearinger, L. H., & Udry, J. R. (1997). Protecting adolescents from harm: Findings from the National Longitudinal Study on Adolescent Health. *Journal of the American Medical Association, 278*(10), 823–832.

Rippetoe, P. A., & Rogers, R. W. (1987). Effects of components of protection–motivation theory on adaptive and maladaptive coping with a health threat. *Journal of Personality and Social Psychology, 52*(3), 596–604.

Sax, L. J. (1997). Health trends among college freshmen. *Journal of American College Health, 45*(6), 252–262.

Schorling, J. B., Gutgesell, M., Klas, P., & Smith, D. (1994). Tobacco, alcohol and other drug among college students. *Journal of Substance Abuse, 6,* 105–115.

Schorling, J. B., Roach, J., Siegel, M., Baturka, N., Hunt, D. E., Guterbock, T. M., & Stewart, H. L. (1997). A trial of church-based smoking cessation interventions for rural African Americans. *Preventive Medicine, 26,* 92–101.

Simpson, T., & Arroyo, J. A. (1998). Coping patterns associated with alcohol-related negative consequences among college women. *Journal of Social and Clinical Psychology, 17*(2), 150–166.

Swaddiwudhipong, W., Chaovakiratipong, C., Ngunttra, P., Khumklum, P., & Silarug, N. (1993). A Thai monk: An agent for smoking reduction in a rural population. *International Journal of Epidemiology, 22*(4), 660–665.

Thoreson, C., Worthington, E. L., Swyers, J. P., Larson, D. B., McCullough, M. E., & Miller, W. R. (1998). Religious/spiritual interventions. In D. B. Larson, J. P. Swyers, & M. E. McCullough (Eds.), *Scientific research on spirituality and health: A consensus report* (pp. 105–128). Rockville, MD: National Institute for Healthcare Research.

Vaughn, C., & Long, W. (1999). Surrender to win: How adolescent drug and alcohol users change their lives. *Adolescence, 34*(133), 9–24.

Wallace, J. M., & Forman, T. A. (1998). Religion's role in promoting health and reducing risk among American youth. *Health Education and Behavior, 25*(6), 721–741.

Wallace, J. M., & Williams, D. R. (1997). Religion and adolescent health-compromising behavior. In J. Schulenberg & J. L. Maggs (Eds.), *Health risks and developmental transitions during adolescence.* (pp. 444–468). New York: Cambridge Press.

Wallston, K. A., Malcarne, V., Flores, L., Hansdottir, I., Smith, C. A., Stein, M. J., Weisman, M. H., & Clements, P. J. (1999). Does God control your health? The God Locus of Health Control scale. *Cognitive Therapy and Research, 23*(2), 131–142.

Wallston, K. A., Wallston, B. S., & DeVellis, R. (1978). Development of the Multidimensional Health Locus of Control (MHLC) scale. *Health Education Monographs, 6,* 161–170.

Wechsler, H., & Issac, N. (1991). Alcohol and college freshmen: Binge drinking and associated problems. *A report to the AAA Foundation for Traffic Safety.* Boston: Harvard School of Public Health, Youth Alcohol Drug Program.

Welton, G. L., Adkins, A. G., Ingle, S. L., & Dixon, W. A. (1996). God control: The fourth dimension. *Journal of Psychology and Theology, 24*(1), 13–25.

Williams, A., & Clark, D. (1998). Alcohol consumption in university students: The role of reasons for drinking, coping strategies, expectancies, and personality traits. *Addictive Behaviors, 23*(3), 371–378.

Willis, A. S. (1999, August). Exploring religiosity, God locus of health control, and religious coping. In K. A. Wallston (Chair), *Research in health psychology and religion.* Symposium conducted at the annual convention of the American Psychological Association, Boston, MA.

Willis, A. S. (2000, August). Religious denomination, outlook, and coping among young adult tobacco users. In A. S. Willis (Chair), *Health and religious denomination affiliation.* Symposium conducted at the annual convention of the American Psychological Association, Washington, DC.

Willis, A. S., Wallston, K. A., Smith, M. S., Plante, T. G., Johnson, K., Christenbery, T., Reeves, J. E., Dutton, G., & Geiger, B. F. (1999, June). *Religious faith and health locus of control predict smoking behaviors in adolescents.* Poster presented at the annual convention of the American Psychological Society, Denver, CO.

Windle, M., & Windle, R. C. (1996). Coping strategies, drinking motives, and stressful life events among middle adolescents: Associations with emotional and behavioral problems and with academic functioning. *Journal of Abnormal Psychology, 105*(4), 551–560.

Worthington, E. L., Kurusu, T. A., McCullough, M. E., & Sandage, S. J. (1996). Empirical research on religion and psychotherapeutic processes and outcomes: A 10-year review and research prospectus. *Psychological Bulletin, 119,* 448–487.

Yarnold, B. M. (1998). The use of alcohol by Miami's adolescent public school students—1992: Peers, risk-taking, and availability as central forces. *Journal of Drug Education, 28*(2), 211–233.

10

RELIGIOUS FAITH AND MENTAL HEALTH OUTCOMES

THOMAS G. PLANTE
NAVEEN K. SHARMA

If one were to type in the keywords "religion," "spirituality," and "health" on various Internet search engines, one would find an exhaustive list of sites, well into the hundreds. Many of these sites publicize clinics that employ spiritual and religious treatments; church organizations promoting health benefits; institutes that educate individuals on the relationship between religion and health; various international religious and spiritual retreats aimed at promoting health; and videos, books, and publications on this topic. As is evident from a simple Internet search, the impact of religion and spirituality on health has become a hot topic among the general public. However, a similar search specifying "mental health" in place of general health results in a comparably smaller number of sites. Although the relationship between religious faith and mental health outcomes may not be as well known among the general public, it has become an increasingly popular subject of investigation among social scientists and professionals in various fields ranging from clinical psychology, to pastoral psychology social work, anthropology, sociology, and medicine.

Recent research on religious faith and mental health outcomes has generally demonstrated a positive association between the two constructs. This research has led to the integration of religious and/or spiritual issues into clinical assessment and treatment of a wide range of mental health issues. Considering that 80% of the world's population belongs to one particular religious tradition or another (Bernstein et al., 1995), it is important to pursue a greater understanding of what role, if any, religion and spirituality play both in fostering positive mental health and in facilitating the recovery from mental illness.

In this chapter we review recent research regarding the relationship between religious faith/spirituality and mental health outcomes, as well as provide directions for future research and discussion. The specific aspects of mental health and illness that we focus on include well-being, depression, anxiety, substance abuse, and schizophrenia. We also briefly discuss research pertaining to religious faith and personality disorders, eating disorders, somatoform disorders, and bipolar disorder.

WELL-BEING

Well-being has been defined as a multidimensional construct including morale, satisfaction with life, congruence with expected and achieved life goals, positive and negative affect, mood, symptoms related to distress (Diener, Suh, Lucas, & Smith, 1999; Levin & Taylor, 1998), self-esteem (Wilcock et al., 1998), and prosocial values and behaviors (Donahue & Benson, 1995). Most studies investigating religious involvement and well-being have uncovered a strong association between the two constructs (Koenig, 1995a; Levin, 1997), though there are studies that have shown either a negative association (Wilcock et al., 1998) or no significantly clear positive or negative association (Donahue & Benson, 1995; Pargament & Park, 1996). In a study using the Santa Clara Strength of Religious Faith Questionnaire, for example, Plante and Boccaccini (1997) found that college students with high strength of religious faith had higher self-esteem, hope, and adaptive coping and less interpersonal sensitivity. Positive associations with well-being may be due to the impact of faith on both positive and negative emotions, such as increased forgiveness and reduced guilt, respectively, which may enhance the individual's development (Ellison, 1998). Idler and Kasl (1997) found that ritualistic religious behavior may likewise promote well-being through such behaviors as cathartic worship services.

Evidence suggests that socialization through religious participation in a congregational setting may also promote prosocial and adaptive qualities, elevating mood and decreasing levels of distress (Donahue & Benson, 1995). For example, in the African American community, church attendance and activities have been found to be an effective coping mechanism, promoting well-being (Blaine & Croker, 1995). Many religious institutions function as sources of social support for youth and families. Informational social support is provided through educating the community on key values and issues ranging from substance abuse and violence prevention to health-compromising behaviors that may influence well-being (Donahue & Benson, 1995). Religious institutions also provide emotional social support by creating a feeling of connectedness for individuals in the congregational community (Blaine & Croker, 1995). Some of the positive effects of religious faith on well-being include increased self-esteem and positive life outlooks, as well as social support networks that may lessen the detrimental effects of stressful life events through religious beliefs, expressions, and support (Koenig, 1995a).

A number of studies have focused on the influence of religion on the well-being of specific populations, such as the elderly, adolescents, and various ethnic groups. These studies have coincided with Levin and Taylor's (1998) view that the relationship between religion and well-being can be accurately estimated only after taking into account such determinants as health, socioeconomic status, age, and ethnicity.

Spirituality has been found to be an integral factor in the African American community. For example, Frame and Williams (1996) termed spirituality the "whole of life" for many African Americans. In a recent study, the well-being components of life purpose and satisfaction were directly related to either or both the individual's relationship with God and an active religious life (Fleming & Anderson, 1998).

In research with adolescents, Varon and Riley (1999) noted that although maternal education, race, type of religion, and frequency of the adolescent's church attendance were not significantly associated with well-being, the social support provided by a mother who attends church at least once a week may be a strong contributor to adolescent well-being. In other investigations among adolescents, religiosity has been found to be a strong inhibitor of maladaptive behaviors that negatively influence well-being (e.g., smoking, alcohol consumption; see Willis, Wallston, & Johnson, Chapter 9, this volume). Religiousness was also observed to be a strong inhibitor of suicide ideation, suicide attempts, alcohol use, and sexual involvement among adolescents, while promoting prosocial behavior, such as volunteer service (Varon & Riley, 1999).

Studies have also examined the relationship between religious coping and well-being. Plante, Saucedo, and Rice (2001) speculated that religious coping might be helpful for individuals experiencing significant trauma but not necessarily for those with moderate daily hassles. They found that religious coping was unrelated to the management of daily hassles among college students. Among caregivers of ill persons, prayer and church attendance emerged as positive coping mechanisms for families of children with disabilities, giving them strength and hope (Bennet, Deluca, & Allen, 1995). Religious coping was also reported as an adaptive coping mechanism among

Salvadoran immigrants migrating to the United States following the civil war in their homeland (Plante, Manuel, Menendez, & Marcotte, 1995).

Selway and Ashman (1998), however, theorized about the possible aversive effects of religion on the well-being of the disabled, recognizing that a number of world religions portray disabled people in a stereotypical and negative manner in many religious texts. In this sense, adherence to these religions may contribute to stigmatization and negatively influence the well-being of church members with disabilities.

To promote well-being, treatment plans have been offered that emphasize the role of spirituality and religiosity in therapy. Richards, Rector, and Tjeltveit (1999) highlighted the value of affirmating clients' core spiritual values, exploring how to live congruently with those values, and accessing the spiritual resources in their lives. Increasing spiritual and/or religious integration in psychotherapy has been found to improve treatment outcome for religious clients (Miller & Thoresen, 1999). Addressing religious issues may also help clients become more aware of goal content and goal conflict, which are associated with well-being (Emmons, Cheung, & Tehrani, 1998). Aside from psychotherapy clients, individuals with chronic medical illnesses, such as HIV/AIDS, frequently seek spiritual and religious resources for well-being (O'Neil & Kenny, 1998).

Many studies that have observed a strong positive association between religiosity/spirituality and well-being reflect variables such as the creation of healthy emotionality, structured rituals, and the belief in a life purpose. For many people, participation in religious or spiritual practices in a congregational setting has also been found to enhance feelings of social support and connectedness with a greater community, as well as inhibit maladaptive behavior such as smoking, excessive drinking, and sexual acting out. Religious coping mechanisms such as prayer and church attendance appear to be helpful in maintaining a sense of well-being. Thus far there is less research about the effectiveness of integrating religious and spiritual perspectives into therapy, but preliminary findings have been promising, and this is becoming an active area of inquiry.

DEPRESSION

Recent research on the relationship between religious faith and depression has generally suggested that religiosity is associated with decreasing levels of depression (Catipovic, Ilakovac, Durjancek, & Amidzc, 1995; Cosar, Kocal, Arikan, & Isik, 1997; Plante & Boccaccini, 1997). However, some studies have found no clear association between depression and religious involvement (Koenig et al., 1997). Most studies that examine the relationship between religion and depression fall into three categories: religiosity as decreasing susceptibility to depression, religion as a coping mechanism for dealing with depression, and the benefits of religious and/or spiritual components in treating depression.

Intrinsic religiosity (religiosity that is based on internal beliefs, such as faith, rather than external benefits, such as social connections) is significantly associated with lower levels of depressive symptoms (Mickley, Carson, & Soeken, 1995; Watson, Milliron, Morris, & Hood, 1994); on the other hand, certain private religious behaviors, such as watching religious television programs and personal prayer, have been found to be positively associated with depression among the elderly (Koenig et al., 1997).

Other studies have focused on "death-depression" (depression related to an increased awareness of the inevitability of death); lower levels of depression were found among individuals who held a belief in some form of an afterlife (Alvarado, Temper, Bresler, & Dobson, 1995). Other studies have noted that depression was less likely among religious individuals with medical illness or religious surgical patients compared with their less religious peers (Richards & Bergin, 2000). Similarly, lower levels of depressive symptoms have been reported among church-attending elderly (Richards & Bergin, 2000), with individuals who attend church being half as likely to be depressed as those who do not (Koenig et al., 1997).

Cross-sectional studies such as these are interesting, but the mixed results are difficult to interpret. It is unclear, for example, whether connections between increased private prayer and increased depressive symptoms (Koenig et al., 1997) mean that greater private religious expression elicits greater distress, that greater distress mobilizes more intensive prayer, or that other unknown variables may be at play. Longitudinal studies, which seek to track these connections over time, are more illuminating. For example, in a 10-year longitudinal study, Miller, Warner, Wickramaratne, and Weissman (1997) found maternal religiosity and maternal–offspring concordance of religiosity to be protective agents against depressive symptoms among their child offspring.

Understanding the role of religion for people of various cultures is integral in appraising the self-assessment and recovery experiences of individuals suffering from depression (Fallot, 1998). Individuals of the same religion around the world have different religious experiences, based on their particular culture. Although Islamic tradition strongly disapproves of suicide, 43% of depressed Muslim women in Turkey repeatedly attempted suicide (Cosar et al., 1997), whereas greater religiosity among Muslim refugees in Afghanistan was associated with lower levels of vulnerability to suicide (Jahangir, ur Rehman, & Jan, 1998). The different cultural contexts of these two Muslim communities may contribute to the dissimilarity of the association between religiosity, depression, and suicide attempts. Similarly, religiosity is associated with low levels of depression and high levels of "happiness" in the Netherlands (Gopal, 1997), whereas it is associated with high levels of depression in employees in Croatia (Catipovic et al., 1995).

As a coping mechanism, religious faith and religious/spiritual practices function to ease the grieving or bereavement process of many individuals experiencing exceptional circumstances who may be at risk for depression. For example, a number of studies have examined the experience of parents grieving the death of their child. The many coping mechanisms employed by individuals whose children had died of sudden infant death syndrome, neonatal death, or stillbirth, reflect, in part, the religiosity of the parents. Parents who regularly attended church prior to the death of their infant continued to attend church as a means of coping after the death, whereas those who previously did not attend church services were still not inclined to do so. Those individuals who did attend church were less likely to report depressive symptoms than those who did not (Thearle, Vance, Najman, Embelton, & Foster, 1995). Self-directed religious behavior, such as going to church, was found to increase under times of high stress and decrease while bereaved parents were suffering symptoms of depression (Bickel et al., 1998). Religiously informed treatment was found to be effective in enhancing the grieving process of parents mourning the loss of their child (e.g., Livneh, Antonak, & Maron, 1995).

Similarly, religious coping mechanisms and religious appraisals played a key role in susceptibility to depression in caregivers responsible for the care of terminally ill family members (Harrington, Lackey, & Gates, 1996; Kazanigian, 1997; Mickley, Pargament, Brant, & Hipp, 1998; Reese & Brown, 1997). Caregivers who appraised their situation of caring for a terminally ill relative as holding meaning in God's greater plan or as a means of spiritual revelation or introspection were less likely to experience depression, whereas those who felt their situation was punishment from God or was unjust were more likely to be depressed. Mickley, Pargament, Brant, and Hipp (1998) found that caregivers who interpreted their difficult situation in terms of "benevolent religious (or secular) reframing" and "God's will" adapted successfully (i.e., displayed fewer depressive symptoms). Unsuccessful appraisals included "apathetic God," "unfair God," and "unjust world."

Other important groups that have been studied with respect to their use of religious or spiritual coping are the elderly and patients with HIV/AIDS. Among the elderly, religiosity was not associated with the incidence of depression but was strongly associated with the improvement of depression (Braam, Beekman, Deeg, Smith, & Tilburg, 1997). In a study by Koenig, Weiner, Peterson, Meador, and Keefe (1997), 43% of a sample of chronically medically ill elderly patients were diagnosed as clinically depressed, with 60% of these depressed patients utilizing religiosity as a coping mechanism and 34% reporting religion to be the most important factor enabling them to cope. Religion was also the most important coping factor for elderly federal inmates. For these men, depression was negatively associated with the inmates' intrinsic religiosity and the perceived importance of religion to the inmate, as rated by their primary caretaker in the facility (Koenig, 1995a). In regard to death-depression, the acceptance of death and decrease of death-depression among many elderly were tied to faith and spiritual values (Hinton, 1999). A decrease in death depression was also negatively associated with the belief in a religious or spiritual afterlife (Alvarado et al., 1995).

As a coping mechanism among patients with HIV/AIDS, religion seems to play a similar role for both men and women patients. For HIV-positive gay men, religious coping was significantly associated with lower levels of depressive symptoms, though religious behavior (e.g., church attendance) was not related to depression (Woods, Antoni, Ironson, & Kling, 1999). For women, religious coping, in the form of prayer and rediscovery or redefining oneself, was the most frequently adopted coping response to their illness (Kaplan, Marks, & Mertens, 1997).

The value of attending to religion in psychotherapy to ameliorate depressive symptoms has been replicated in various studies, though it is not evident in all empirical findings (McCullough, 1999). Hood-Morris (1996) proposed a spiritual well-being model for providing holistic treatment for depression in older women. She described holism as "an integrated dynamic, evolutionary, and vital conceptualization of the biological, psychological, social and spiritual aspects of human nature" (p. 440). Though her model emphasizes the use of holism in regard to depressed elderly women, this type of biopsychosociospiritual model is advocated by many other health professionals for assessment and therapy (e.g., Cornet, 1998; Kok & Jongsma, 1998). A multidimensional model such as this is also beneficial in acknowledging the potential role of the pastor as a provider of treatment, along with family and the medical community (Gilbert, 1998). Research has also shown the beneficial effects of religiously oriented treatment with depressed disabled elderly patients (Chang, Noonan, & Tennstedt, 1998), as well as with depressed students (Shapiro, Schwartz, & Bonner, 1998).

Religiousness and spirituality appear to reduce the incidence of depressive symptoms, though religious practices sometimes have been positively associated with depression. Intrinsic religiosity, maternal–offspring concordance of religiosity, and church attendance are a few religious factors that have been shown to reduce the incidence of depression. Religious coping mechanisms such as church attendance and healthy religious appraisals have been helpful to buffer the effects of or reduce the susceptibility to depression among bereaved individuals, caregivers, and the terminally ill. Holistic treatment strategies that integrate religious and spiritual factors into therapy appear to be beneficial for many people suffering from depression.

ANXIETY

Religious faith has been shown to possibly both contribute to (Shooka, Al-Haddad, & Raees, 1998; Trenthold, Trent, & Compton, 1998) and inhibit the incidence of anxiety symptoms (Ita, 1995–1996; Kaplan et al., 1997). Positive mental health outcomes among anxiety patients have been noted among individuals who are intrinsically religious and among individuals who employ religious or spiritual coping mechanisms, as well as among both religious and nonreligious individuals who participate in religion or spirituality-based treatment (Jahangir, 1995). Negative outcomes among anxious persons have been found among individuals who were raised with strict religious upbringings and among religious individuals with obsessive–compulsive disorder (Shooka et al., 1998). In a multiethnic, multireligious sample, the majority of patients with obsessive–compulsive disorder identified themselves with a religious affiliation, but no clear relationship could be found between the type of obsessive–compulsive symptoms and the specific religious affiliations of the patients with obsessive–compulsive disorder (Rapheal, Rani, Bale, & Drummond, 1996).

Research has also shown that panic patients may overemphasize religious concepts such as sin. This overemphasis may lead to hyperbolic feelings of guilt and shame, causing additional panic (Barr, 1995). Trenthold, Trent, and Compton (1998) broaden the definition of panic disorder to include one who "is fraught with anxiety that is fueled by cognitions about her needs for both approval and perfection, someone whose failures are associated with thoughts about blame and punishment, someone who is in conflict about her ability to meet the standards set by her religion which, in turn, is associated with guilt" (p. 63). Specific examples of the moral transgressions and conflict experienced consciously or unconsciously by panic sufferers raised with strict religious upbringings include anger toward God during periods of bereavement and questioning one's sexuality. Interestingly, religious conflicts regarding moral transgressions are significant predictors of panic disorder but not of other psychological disorders (Trenthold, Trent, & Compton, 1998).

However, as in depression, a normal, healthy religious life appears to be a predictor of positive mental health outcomes and negatively associated with anxiety disorders. Intrinsic religiosity has been associated with low levels of general anxiety in various populations (Lotufo-Neto, 1996; Mickley et al., 1995; Richards & Bergin, 2000) and low levels of death-anxiety when compared with individuals who were extrinsically religious (Clements, 1998; Richards & Bergin, 2000). Intrinsic religiosity was also negatively associated with neurotic guilt (Richards & Bergin, 2000). In a proposed causal path model, Ita (1995–1996) attributed the negative correlation between age and death-anxiety to the increasing importance of spirituality for individuals throughout the lifespan. Death-anxiety among terminally ill patients with HIV/AIDS was negatively correlated with utilization of religious and spiritual coping mechanisms (Woods et al., 1999), specifically with the use of prayer and self-discovery (Kaplan et al., 1997).

Though most research on the relationship between intrinsic religiosity and anxiety demonstrates an overwhelmingly negative association, research examining this relationship within particular socioreligious contexts suggests important cultural differences. In a cross-cultural study by Tapanya, Nicki, and Jarusawad (1997), intrinsic religiosity among Christian and Buddhist individuals was inversely associated with anxiety. However, extrinsic religiosity was associated with high levels of anxiety for Buddhists but not associated with anxiety for Christians. One possible explanation for this difference is the different notions of the afterlife and means toward enlightenment in these religions. Extrinsic religiosity among Buddhists, theoretically, could hinder a person's path toward enlightenment, which ideally is gained through intrinsic religiosity and inner awareness. For Christianity, extrinsic religiosity would not necessarily prevent a person from attainment of a positive afterlife experience.

Religious and spiritual involvement among people experiencing high levels of stress is significantly associated with lower levels of anxiety (Holtz, 1998). For example, high strength of religious faith was associated with lower anxiety among substance abusers (Plante, Yancey, Sherman, Guertin, & Pardini, 1999). For HIV individuals who were preparing for or experiencing the death of a partner, various personal and traditional religious rites for the spirit and body of the dying helped them cope and obtain closure with the loss of the loved one (T. Richards & Folkman, 1997). Though religious and spiritual coping mechanisms were reported as highly comforting for the bereaved, the experience of spiritual phenomena, such as feeling the presence of the deceased, was related to higher short-term anxiety.

Psychotherapy that integrates issues of religion and spirituality for individuals with an anxiety disorder has been productive for religious individuals (Razali, Hasanah, Aminah, & Subramaniam, 1998). During psychotherapy, therapists may also suggest that a client create a personal sense of religious meaning (or set of spiritual beliefs, if the client is not affiliated with any formal religion) and rituals that may serve as coping mechanisms (T. Richards & Folkman, 1997). For those individuals whose anxiety disorder is assessed to be related to strict religious upbringing, possible directions for therapy may include positive self-talk assignments to counter feelings of guilt and shame (Barr, 1995) and addressing topics of forgiveness of sin and salvation (Trenholm, Trent, & Compton, 1998).

Because religion and spirituality have been both positively and negatively associated with anxiety, further research needs to be conducted to investigate the nature of the religious or spiritual factors that may influence the incidence and treatment of anxiety. Recent research presents the possibility that the positive association between religion and anxiety occurs among individuals experiencing unusually strict religious upbringings or among individuals with underdeveloped, vague, or overemphasized ideas of religion or spirituality. Research investigating the particular nature of religion and spirituality among anxiety sufferers may shed light on why a positive association exists. At the same time, we cannot dismiss the wealth of research that demonstrates a negative association between religion/spirituality and anxiety among individuals with "healthy" religious and spiritual beliefs and practices.

SUBSTANCE ABUSE

Though some researchers have theorized that a lack of a sense of spirituality may contribute to alcoholism (Warfield & Goldstein, 1996), it is difficult to ascertain whether alcoholism is directly related to the nature of one's spirituality (Chapman, 1996; Wing, Crow, & Thompson, 1995). Many studies have examined the association between religiosity and spirituality and alcoholism and the effectiveness of spiritual interventions in the recovery process. Religion plays a significant role in one's decision to use alcohol (Rajarathinam & Muthusamy, 1996). Intrinsic religiosity is a predictor of low levels of substance use or abuse (Fischer & Richards, 1998), whereas predictors of substance abuse include a feeling of disconnectedness with one's religion (Gillis, & Mubhashar, 1995) and one's specific religious affiliation (Peele, 1997). Likewise, individuals who were substance abusers or users generally have low levels of religious involvement (Miller, 1998).

In a study examining the religious dimensions of personal devotion, personal conservatism, and institutional conservatism, Kendler, Gardner, and Prescott (1996) found religiosity to be significantly and negatively associated with substance abuse and a lifetime history of alcoholism. Though religious beliefs influenced a person's tendency ever to use a substance, one's religious devotion or spirituality influenced one's ability to quit or maintain low levels of substance use (Kendler et al., 1997; Miller, 1998). Similarly, higher levels of religiosity or spirituality among individuals recovering from substance abuse are also associated with enhanced coping, greater resilience to stress, an optimistic life orientation, greater perceived social support, and lower levels of anxiety among inpatient and halfway-house substance abusers (Pardini, Plante, & Sherman, 2001).

Religious and spiritual treatments have been effective in the recovery process of some individuals suffering from alcoholism (Navarro, Wilson, Berger, & Taylor, 1997; Schaler, 1996). Green, Fullilove, and Fullilove

(1998) describe the recovery experience for many substance abusers as an intense spiritual journey in which the individual embraces a higher power and undergoes a personal transformation. Carroll (1997) incorporates understanding of the self and others, as well as a higher power, in describing the spiritual journey of the substance abuser, emphasizing the importance of recognizing the relationship between one's spirituality and psychosocial functioning.

In a proposed sociospiritual approach to treating substance abuse addiction, Morrell (1996) identifies substance abuse as a condition dominated by a spiritual or social condition. Spiritual world views, along with political world views, serve to provide the individual with the conviction that human beings are interconnected through their beliefs in a higher power, decreasing feelings of separation and suffering.

Individuals treating clients with addictive disorders should take the spirituality of the client into account in using treatment strategies that properly reflect the needs of the client (Jackson, 1995). In a study comparing individuals in a substance abuse program with medical students in their attitudes toward issues of spirituality and the perceived importance of spirituality in treatment, it was found that the students significantly misassessed the value of spirituality in treatment for the clients (Goldfarb, Galanter, McDowell, Lifshutz, & Dermatis, 1996). The medical students in the study were found to be significantly less spiritually oriented than the clients (whose spirituality was representative of the population as a whole), and this factor may have contributed to the underestimation of their clients' desire or need for spiritual aspects of treatment. The authors suggest that medical students and other professionals whose careers are focused on biological sciences may need added training to adequately treat individuals who require spiritual components in therapy.

Alternatives to medically oriented therapy include intervention programs such as Alcoholics Anonymous and Narcotics Anonymous, which concentrate on such themes as accepting and relying on a higher power. In a study conducted by Pardini, Plante, and Sherman (2001), individuals recovering from substance abuse reported themselves as being more spiritual than religious, though they were found to have high levels of religiosity as well. Membership in the spirituality-based program Alcoholics Anonymous (AA) has been negatively associated with alcohol consumption, suggesting that it may be an effective method in modifying drinking behavior (Peele, 1997), although it has been difficult to conduct appropriate clinical trials to establish the efficacy of AA. Many individuals who are members of Alcoholics Anonymous found comfort in placing trust and responsibility for positive and negative events in their lives onto a higher power. Individuals in AA also expressed the desire to maintain their spirituality throughout their lives (Sommer, 1997).

However, there is controversy as to whether the apparent effectiveness of programs such as AA is due to their spiritual focus as opposed to other important elements, such as the social support offered through membership or the specific guidelines they provide concerning recovery (Vick, Smith, & Herrera, 1998). In a study examining the attitudes of individuals in a 12-step program (Nealon-Woods, Ferrari, & Jason, 1995), 71% of the individuals who attended weekly meetings indicated that they were not motivated by spiritual aspects of the meeting. Eighty-eight percent indicated that they benefited from working with a sponsor, and 53% indicated that they were involved with the program because it offered a sense of fellowship with others in need of similar recovery. Contrary to the belief that spirituality is a necessary component in treating addictive disorders, individuals attending meetings of secular programs, such as Secular Organizations for Sobriety (SOS) or secular professional addictions treatment, regard these programs as effective in achieving and maintaining abstinence (Connors & Dermen, 1996). When comparing the spirituality of individuals in a religious therapy group (12-step) with that of those in a nonreligious therapy group, spirituality levels of both groups were found to increase, regardless of treatment style (Borman & Dixon, 1998).

The issue of whether spirituality is a necessary component in the treatment of substance abuse is a difficult one to assess. Though some individuals purposefully choose treatment plans that are secular in nature, it is unclear whether the increased level of spirituality they may develop is due to the inherent spirituality of the individual substance abusers or whether the secular programs also offer spiritual support. Further research comparing secular and religious therapy and individuals who choose these various treatment programs needs to be conducted to gain more insight into the role that religion and spirituality play in the process of recovery from substance abuse.

SCHIZOPHRENIA

Whereas past research has suggested that religiosity may be positively associated with the incidence of schizophrenia, recent research has focused on the possibility that some religious individuals are misdiagnosed with schizophrenia. Behaviors or ideology that reflect normal religious functioning may overlap with schizophrenic characteristics. Wahass and Kent (1997b) highlight two case studies in which the clients' normal religious behaviors were assessed as schizophrenic, asserting that even the third revised edition of the *Diagnostic and Statistical Manual of Mental Disorders* might tend toward such misdiagnoses. A proper assessment for schizophrenia in religious patients can only be completed when taking into consideration the premorbid religious or spiritual ideology of the client. Whereas a therapist may assess a client's psychopathology as schizophrenia, a religious client may diagnose himself or herself as struggling with spirit or demon possession. Understanding the client's perceptions of the phenomenon and his or her religious background may be helpful for therapists in both assessment and intervention strategies (Gopal & Sharon, 1997; Schneider, 1997; Wahass & Kent, 1997c).

In addressing the religious beliefs and background of an individual who is self-diagnosed with possession, intervention strategies may include more than the traditional administration of psychotropic medicine (Azaunce, 1995). For example, in many Middle Eastern cultures, psychiatric symptoms such as hallucinations are sometimes attributed to possession by demons or to God's will (Wahass & Kent, 1997a). When antipsychotic medication showed no positive outcome among Islamic schizophrenic clients, the integration of religious doctrine into therapy was effective with two-thirds of the clients (Wahass & Kent, 1997b). One possible treatment strategy for individuals of various religious beliefs includes the combined efforts of the psychotherapist and a religious or spiritual healer from the client's religious background, such as an exorcist, voodoo doctor, obeahman, or faith healer (Azaunce, 1995).

Schneider (1997) describes the "paranoid" religious thoughts of some schizophrenics "as an expression of healthy searching in the therapeutic process and not necessarily as a psychotic and unhealthy delusion" (p. 379). When religious delusions that are used as tools for fostering a normal sense of reality are perceived as psychotic, the person tends to create more delusions and appear more psychotic (Schneider, 1997).

Religious coping methods have been shown to have positive effects on individuals who are diagnosed with schizophrenia, as well as with their families (Wahass & Kent, 1995). The religious disposition of schizophrenic individuals tends to be consistent with their previous religious affiliation, even though their perceptions of the world may have become significantly impaired. For individuals who have the same religious affiliation as their families, religion can serve as a unifying force for all parties through the practice of traditional rituals and symbols which reflect the family's value system (Walsh, 1995). For the schizophrenic individual, religious worship with the family or with a congregation may serve to integrate the person into a greater community during times in which he or she is most likely feeling isolated. For the family, religious worship with the schizophrenic family member serves as a means of feeling connected with the individual who has lost touch with reality. The therapist's understanding and respect for the religious beliefs and practices of the client and the client's ability to use his or her natural coping mechanism have been helpful in treatment for Christian clients (MacGreen, 1997). In a cross-cultural study by Wahass and Kent (1997a) examining the use of coping mechanisms of Western and non-

Western schizophrenic clients, culture was related to the choice of coping mechanism employed.

The use of treatment strategies that include religious or spiritual components for schizophrenic clients seems to be important in providing optimum treatment outcomes. Cultural and religious differences among clients may dramatically vary the treatment methods that could be employed by therapists. The role of religion and the nature of the illness, the client's perceptions of the illness, and cultural differences should be taken into consideration for assessment and treatment (Fallot, 1998; Wahass & Kent, 1997a, 1997b).

PERSONALITY, EATING, SOMATOFORM, AND BIPOLAR DISORDERS

Few studies have been conducted regarding the relationship of religion/spirituality and personality, eating, somataform, dissociative, or bipolar disorders. In relation to treating borderline patients, Vitz and Mango (1997) discuss the role of Kernbergian psychodynamics and religious aspects of forgiveness, emphasizing how repentance and forgiveness cannot be offered through psychotherapy but rather through religious and morality-based treatment approaches. Other research on personality disorders has been similar to recent research on schizophrenia. The increase in studies focusing on the misdiagnosis of schizophrenia in normal-functioning religious individuals is similar to research that presents the possibility that normal functioning religious individuals are misdiagnosed with schizotypal personality disorder (Day & Peters, 1998; Jackson & Fulford, 1997; McCreery & Claridge, 1995). McCreery and Claridge (1995) term individuals who are well adjusted but score high on scales measuring positive symptomatology for schizotypal personality disorder as "happy schizotypes." In studying new religious movements and schizotypy, Day and Peters (1998) found that an overlap existed between the experiences of individuals in these new religions and positive symptomatology. However, individuals in these new religions were not found to be distressed overall (Day & Peters, 1998; Jackson & Fulford, 1997). Abnormal religious experiences such as out-of-body sensations (McCreery & Claridge, 1995) and intense religious moments (Jackson & Fulford, 1997) may be common among individuals who are "happy schizotypes," but these types of experiences do not necessarily indicate the presence of mental illness or maladjustment (McCreery & Claridge, 1995).

Religion and spirituality have also been examined with respect to the etiology and treatment of eating disorders. In assessing possible causal factors of eating disorders, McCourt and Waller (1996) discuss how religion, along with other factors such as gender and acculturation, may have an impact on eating disorders or disturbed eating attitudes. Some religious and spiritual beliefs that have been common among individuals with eating disorders include feelings of spiritual unworthiness, shame, fear of abandonment by God, and negative perceptions of God (P. Richards et al., 1997). Spiritual interventions have been found to be helpful with obese, overweight (Davis, Clance, & Gailis, 1999) and anorexic individuals (Garret, 1996; Banks, 1997). Obese women who attended meetings for Overeaters Anonymous, which focuses on abstinence and spirituality as emphasized in Alcoholics Anonymous, reported success rates that were significantly associated with the importance they attributed to abstinence and spirituality. Treatment interventions that integrate religious or spiritual components might also be employed in psychotherapy for obese individuals who either identify themselves as religious or are from religious or spiritual cultures, such as the African American community (Davis et al., 1999).

In an article highlighting a case study of somatization, Ruiz (1998) discusses the roles of religion in the client's conceptualization of the illness, the process of somatization, the client's difficulties with treatment compliance, and the integration of religion in the treatment process. In Ruiz's case study, a middle-aged immigrant woman who was experiencing a major depressive episode in conjunction with somatization disorder believed that she was not depressed but was being punished by God. She was administered antidepressants but refused to comply with any treatment by her psychiatrist until she was advised to do so by a priest in her local church. Religious or spiritual treatment plans were also considered to be important in the care of religious individuals with bipolar disorder (Fallot, 1998).

CONCLUSION AND FUTURE DIRECTIONS

Most research examining the relationship between religion and spirituality and mental health outcomes shows positive associations. Healthy religious functioning or a spiritual outlook on life has been clearly associated with mental well-being and negatively associated with depression, anxiety, and substance abuse. However, there are both positive and negative associations of religion and spirituality with anxiety and schizophrenia. More research needs to be conducted on whether the elevated incidence of these disorders among religious individuals is specific to those who have experienced strict or abnormal religious upbringings or whether these disorders are also found disproportionately among individuals with healthy religious upbringings. Likewise, more research needs to be conducted to understand the role of religion and spirituality in the incidence of other mental disorders, such as bipolar, somatoform, eating, or personality disorders.

Also, nearly all research has emphasized the importance of considering the religious or spiritual background of individuals with mental illness to aid in assessment and the construction of effective treatment plans. Useful tools for assessment are vital in developing effective treatment strategies. One should take into account the relationship between sociodemographic factors and individuals' religious or spiritual beliefs. Likewise, it is also important to consider the specific cultural backgrounds of the individuals. Though many people around the world may have the same religious affiliation, religious beliefs and practices vary based on factors such as ethnic culture and family culture. To do a proper assessment, a therapist should investigate these influences. Integrating religion and spirituality into treatment may include the aid of religious professionals, such as clergy. Because trust is important to many individuals seeking therapy, religious individuals may feel most comfortable when treated by a trusted religious professional along with a psychotherapist.

Because religion and spirituality may play an important role in the etiology, assessment, and recovery process of some individuals with mental illness, holistic models that encompass religion and spirituality may be more useful than traditional models.

REFERENCES

Alvarado, K., Temper, D., Bresler, C., & Dobson, D. (1995). The relationship of religious variables to death depression and death anxiety. *Journal of Clinical Psychology, 51,* 202–204.

Azaunce, M. (1995). Is it schizophrenia or spirit possession? *Journal of Social Distress and the Homeless, 4,* 255–263.

Banks, C. (1997). The imaginative use of religious symbols in subjective experiences of anorexia nervosa. *Psychoanalytic Review, 84,* 227–236.

Barr, C. (1995). Panic disorder: "The fear of fearful feelings." *Journal of Psychology and Christianity, 14,* 112–125.

Bennet, T., Deluca, D. A., & Allen, R. W. (1995). Religion and children with disabilities. *Journal of Religion and Health, 34,* 301–311.

Bernstein, E., Calhoun, D., Cegielksi, C., Latham, A., Shepherd, M.C., Sparks, K. J., Bickel, C., Ciarrocchi, J., Sheers, N., Estadt, B., Powell, D., & Pargament, K. (1995). Perceived stress, religious coping styles, and depressive affect. *Journal of Psychology and Christianity, 17,* 33–34.

Bickel, C. O., Ciarrocchi, J. W., Sheers, N. J., Estadt, B. K., Powell, D. A., & Pargament, K. I. (1998). Perceived stress, religious coping styles, and depressive affect. *Journal of Psychology and Christianity, 17*(1), 33–42.

Blaine, B., & Croker, J. (1995). Religiousness, race, and psychological well-being: Exploring social psychological mediators. *Personality and Social Psychology Bulletin, 21,* 1031–1041.

Borman, P. D., & Dixon, D. N. (1998). Spirituality and the 12 steps of substance abuse recovery. *Journal of Psychology and Theology, 26,* 287–291.

Braam, A., Beekman, A., Deeg, D., Smith, J., & Tilburg, W. (1997). Religiosity as a protective prognostic factor of depression in later life: Results from a community survey in the Netherlands. *Acta Psychiatrica Scandinavica, 96,* 199–205.

Carroll, M. M. (1997). Spirituality, alcoholism, and recovery: An exploratory study. *Alcoholism Treatment Quarterly, 15,* 89–100.

Catipovic, V., Ilakovac, V., Durjancek, J., & Amidzc, V. (1995). Relationship of eight basic emotions with age, sex, education, satisfaction of life needs, and religion. *Psychological Reports, 77,* 115–121.

Chang, B., Noonan, A., & Tennstedt, S. (1998). The role of religion/spirituality in coping with caregiving for disabled elders. *Gerontologist, 38,* 463–470.

Chapman, R. J. (1996). Spirituality in the treatment of alcoholism: A worldview approach. *Counseling and Values, 41,* 39–50.

Clements, R. (1998). Intrinsic religious motivation and attitudes toward death among the elderly. *Current Psychology: Developmental, Learning, Personality, and Social, 17,* 237–248.

Connors, G. J., & Dermen, K. H. (1996). Characteristics of participants in Secular Organizations for Sobriety (SOS). *American Journal of Drug Alcohol Abuse, 22,* 281–295.

Cornet, C. (1998). *The soul of psychotherapy: Recapturing the spiritual dimensions in the therapeutic encounter.* New York: Free Press.

Cosar, B., Kocal, N., Arikan, Z., & Isik, E. (1997). Suicide attempts among Turkish psychiatric patients.*Canadian Journal of Psychiatry, 42,* 1072–1075.

Davis, N., Clance, P., & Gailis, A. (1999). Treatment approaches for obese and overweight African American women: A consideration of cultural dimensions. *Psychotherapy, 36,* 27–35.

Day, S., & Peters, E. (1998). The incidence of schizotypy in new religious movements. *Personality and Individual Differences, 27,* 55–67.

Diener, E., Suh, E. M., Lucas, R. E., & Smith, H. L. (1999). Subjective well-being: Three decades of progress. *Psychological Bulletin, 125,* 276–302.

Donahue, M. J., & Benson, P. L. (1995). Religion and the well- being of adolescents. *Journal of Social Issues, 51,* 145–160.

Ellison, C. G. (1998). Introduction to symposium: Religion, health, and well-being. *Journal for the Scientific Study of Religion, 37,* 692–694.

Emmons, R., Cheung, C., & Tehrani, K. (1998). Assessing spirituality through personal goals: Implications for research on religion and subjective well-being. *Social Indicators Research, 45,* 391–422.

Fallot, R. (1998). The place of spirituality and religion in mental health services. In R. Fallot (Ed.), *Spirituality and religion in recovery from mental illness: New directions for mental health services* (pp. 3–12). San Francisco: Jossey-Bass.

Fischer, L., & Richards, P. S. (1998). Religion and guilt in childhood. In J. Bybee (Ed.), *Guilt and children* (pp. 139–155). San Diego, CA: Academic Press.

Fleming, M., & Anderson, B. (1998). Spiritual Well-Being Scale: Ethnic differences between Caucasians and African-Americans. *Journal of Psychology and Theology, 26,* 358–364.

Frame, M. W., & Williams, C. B. (1996). Counseling African Americans: Integrating spirituality in therapy. *Counseling and Values, 41,* 2–16.

Garret, C. (1996). Recovery from anorexia nervosa: A Durkheimian interpretation. *Social Science and Medicine, 43,* 1489–1506.

Gilbert, B. (1998). *The pastoral care of depression: A guidebook.* New York: Haworth Pastoral Press.

Gillis, J. S., & Mubhashar, M. H. (1995). Risk factors for drug abuse in Pakistan: A replication. *Psychological Reports, 76,* 99–108.

Goldfarb, L. M., Galanter, M., McDowell, D., Lifshutz, H., & Dermatis, H. (1996). Medical student and patient attitudes toward religion and spirituality in the recovery process. *American Journal of Drug and Alcohol Abuse, 22,* 549–561.

Gopal, M. (1997). The role of religion in psychotherapy: A cross-cultural examination. *Journal of Contemporary Psychotherapy, 27,* 34–48.

Green, L. L., Fullilove, M. T., & Fullilove, R. E. (1998). Stories of spiritual awakenings: The nature of spirituality in recovery. *Journal of Substance Abuse Treatment, 15,* 325–331.

Harrington, V., Lackey, N. R., & Gates, M. F. (1996). Needs of caregivers of home and hospice care patients. *Cancer Nursing, 19,* 118–125.

Hinton, J. (1999). The progress of awareness and acceptance of dying assessed in cancer patients and their caring relatives. *Palliative Medicine, 13,* 19–35.

Holtz, T. (1998). Refugee trauma versus torture trauma: A retrospective controlled short study of Tibetan refugees. *Journal of Nervous and Mental Diseases, 186,* 24–34.

Hood-Morris, L. E. (1996). A spiritual well-being model: Use with older women who experience depression. *Issues in Mental Health Nursing, 17,* 439–455.

Idler, E. L., & and Kasl, S. V. (1997). Religion among disabled and non-disabled elderly persons: II. Attendance at religious services as a predictor of the course of disability. *Journal of Gerontology Series B—Psychological Sciences and Social Sciences, 52B,* S306–S316.

Ita, D. (1995–1996). Testing of a causal model: Acceptance of death in hospice patients. *Omega, 32,* 81–82.

Jackson, M. S. (1995). Afrocentric treatment of African American women and their children in residential chemical dependency program. *Journal of Black Studies, 26,* 17–30.

Jackson, M. C., & Fulford, K. W. M. (1997). Spiritual experience and psychopathology. *Philosophy, Psychiatry, and Psychology, 1,* 41–65.

Jahangir, F. (1995). Third force therapy and its impact on treatment outcome. *International Journal for the Psychology of Religion, 5,* 125–129.

Jahangir, F., ur Rehman, H., & Jan, T. (1998). Degree of religiosity and vulnerability to suicidal attempt/plan in depressive patients among Afghan refugees. *International Journal for the Psychology of Religion, 8,* 265–269.

Kaplan, M., Marks, G., & Mertens, S. (1997). Distress and coping among women with HIV infection: Preliminary findings from a multiethnic sample. *American Journal of Orthopsychiatry, 37,* 80–91.

Kazanigian, M. A. (1997). The spiritual and psychological explanation for experience. *Hospice Journal, 12,* 17–27.

Kendler, K. S., Gardner, C. O., & Prescott, C. A. (1996). Religion, psychopathology, and substance use and abuse: A multimeasure, genetic-epidemiologic study. *American Journal of Psychiatry, 154,* 322–329.

258   FAITH AND HEALTH IN SPECIAL POPULATIONS

Koenig, H. (1995a). Religion and older men in prison. *International Journal of Geriatric Psychiatry*, 10, 219–230.

Koenig, H. (1995b). *Research on religion and aging: An annotated bibliography.* Westport, CT: Greenwood Press.

Koenig, H., Hays, J., George, L., Blazer, D., Larson, D., & Landerman, L. (1997). Modeling the cross-sectional relationship between religion, physical health, social support, and depressive symptoms. *American Journal of Geriatric Psychiatry*, 5, 131–144.

Koenig, H., Weiner, D., Peterson, B., Meador, K., & Keefe, F. (1997). Religious coping in the nursing home: A biopsychosocial model. *International Journal of Psychiatry in Medicine*, 27, 365–376.

Kok, J., & Jongsma, A. (1998). *The pastoral counseling treatment planner.* New York: Wiley.

Levin, J. (1997). The role of the Black Church in community medicine. *Journal of the National Medical Association*, 76, 477–483.

Levin, J., & Taylor, R. (1998). Panel analyses of religious involvement and well-being in African-Americans: Contemporaneous vs. longitudinal effects. *Journal for the Scientific Study of Religion*, 37, 695–709.

Livneh, H., Antonak, R., & Maron, S. (1995). Progeria: Medical aspects, psychosocial perspectives, and intervention guidelines. *Death Studies*, 19, 433–452.

Lotufo-Neto, F. (1996). The prevalence of mental disorders among clergy in Sao Paulo, Brazil. *Journal of Psychology and Theology*, 24, 313–322.

MacGreen, D. (1997). Spirituality as a coping resource. *Behavior Therapist*, 20, 28.

May, A. (1997). Psychopathology and religion in the era of "enlightened science": A case report. *European Journal of Psychiatry*, 11, 14–20.

McCourt, J., & Waller, G. (1996). The influence of sociocultural factors on the eating psychopathology of Asian women in British society. *European Eating Disorders Review*, 4, 73–83.

McCreery, C., & Claridge, G. (1995). Out of body experiences and personality. *Journal of the Society for Psychological Research*, 60, 129–148.

McCullough, M. (1999). Research on religion-accommodative counseling: Review and meta-analysis. *Journal of Counseling Psychology*, 46, 92–98.

Mickley, J., Carson, V., & Soeken, L. (1995). Religion and adult mental health: State of the science in nursing. *Issues in Mental Health Nursing*, 16, 345–360.

Mickley, J., Pargament, K., Brant, C., & Hipp, K. (1998). God and the search for meaning among hospice caregivers. *Hospice Journal*, 13, 1–17.

Miller, L., Warner, V., Wickramaratne, P., & Weissman, M. (1997). Religiosity and depression: Ten-year follow-up of depressed mothers and offspring. *Journal of the American Academy of Child and Adolescent Psychiatry*, 36, 1416–1425.

Miller, W. R. (1998). Researching the spiritual dimensions of alcohol and other drug problems. *Addiction*, 93, 979–990.

Miller, W., & Thoresen, C. (1999). Spirituality and health. In W. Miller (Ed.), *Integrating spirituality into treatment: Resources for practitioners* (pp. 6–19). Washington, DC: American Psychological Association.

Morell, C. (1996). Radicalizing recovery: Addiction, spirituality, and politics. *Social Work*, 41, 306–312.

Navarro, J., Wilson, S., Berger, L., & Taylor, T. (1997). Substance abuse and spirituality: A program for Native American students. *American Journal of Health Behavior, 21,* 3–11.

Nealon-Woods, M. A., Ferrari, J. R., & Jason, L. A. (1995). Twelve-step program use among Oxford house residents: Spirituality or social support in sobriety? *Journal of Substance Abuse, 7,* 311–318.

O'Neil, D., & Kenny, E. (1998). Spirituality in chronic illness. *IMAGE: Journal of Nursing Scholarship, 30,* 275–280.

Pardini, D., Plante, T. G., & Sherman, A. (2001). Strength of religious faith and its association with mental health outcomes among recovering alcoholics and addicts. *Journal of Substance Abuse Treatment, 19,* 347–354.

Pargament, K. I., & Park, C. L. (1996). Merely a defense? The variety of religious means and ends. *Journal of Social Issues, 51,* 13–32.

Peele, S. (1997). Utilizing culture and behavior in epidemiological models of alcohol consumption and consequences for Western nations. *Alcohol and Alcoholism, 32,* 51–64.

Plante, T. G., & Boccaccini, M. (1997). The Santa Clara Strength of Religious Faith Questionnaire. *Pastoral Psychology, 45,* 375–387.

Plante, T. G., Manuel, G., Menendez, A., & Marcotte, D. (1995). Coping with stress among Salvadoran immigrants. *Hispanic Journal of Behavioral Sciences, 17,* 471–479.

Plante, T. G., Saucedo, B., & Rice, C. (2001). The association between religious faith and coping with daily stress. *Pastoral Psychology, 49,* 291–300.

Plante, T. G., Yancey, S., Sherman, A., Guertin, M., & Pardini, D. (1999). Further validation for the Santa Clara Strength of Religious Faith Questionnaire. *Pastoral Psychology, 48,* 11–21.

Rajarathinam, R. M., & Muthusamy, R. (1996). Pattern of substance abuse in Salem: A three-year study. *International Medical Journal, 3,* 309–312.

Rapheal, F., Rani, S., Bale, R., & Drummond, L. (1996). Religion, ethnicity and obsessive–compulsive disorder. *International Journal of Social Psychiatry, 42,* 38–44.

Razali, S., Hasanah, C., Aminah, K., & Subramaniam, M. (1998). Religious sociocultural psychotherapy in patients with anxiety and depression. *Australian and New Zealand Journal of Psychiatry, 32,* 867–872.

Reese, D., & Brown, D. (1997). Psychosocial and spiritual care in hospice: Differences between nursing, social work, and clergy. *Hospice Journal, 12,* 29–41.

Richards, P., & Bergin, A. (Eds.). (2000). *Handbook of psychotherapy and religious diversity.* Washington, DC: American Psychological Association.

Richards, P., Hardman, R., Frost, H., Berrett, M., Clark-Sly, J., & Anderson, D. (1997). Spiritual issues and interventions in treatment of patients with eating disorders. *Eating Disorders: The Journal of Treatment and Prevention, 5,* 261–279.

Richards, P., Rector, J. M., & Tjeltveit, A. (1999). Values, spirituality, and psychotherapy. In W. Miller (Ed.), *Integrating spirituality into treatment: Resources for practitioners* (pp. 133–160). Washington, DC: American Psychological Association.

Richards, T., & Folkman, S. (1997). Spiritual aspects of loss at the time of a partner's death from AIDS. *Death Studies, 21,* 527–552.

Ruiz, P. (1998). The role of culture in psychiatric care. *American Journal of Psychiatry, 155,* 1763–1765.

Schaler, J. A. (1996). Spiritual thinking in addiction-treatment providers: The Spiritual Belief Scale. *Alcoholism Treatment Quarterly, 14,* 7–33.

Schneider, S. (1997). Jerusalem, religious awakenings and schizophrenia. *Group Analysis, 30,* 379–393.

Selway, D., & Ashman, A. F. (1998). Disability, religion and health: A literature review in search of the spiritual dimensions of disability. *Disability and Society, 13,* 429–439.

Shapiro, S., Schwartz, G., & Bonner, G. (1998). Effects of mindfulness-based stress reduction on medical and premedical students. *Journal of Behavioral Medicine, 21,* 581–599.

Shooka, A., Al-Haddad, M., & Raees, A. (1998). OCD in Bahrain: A phenomenological profile. *International Journal of Social Psychiatry, 44,* 147–154.

Sommer, S. M. (1997). The experience of long-term recovering alcoholics in Alcoholics Anonymous: Perspectives of therapy. *Alcoholism Treatment Quarterly, 15,* 75–80.

Tapanya, S., Nicki, R., & Jarusawad, O. (1997). Worry and Intrinsic/extrinsic religious orientation among Buddhist (Thai) and Christian (Canadian) elderly persons. *International Journal of Aging and Human Development, 44,* 73–83.

Thearle, M. J., Vance, J., Najman, J., Embelton, G., & Foster, W. (1995). Church attendance, religious affiliation and parental responses to sudden infant death, neonatal death and stillbirth. *Omega, 31,* 51–58.

Trenholm, P., Trent, J., & Compton, W. C. (1998). Negative religious conflict as a predictor of panic disorder. *Journal of Clinical Psychology, 54*(1), 59–65.

Varon, S. R., & Riley, A. W. (1999). Relationship between maternal church attendance and adolescent mental health and social functioning. *Psychiatric Services, 50,* 799–805.

Vick, R. D., Smith, L. M., & Herrera, C. I. (1998). The healing circle: An alternative path to alcoholism recovery. *Counseling and Values, 42,* 133–141.

Vitz, P., & Mango, P. (1997). Kernbergian psychodynamics and religious aspects of the forgiveness process. *Journal of Psychology and Theology, 25,* 72–80.

Wahass, S., & Kent, G. (1997a). Coping with auditory hallucinations: A cross-cultural comparison between Western (British) and non-Western (Saudi Arabian) patients. *Journal of Nervous and Mental Disease, 185,* 664–668.

Wahass, S., & Kent, G. (1997b). The modification of psychological interventions for persistent auditory hallucinations to an Islamic culture. *Behavioral and Cognitive Psychotherapy, 24,* 351–364.

Wahass, S., & Kent, G. (1997c). The modification of psychological interventions for persistent auditory hallucinations to an Islamic culture. *Behavioral and Cognitive Psychotherapy, 25*(4), 351–364.

Walsh, J. (1995). The impact of schizophrenia on clients' religious beliefs: Implications for families. *Families in Society, 76,* 551–558.

Warfield, R. D., & Goldstein, M. B. (1996). Spirituality: The key to recovery from alcoholism. *Counseling and Values, 40,* 196–205.

Watson, P., Milliron, J., Morris, R., & Hood, R. (1994). Religion and rationality: II. Comparative analysis of rational-emotive and intrinsically religious irrationalities. *Journal of Psychology and Christianity, 13,* 373–384.

Wilcock, A., Van Der Arend, H., Darling, K., Scholz, J., Siddaly, R., Snigg, C., & Stephens, J. (1998). An exploratory study of people's perceptions and experiences of well-being. *British Journal of Occupational Therapy, 61,* 75–82.

Wing, D. M., Crow, S. S., & Thompson, T. (1995). An ethnonursing study of Muscogee Indians and effective health care practices for treating alcohol abuse. *Family and Community Health, 18,* 52–64.

Woods, T., Antoni, M., Ironson, G., & Kling, D. (1999) Religiosity is associated with affective and immune status in symptomatic HIV-infected gay men. *Journal of Psychosomatic Research, 46,* 165–176.

PART III

◄O►

FAITH AND HEALTH
IN THE CLINIC

11

‑<O>‑

ASSESSING RELIGIOUS AND SPIRITUAL CONCERNS IN PSYCHOTHERAPY

JOHN T. CHIRBAN

Many clinicians are beginning to recognize the value of religion and spirituality in the lives of their patients, as well as the significance of these factors for emotional and physical well-being. Research on this subject is, however, only in its infancy, and assessment remains complicated in a clinical setting. This chapter explains the importance of addressing and assessing religion and spirituality in treatment and examines problems inherent to this task. It also identifies specific dimensions that are relevant to explore in psychotherapy. Following the proposal of the Religion and Spiritual History Inventory, which identifies salient components for assessing the roles of religion and spirituality in a patient's life, this chapter addresses challenges regarding the clinician's role.

CHANGING ATTITUDES ABOUT ASSESSING RELIGIOUS AND SPIRITUAL ISSUES IN PSYCHOTHERAPY

At the dawn of the third millennium, a truce has been called in the historical standoff between psychology and religion. Vande Kemp (1996) reports that while most prominent psychologists have examined religion, it has not been integrated into the mainstream of psychotherapy. Psychologists today are beginning to recognize the significance of attending to religious and spiritual concerns, both generally in their work and more specifically within psychotherapeutic settings. Now the voices calling for psychologists to address religious concerns are overcoming those of critics who assess this endeavor as "unscientific" and "nonpsychological." Opponents argue that religion and spiritual factors can, among other things: (1) confuse treatment by introducing nonscientific phenomena; (2) create conflicts between therapist and patient, both in cases in which they share common beliefs and in which their beliefs are divergent; (3) introduce different goals and criteria that confound treatment; and (4) introduce phenomena unrelated to the goals of psychology, which is appropriately driven by the scientific method (Aguinis & Aguinis, 1995; Hoshmond, 1995; Ward, 1995). And yet, despite these criticisms, psychology has inaugurated an active partnership with religion and spirituality, adding a spiritual dimension to therapy.

In fact, while we are witnessing a renaissance of the holistic, psychosomatic view of the person, which introduces or reintroduces the φυχή (*psyche*, the Greek for "soul") into psychology and psychiatry (Chirban, in press), these fields have further extended their reach to include religious concerns in psychotherapy. Psychology is now addressing religious issues with fervor. Hill and Hood's volume (1999) provides reviews of 126 assessment measures of psychology and religion dating from 1935, and the authors promise a companion volume on measures of spirituality. Several recent texts (including works published by the American Psychological Association) discuss the importance of addressing religion and spirituality in therapy and advocate screening this dimension (Kelly, 1995; Miller, 1999; Shafranske, 1996; see also Tan & Dong, Chapter 12, this volume). Such works represent a significant shift in psychology's treatment of religion.

Nevertheless, the absence of attention to spirituality and religion in psychotherapy in the past has left clinicians uncertain about how to approach these issues. They are now encouraged to consider concerns that heretofore have been perceived as taboo or unrelated to their task. Clinicians admit discomfort with this area, as 85% of clinical psychologists report having little or no training in psychology in relation to religion (Shafranske, 2000; Shafranske & Malony, 1990; see also Shafranske, Chapter 13, this volume). Currently, few therapists systematically seek information about their clients' religiosity and spirituality (Richards & Bergin, 1997).

Radical changes in attitudes concerning the use and role of religion and spirituality in psychology, coupled with clinicians' lack of training in addressing these issues, present serious questions:

1. Is entertaining religious or spiritual concerns consistent with the clinician's theoretical perspective and therapeutic stance?
2. How does the clinician's response to these issues affect treatment?

3. What is an appropriate approach for addressing religious and spiritual concerns?

Assessing this area in therapy requires discernment of the impact of religion and spirituality in the life of a patient. As with other clinical assessments, it accounts for both resources and problems and attends to the impact of the clinician in the process of evaluation. The first part of this chapter offers guidelines for assessing spiritual and religious concerns in psychotherapy: What are the benefits of assessing these issues, and which specific areas should the clinician address? The second part considers the process of assessment: What problems might arise during assessment? How is the evaluation shaped by the person of the clinician and the therapeutic relationships? What guidelines might help direct the inquiry?

TREATMENT CONCERNS

Why Assess Spiritual Issues in Psychotherapy?

There are several reasons why religious and spiritual issues are significant for psychotherapy. First, the shift in psychology's reception of religion and spirituality, from skeptical to enthusiastic, is driven by compelling health-outcome research that shows the potential benefits of religion and spirituality for psychological well-being and for the reduction of physical, emotional, and spiritual illness (Benson & Stark, 1996; Larson & Milano, 1995; Merwick, 1995). As discussed elsewhere in this volume, people with stronger religious or spiritual involvement appear to demonstrate lower mortality rates, a lower frequency of certain illnesses, and better mental health than their nonparticipatory counterparts (Gorsuch, 1994; Levin & Chatters, 1998, McCullough & Larson, 1999; see also Thoresen, Harris, & Oman, Chapter 2, McCullough, Chapter 3, and Plante & Sharma, Chapter 10, this volume). This empirical factor may be the catalyst for greater acceptance of religion and spirituality in psychology.

Second, religion and spirituality express existential needs. Therefore, one's faith may promote the determination and integration of one's goals, providing meaning and purpose. In this process, the values and commitment of one's faith may provide guidance for coping with and peacefully managing daily life. Psychological problems are often manifestations of existential sickness (Maddi, 1970).

Third, by engaging and understanding religion and spirituality, the clinician enters an area of central concern and passion. Quite often, the patient's most intense positive and negative feelings are connected to his or her religious and spiritual experiences. Tapping such experiences may reveal significant clinical information about a patient: values, relationships, personality, goals, and emotional resources.

Fourth, appreciation of patients' religious and spiritual dimension is essential to the assessment process because it allows clinicians to determine whether patients' religious views are idiosyncratic and possibly diagnostic, conventional and reflective of the patients' traditions, or both. Whereas in one person's history psychological problems may stem from religious and spiritual concerns, for another person religion and spirituality may provide a resource for healing from an emotional difficulty. Identification of resources, strengths, and supports constitutes a standard part of an initial interview. On the other hand, religious traditions may lead people in conflicting directions. One clergyman directed his parishioner, who was depressed, to stop seeing the psychiatrist to whom I had referred him; the clergyman argued that faith in God would be his parishioner's long-term cure. Not knowing that the patient was suicidal nor understanding the potential risks of such advice, the clergyman advocated an action that could have been fatal. Unless clinicians attend to patients' religious and spiritual issues, they will not know of such conflicts or have the opportunity to resolve them.

Fifth, although psychologists themselves continue to be less involved in religion and spiritual practices than most Americans, the sociocultural changes of a "spiritual renaissance" have dramatically increased Americans' spiritual activity. One survey found that over 80% of the population believed in God or a spiritual force but that they did not necessarily practice religion or hold religious beliefs (Lukoff, Francis, & Turner, 1992). Additionally, it is noteworthy that under the umbrella of spirituality fits a wide range of practices—from traditional customs to New Age religion and goddess circles to meditation and the martial arts. Lukoff, Lu, and Turner (1998) speculated that the increasing percentages of people who report contact with the dead, visions, extrasensory perception, mystical experiences, and other unusual occurrences may forecast an increase in spiritually related problems in psychotherapy. Here, it is noted that the term "religious" becomes so broadly inclusive that it may lose its meaning.

Obviously, religious and spiritual affiliation or participation does not provide automatic health improvements for all. For example, religion may subsume followers, suppressing their self-concept and self-esteem. It appears that such factors as restrictive religious forces or a condemning deity sometimes exert a negative influence on participants (Gorsuch & Miller, 1999). Kate Lowenthal (1995, p. 121) writes that religion may be associated with poor mental health:

> Fanaticism, persecution, and indifference to suffering all have a common feature—cruelty. They may also have similar psychological roots. They are also held up, rightly, as a shameful and all too frequent feature of orga-

nized religion. Holy wars, martyrs, inquisition, crusade, pogrom . . . the worst atrocities in human history are carried out in the name of religion, supposedly justified by religion.

At times, religion has been shown to contribute to poor social adjustment or increased health risks (Fitchett & Handzo, 1998; Gorsuch, 1994). So it is not religion or spirituality in the broad sense (i.e., generalized identification) but rather particular experiences of religion and spirituality (e.g., prayer, connectedness), that promote well-being—or, conversely, that can cause unhealthy experiences and account for the negative attitudes toward religion that have characterized the field of psychology.

Religions and spiritualities vary widely—even within particular denominations. Conceptual differences, methodological problems, and measurement difficulties have resulted in little consensus about standardized measures for assessing religion and spirituality. In view of these complications, some find good reason to challenge the entire endeavor of attending to spiritual concerns in health care, regrettably throwing out the baby with the bathwater. It is fair to say that such concerns need to be ironed out; however, it does not appear prudent to disavow or disregard that which one does not fully understand. So, in the clinical setting, in which one inevitably encounters both the multiplicity of variables that define religion and spirituality and the complexity involved in addressing the patient's growth and development, the clinician must determine the basis and plan for his or her own work in this area.

Different Meanings of Religion among Different Clinicians: The Case of B. F. Skinner

In my professional psychological development, B. F. Skinner provided the principal challenge to my beliefs and my approach to psychology. Our first discussions, which began in the early 1970s, reflected our very different histories and polarized understandings of human nature—both psychologically and spiritually. Skinner was an experimental scientist, the father of strict behaviorism; his religious roots stemmed from Presbyterianism and out of the theology of Jonathan Edwards. Before studying psychology, I was a student of Greek Orthodox theology; although ecclectic in my approach to psychology, psychodynamic principles undergirded my orientation. Skinner had low expectations of religion; I had high expectations. He found no nurturance through faith or God; I found that faith and God were strengthening and sustaining. Our lenses were different.

In the mid-1980s, when Skinner was working on a book concerning ethics and behavior, we embarked on weekly conversations over several years, this time collaboratively, to analyze and to explore our understanding of "the spiritual" from our different perspectives. Skinner previously had presented himself as antireligious and even atheistic. Our discussions revealed the origins of his psychology—as well as his curious preoccupation as a utopian philosopher. Our weekly systemic discussions over the last 5 years of his life provide a case example of how striking the effects of religious experiences may be, even for an avowed nonbeliever.

I learned that, in fact, Skinner's early religious experiences were powerful. In his autobiography, *Particulars of My Life* (1976), he wrote:

> The first religious teaching I can remember was at my grandmother Skinner's. It was her desire that I should never tell a lie, and she attempted to fortify me against it by vividly describing the punishment for it. I remember being shown the coal fire in the heating stove and told that little children who told lies were thrown in a place like that after they died. . . . Some time later I went to a magician's show the final act of which concerned the appearance of a devil. I was terrified. I questioned my father as to whether a devil just like that threw little boys to Hell and he assured me it was so. I suppose I have never recovered from that spiritual torture. Not long afterward I did tell a real lie to avoid punishment and that bothered me for years. I remember lying awake at night sobbing, refusing to tell my mother the trouble, refusing to kiss her goodnight. I can still feel the remorse, the terror, the despair of my young heart at the time. . . . (Skinner, 1976, p. 60)

His family's literalistic, punitive image of religion was averse to the spirit as I understand it. To what extent did such experiences affect his perception that religion is negative and aversive?

As we spoke, it became more and more evident how our beliefs shaped our psychology. In *A Matter of Consequences*, Skinner (1983) openly acknowledged that much of his scientific position had its roots in Presbyterian theology. His point of view in psychology that there is no choice and no freedom and the importance he placed on external control found a conspicuous parallel with the theology of the Congregation of Jonathan Edwards.

In one of our conversations, Skinner shared the following:

> There was always a certain element of fear. Not exactly that I might have the wrong religion . . . [such as] be a Presbyterian instead of Catholic. I went to Sunday school, but I never stayed on. I had a certain amount of fear of religion, I suppose. So that when I finally escaped, it would have been an element of relief, although it took me a long time. I remember when I was a freshman in college I was still somewhat bothered by . . . worried . . . about religion. I remember going to the professor of philosophy and telling him that I had lost my faith. The fact that the biologist, whom I liked and admired very much, taught Sunday school bothered me. These were problems. (in Chirban, 1992)

As we spoke, I recognized that Skinner's argument was not against what I called "spirituality"; his suspicion of spirituality resulted from the abuses in religion that he personally felt. Moreover, his own yearnings fueled his fervor to understand and to create the positive that he could not find. This hopeful wish asserted itself in his identity as a utopian visionary (Skinner, 1983). He told me, "what you say does not sound like religion . . . [it] seems to me very close to what I've been working on" (in Chirban, 1996a, p. 82). His understanding of the term "spirituality" depended on callow images and childhood associations. He did not equate religion with spiritual experiences. In our discussions, he stated that heretofore he had not seen the religious experiences that I reported as having anything to do with spirituality, yet these spiritual experiences he called "feeling states," which he judged as very significant for psychology. For example, he elaborated on his commitment to psychology's role in creating a better future for humanity and was interested in how spiritual paths might support that through cultural conditioning. In the end, we considered how the integration of the viable expression of the spirit was critical for both faith and science.

So our challenge as therapists is to understand and to discern how and why religion and the spiritual are understood and experienced by the patient. Much may be inferred when patients or therapists refer to the general constructs of "religion" and "spirituality." However, little is really understood by these terms unless we take the time necessary to find out what such terms mean spiritually and imply psychologically for the particular person.

Approaches for Understanding Religion and Spirituality

Although researchers have developed and refined several quantitative measures to assess religion and spirituality over several decades (Gorsuch & Miller, 1999; Hill & Hood, 1999; see also Sherman & Simonton, Chapter 6, this volume), an adequate or comprehensive measurement of this dimension for the clinical setting does not exist. Additionally, structured questionnaires are not optimal for generating personal explorations and in-depth introspection consistent with therapy. The clinician's primary concern is to consider the individual's own perception of religion and spirituality in view of the multiplicity of variables associated with a religious and spiritual framework. Therefore, an open-ended interviewing approach is proposed for clinical settings—the Religion and Spiritual History Inventory (RSHI). This approach engages a deeper, more extensive understanding than brief research questionnaires and highlights particular experiences that have implications for the patient's psychological well-being.

Within the medical setting, several interviews have been developed to address aspects of religion and spirituality as a legitimate and purposeful area for inquiry (Fitchett & Handzo, 1998; Kuhn, 1988; Maugans, 1996). Some of these clinical assessments may be relevant for psychotherapy as well. For example, a functional six-stage assessment of spiritual needs was developed by Stoddard (1993) to identify levels of spiritual concerns based on specific symptoms and to assist with directing referrals to chaplains.

In contrast, the RSHI was developed for use in psychotherapy and was intended to allow for a richer, more comprehensive exploration than is usually feasible in medical settings. This interview provides a broad framework for understanding the patient's religion and spirituality and offers an opportunity for the patient's self-assessment of this matter.

Religion and Spiritual History Interview

The RSHI is outlined in the appendix to this chapter. As with most clinical evaluations, this interview evolves in conjunction with the patient's needs and treatment questions. It is recommended that during initial screening, general inquiries be made of patients regarding their religious and spiritual affiliations and current participation. A clinical determination is required to assess the extent to which the RSHI should be implemented and the appropriateness of using standardized assessment in this area. For example, much of the interview may be used with a patient who is struggling with existential concerns, identity and self-concept, or depression; yet it may be contraindicated and counterproductive for someone with paranoid personality disorder or psychotic processes.

As with most treatments, religious and spiritual matters should be addressed in accordance with the patient's intent and motivation. Therefore, a religious and spiritual history must be tailored to the patient, drawing out psychologically relevant religious and spiritual themes based on clinical judgment of the patient's needs.

This interview concerns issues relating to most patients, whether or not they describe themselves as religious, agnostic, atheistic, spiritual, or uninterested in spirituality. The inventory explores a wide range of interpretations and understandings of the words "spirituality" and "religion" that relate to the patient's meaning, self-awareness, and relationships. Additionally, the inventory prompts discussion of the common boundary between religious and spiritual issues and existential concerns. Therefore, this assessment merits similar attention if the patient is spiritually oriented and expressing overt religious conflicts or is having spiritual conflicts but is unaware of their connection with his or her clinical problems and is overtly spiritually uninterested.

The RSHI invites exploration of several themes that research has shown to be significant. These include, among others, the following:

Family History. Most people retain the tradition with which they were raised. The appropriation of one's family's religious tradition—particularly as one embraces intrinsic values of faith that are expressed, shown, and celebrated in the family—influences one's convictions and identity formation more generally. Alternatively, whether or not a patient has rebelled against the family may also correspond to his or her religious and spiritual choices. Therefore, it is important to distinguish between religious preference, church affiliation, and involvement in organized religion.

Religious Affiliation. Worldwide, the majority of people are associated with a religious denomination (Richards & Bergin, 1997). One's religious tradition informs both religious symbols and language and also heightens one's sensitivity to particular experiences and concerns in life. For example, a religious Hindu who suffers a difficult phase in his or her life may accept this as a test of his or her ability to respond to a Divine challenge, leading him or her to be rewarded in the next life. In contrast, a Reform Jew may feel that God's challenge is for all people to achieve everything that is within their power in the here and now; therefore, his or her attitude toward difficult phases of life may differ from the Hindu's. In this way, different religious traditions may direct the patient to a different framework of meaning and actions.

Religious and Spiritual Development. In James Fowler's work (Fowler 1981, 1996; Fowler & Keen, 1985), which is based on both theology and psychology, expression of religiousness and spirituality is viewed as moving through discrete, universal stages. For example, although an adult's formal education about God may stem from a third-grade Sunday School class, his or her expression of faith may demonstrate a far more evolved understanding reflective of his or her growth and change. Fowler's structural/developmental paradigm describes an individual's progression in faith across seven variables that characterize his or her faith system: (1) form of logic, (2) form of world coherence, (3) role taking, (4) boundaries of social awareness, (5) moral judgment, (6) role of symbols, and (7) locus of authority. The RSHI may be helpful in drawing out pertinent information to assess the patient's stage of faith.

Intrinsic/Extrinsic Religious Motivation. Allport's (Allport & Ross, 1967) research in intrinsic and extrinsic religion describes intrinsic faith as part of personality, by which one is spiritual and devout by nature. Those with a mature, intrinsic orientation find their master motive in religion. By contrast, extrinsic faith fulfills external or peripheral needs. Those with an extrinsic orientation use religion for their own ends; they turn to God but without turning away from self. Patients' comments about what gives life meaning and purpose and about their commitment to and experiences with faith help the clinician to understand patients' psychological goals within a broader context of values, faith, and commitments that are internally or externally driven (Chirban, 1981). Intrinsicness is a mature religious orientation that has been positively linked with emotional and social adjustment, whereas extrinsic, immature religious adjustment has been correlated negatively with adjustment (Richards & Bergin, 1997). Additionally, the clinician may find a relationship between the patient's internalized and externalized faith orientation and his or her personality style (Axis II in the *Diagnostic and Statistical Manual of Mental Disorders* [DSM IV-TR], American Psychiatric Association, 2000). Specific personality styles may contribute to a more or less intrinsic or extrinsic orientation. For example, those with hysterical traits may be driven to an extrinsic religious orientation, whereas those with avoidant traits may adopt better to an internal religious orientation.

God's Image. Research suggests that several factors influence one's image of God, including parental relationships, relationships with significant others, self-esteem, religious instruction, and religious practices. It appears that parental relationships and self-esteem affect one's image of God most strongly. Those who experienced loving, nurturing relationships and possessed positive self-esteem tended to view God as accepting, forgiving, and loving (Richards & Bergin, 1997). The perception of God, as both a physical and a spiritual being, is often "exquisitely particular" (Rizzuto, 1992, p. 57) as a function of one's religion, culture, and emotional development (Rizzuto, 1979). God images are held both consciously and unconsciously as one may not be aware of the functions of an internal representation. Thus a child's perception of God may reflect his or her self-interpretive processes, serving as a major element in the child's view of self, others, and the world.

Problem Solving and Coping. Pargament (1997; Pargament et al., 1988) identified three styles of religious problem solving that characterize basic approaches to standard life events: deferring, self-directing, and collaborative. Those with a deferring style "defer" responsibility to God; those with a self-directing style favor an active problem-solving approach in which God is not directly involved; those with a collaborative style maintain a posture jointly with God in problem solving. Research on coping has focused on the role of religion in an individual's search for meaning and efforts to meet life's challenges. Pargament's (1997) work suggests that different types of religious coping may yield various results: On the helpful end of the spectrum were coping strategies such as spiritual support, collaborative religious coping, benevolent religious reframing, and congregational support; harmful strategies included expressions of discontent with congregation and God and negative reframing. Some coping strategies had mixed implications (religious rituals, self-directing and deferring religious coping, and religious conversion).

Religious Practices. Most religious traditions encourage specific rituals and activities and prohibit others. For example, prayer and meditation have been particularly linked with health and well-being (Goldbourt, Yaeri, & Madalie, 1993). Also, religious fasting and dietary requirements have been linked with beneficial effects on health. Conversely, religious prohibitions may also affect health. Note the proscription against blood transfusions for Jehovah's Witnesses and allopathic medical care by Christian Scientists (Maugans, 1996).

Spiritual Experience. Personal spiritual experiences may be another important area for assessment. Research by Kass and colleagues (1991) focused on "core spiritual experiences," involving a sense of closeness to God or perceptions that God dwells within. They found that medical patients who reported these experiences demonstrated greater life purpose and satisfaction and less frequent medical symptoms than those who did not.

Other dimensions of religiousness and spirituality that are assessed by the RSHI can be found in the Appendix to this chapter.

THE CHALLENGE THE CLINICIAN FACES IN ASSESSING RELIGION AND SPIRITUALITY

The Process of Addressing Religious and Spiritual Material

Discussing religion and spirituality is often difficult, even for a religious clinician. Nevertheless, to a great extent, it is the therapist who determines how the concerns and questions of religion and spirituality will be approached and examined, and, indeed whether they will be approached at all. Therefore, whether the patient's problems center on religious issues or whether religion might simply serve as a vehicle for understanding the patient's psychology, the therapist must make the critical decision of whether and how to deal with religion.

Religion and spirituality are expressed in many facets of a person's life (biological, psychological, relational, intimate, familial/sociological, and spiritual); each expression reveals a different aspect of his or her psychic and relational self. In order to address an individual's psychology, clinicians should consider all these dimensions and be trained to treat them. When clinicians are attuned to the various nuances of religion and spirituality, they deepen their understanding of their patients' problems and of the different modalities through which religion and spirituality are expressed. So how does one know which dimensions of religion and spirituality are at issue? What does one assess?

The Multimodal Perspective

Sometimes, because one has a hammer, every problem looks like a nail. If a clinician has been trained to approach an issue in only one way or to see only a specific problem or use only a particular tool—as some have with regard to religious and spiritual issues—he or she may not be open to other effective perspectives or options.

The hammer may be the clinician's theoretical model, theological position, or attention to single variables and partial aspects of religion and spirituality to the exclusion of wider considerations. There is no magic bullet, no all-purpose strategy to assess religion and spirituality, so the clinician needs to stay alert to what shapes religious or spiritual concerns or problems for the patient.

A multimodal assessment of religion and spirituality requires attunement to a multilevel interlocking cycle. I approach religious and spiritual concerns by generally examining five areas: biological dimensions (age, sex, and health); psychological dimensions (emotional issues, developmental issues, and personality styles); relational dynamics (personal and familial relationships); sociological dimensions (culture, social group, norms, traditions, and customs); and spiritual dimensions (values, beliefs, and faith system). Although these areas are not mutually exclusive, they provide important information about the different sources and influences of religion and spirituality in the patient's life. For example, consider these important aspects of the five areas:

- *Biological*: Health- and life-threatening experiences may play a significant role in existential concerns.
- *Emotional*: Developmental needs, personality, and mental health may lead one to gravitate to specific religious or spiritual solutions.
- *Relational*: Dyadic dynamics with others, especially family members, may significantly affect the patient's choice in religion.
- *Sociological*: The patient's cultural experiences may have played a significant role in his or her religious identity. Also, cultural expectations may create internal and relational conflicts when one confronts different customs.
- *Spiritual*: Religion and spirituality potentially contain both numerous positive and negative elements. Religion and spirituality may engender feelings of guilt, fear, and denial of self and life; or they may establish meaning and value that enhance life.

Any of these areas may be the focus of clinical concern—and all of these dimensions may play a role. The challenge for the clinician is to assess related areas and pursue a plan that is integrative. To determine which area or areas to focus on, the clinician should review the patient's history of religion and spirituality, in conjunction with the clinical question or diagnosis. Such a history assesses the areas of the multimodal model outlined here and directs the clinician to the system most implicated. The clinician's skill, perceptiveness, and art are called on equally for the assessment and treatment plan.

The Interactive–Relational Perspective

As patients discuss issues of religion and spirituality with the clinician, they may reveal some of their most private experiences—even ones they have never shared with another person. If the clinician displays attention and respect, patients will become more open. Patients present their religious and spiritual concerns as a function of their urgency and of the level of comfort or understanding that they perceive in their relationship with the clinician.

The interactive–relational approach (Chirban, 1996a; in press) proposes a helpful perspective for assessing religious issues in therapy by emphasizing the impact of the clinician on the therapeutic process. It emphasizes the importance of the clinician's empathetic qualities and what the clinician brings, through his or her person, to the therapeutic encounter. The clinician's own personal characteristics (both positive and negative), beliefs, and values are recognized as significant to the treatment process with respect to the clinician's conscious and unconscious self-disclosure. Furthermore, while it is important to recognize the relationship of the clinician and patient in terms of transfer-- ence and countertransference, these do not account for the real, genuine dimensions of the relationship that are critical for treatment. The clinician's role is important not only with regard to his or her professional intervention but also with regard to who he or she is and how his or her particular relationship with the patient affects the treatment. The interactive–relational perspective provides one way of addressing religious issues in the therapeutic relationship; it underscores how both client and clinician are affected by the vulnerability that comes with addressing sensitive concerns.

Before proposing specific recommendations for addressing religious and spiritual material in the therapeutic setting, I identify five broad goals for clinicians regarding their approach to these issues.

First, express openness about and engage the patient's religion, spirituality, and existential concerns. During the initial consultation, inquire about the patient's religious identification and involvement. Religion and spirituality constitute a basic area that a clinician should address, regardless of the presenting problem, just as he or she addresses the patient's general health, education, and family background. The mere question signals the clinician's openness to discuss such material. On the basis of the patient's response, other questions may follow, regarding whether he or she participates in religious activities and the perceived meaning or values of those experiences. The intention here is to clarify the role of spirituality in the patient's life. In my experience, it has not been unusual for a patient to respond, "Oh, you're asking about that," implying, "That's actually very important to me, but I never thought we'd discuss it here." Patients have learned to separate treatments for body, mind, and soul, and they present themselves according to what they anticipate various professionals will expect. Such fragmentation often leads the patient to edit out critical information and, more disturbingly, to feel isolated and alone. By expressing openness to religious and spiritual concerns, the clinician conveys that all aspects of the patient's life are of concern.

On the other hand, in my view, it is not the task of the clinician especially to nurture faith but rather to consider it and understand it in view of the clinical objectives. An article (Sloan, Bagiella, & Powell, 1999) quoting an American Medical Association publication discussed the fact that clinicians were being asked to inquire of patients, "What can I do to *support* [emphasis added] your faith or religious commitment?" This question implies that the clinician is knowledgeable and trained to "support" the patient's religious commitment, which sets up expectations that the clinician may not be able to fulfill. Additionally, this question suggests that the authority of the clinician's professional role transfers to the religious field. I feel that this may cross the line of professional responsibility. The professional concern regarding the patient's religion and spirituality may be more supportively expressed in the question, "How can we understand your problem in view of your faith?"

I have found that many clergy and faithful laity often prefer psychological counseling of spiritual and emotional concerns to pastoral counseling because of their apprehension regarding confidentiality, judgment, and role confusion. I feel that therapists should respond affirmatively to the question "Does the patient feel free to share concerns, feelings, or experiences about religious and spiritual issues?"

Second, recognize the integrity of the patient's religion and spirituality and do not reduce them with psychological interpretations. The anticipated lack of support for religious and spiritual issues on the part of mental health professionals often dissuades patients from revealing their spiritual side, precluding a potential treatment resource and potentially masking significant issues of the patient's life in general. Assessing the patient's religious and spiritual dimension allows the clinician both to learn about the patient's traditions and to relate the patient's faith and culture to his or her psychological concerns. Does the patient feel that his or her beliefs are understood or merely psychologized, pathologized, or interpreted in reductionist categories?

Third, appreciate the intrinsic, passionate, and formative value of the patient's religion and spirituality. Engaging a patient in a discussion of his or her religion and spirituality may tap a wellspring of deep personal experiences, influences, and wishes. How do the patient's religious and spiritual concerns affect daily life?

Fourth, explore the impact of the religious and spiritual dimension for the patient. The clinician may explore enhancements, as well as problematic aspects, of integrating the patient's religious and spiritual life with the other dimensions of his or her life. How do religion and spirituality relate to his or her psychological functioning?

Fifth, understand the impact of religion and spirituality on the therapeutic relationship. As treatments that engage religion and spirituality promote appreciation of the patient's most personal and passionate concerns, the clinician cultivates a connection with the patient, affirming the individual, reducing feelings of isolation, and understanding the patient as more than merely a psychological case. By understanding how spiritual values enhance the patient's relationships with others, the clinician enhances his or her connection with the patient (Chirban, 1996b). Does the discussion of religion enhance this therapeutic relationship?

The Clinician's Perspective

Although psychologists today feel more free to assess religion in psychotherapy, there is little uniformity, much less standardized guidelines, in this assessment. Over the years, in fact, several distinct clinical approaches have evolved. Albert Einstein (Watzlawick, 1977) noted, "It is theory which decides what we observe." Our values influence what we understand as fact.

Freud (1927/1961) and Skinner (1953), whose models guided traditional mental health care, maintained a negative and reductionist approach, which was skeptical of religion and spirituality and explained them exclusively in terms of these men's own respective theoretical perspectives. Rizzuto (1979) and Meissner (1984), demonstrating a neutral perspective, presented a descriptive approach that sought to explain why individuals develop and how they process religious concerns. Jung (1933) and Frankl (1962) embraced a positive approach to spiritual issues, considering this dimension essential and innate. Most recently, Richards and Bergin (1997) advocated a theistic approach, which proposes a spiritual strategy for mainstream psychology and psychotherapy. This posture assumes that "God exists, that human beings are the creations of God, and that there are unseen spiritual processes by which the link between God and humanity is maintained" (Richards & Bergin, 1997).

To address the religious and spiritual dimension, the clinician must feel both personally and professionally prepared. It is one thing to require psychologists to be sensitive to religious issues (as required by the ethical guidelines of the American Psychological Association, 1992) and another to expect that psychologists will assess these concerns uniformly or in ways that are not affected by their own beliefs. Because of the personal, educational, psychophilosophical, and psychotheoretical issues involved, clinicians should clarify their readiness in the following four areas.

First, clinicians should clarify their own psychoreligious stance. Although clinicians are not expected to be religious or spiritual guides or to specialize in this area, they cannot pursue this critical dimension effectively without having a consistent perspective. Various approaches have been advanced. Tan (1996) notes that clinicians have addressed religion in psychotherapy through either an implicit or explicit integration. An *implicit* integration describes the clinician who does not initiate discussion of religious and spiritual content, such as prayer, Scripture, or other religious practices, but who is open to discussing spiritual concerns raised by the patient; an *explicit* integration describes the clinician who proactively introduces this discussion. The clinician should establish an approach that corroborates his or her personal and theoretical beliefs but does not limit attention to the broader possibilities and dimensions of religious matters. In this process, the clinician should also take an inventory of his or her own religious and spiritual history. By such an exploration, through the RSHI proposed here, for example, the clinician may clarify issues for himself or herself. Such self-examination may not resolve one's beliefs, but it may at least create an awareness of personal issues, thereby reducing countertransference, if not enhancing the clinician's own self-awareness.

Second, clinicians should acquire a basic knowledge of patients' religion and spirituality. In order to interpret and understand the role and function of religion and spirituality in a patient's life, the clinician must have a basic appreciation of the patient's traditions, rituals, and beliefs. Several books have been written providing guidance for clinicians about the implications of specific religious traditions for counseling and psychotherapy (Kelly, 1995; Richards & Bergin, 2000).

Third, clinicians should differentiate between legitimate and problematic uses of religion and spirituality. Multicultural sensitivity has encouraged a psychological climate that is open to a wide range of human experiences and behaviors (Bhugra, 1996), as well as an unbiased objectivity that transfers well to normative religious and spiritual expression. However, the clinician must balance the goals of supporting the values held by the patient and resolving conflicts within these values.

Fourth, clinicians should address the transferential and countertransferential dimensions of religion and spirituality. Spiritual material inevitably intensifies transference, resistance, and countertransference, which may complicate the therapeutic process. Just as with other personally sensitive themes, such as sexuality and politics, the clinician must feel personally and professionally comfortable and proceed with vigilance. Although spiritual issues provide opportunities for understanding the patient in greater depth, the mismanagement of such issues creates the possibilities of confusing boundaries and roles and of misunderstanding the patient's struggle.

Countertransference

The words "religion" and "spirituality" have different meanings for and stir different responses in both patient and clinician. So the clinician is susceptible to unconscious forces out of his or her own history that may affect treatment regardless of well-meaning intentions. In view of the power of the clinician to attend to, pursue, and direct—as well as curtail or disengage—exploration of religion and spirituality, the clinician must monitor countertransference.

Even before commencing treatment the clinician should consider the following:

1. Clarify his or her approach to addressing religion and spirituality in therapy. It can be helpful to patients if, when asked, the clinician articulates his or her clinical approach to and treatment plan for addressing these issues.
2. Assess the degree to which his or her understanding of and interest in pursuing religious and spiritual material matches the patient's objectives. Additionally, when the clinician has a clear understanding of his or her objectives in addressing religion and spirituality, the ethical boundaries of treatment must remain focused.
3. Recognize his or her basic prejudices, biases, and values regarding the nature of "healthy" spirituality. It is important to identify one's own religious and spiritual values separate from those of the patient.
4. Modulate language so that it is genuine, professional, and in synchrony with the patient's. The clinician may need to clarify his or her use of terms and express sensitivity to the meanings that religion and spirituality hold for the patient.

The assessment and understanding of religion and spirituality should be driven by the pursuit of identified psychological objectives and the religious needs of the patient and not engaged in or curtailed because of the clinician's personal issues. Psychoanalysts have drawn attention to the concept of "intersubjectivity" (Stolorow, 1991) to emphasize how each party in the therapeutic relationship necessarily evokes personal responses, fundamental values, and beliefs.

The Vulnerability of Talking about Religion and Spirituality

Guided by multidimensional assessment models and an integrative perspective, a broad range of clinicians who do not consider themselves pastoral psychologists are in a position to treat religious issues. Yet some clinicians still do not feel comfortable discussing these matters, even after engaging in appropriate training and supervision, and refer patients with such concerns to specially trained clinicians for particular interventions. It is always appropriate to refer patients to other specialists when their concerns are beyond the clinician's ability to address them; however, sometimes the precipitant of this decision stems from the clinician's vulnerability in addressing religion and spirituality.

Religion and spirituality constitute an arena that is very private and one in which patients and clinicians may be psychologically vulnerable. These issues raise particularly important questions for clinicians regarding comfort:

- How has the clinician's own religious and spiritual experiences affected his or her ability to treat these issues?
- Given that one's thoughts and feelings about religion and spirituality tend to be kept personal and are revealed only when one feels profound trust, at what point does the clinician address the religious or spiritual feelings and countertransference that are elicited in therapy?

For both patient and clinician, longings for connectedness and meaning elicit reactions that lie along a continuum from collusions to subtle verbal and nonverbal encouragement, discouragement, and judgment of particular material in therapy. Conscious discomfort with religion and spirituality on the part of the clinician is often conveyed through inappropriate management of religious and spiritual topics (directing, minimizing, and evading religious material). Unconscious discomforts are often expressed through nonverbal communication, including body responses, silence, tone of voice, particular choices of words, laughter, and interpretations. Patients sense these messages (Chirban, 2001).

Spero (1981) offers specific suggestions for therapists to increase their awareness of religious and spiritual countertransference by recognizing: (1) counselor–client similarities in religious and spiritual values that do not have the same origin and function in the client as in the counselor; (2) shared religious and spiritual values that may lead to collusive avoidance rather than to clarifying and perhaps challenging exploration of beliefs and practice; (3) clinician–client dissimilarities in religious and spiritual beliefs, practices, and development that lead to the counselor's negative or dismissive reaction to the religious/spiritual dimension of clients' behavior; (4) clinician's religious enthusiasm that may lead to misfocusing on religious and spiritual issues at the expense of more pertinent dynamic factors; and (5) intrusions of interested third parties (e.g., clergy, relatives, teachers) whose religious and spiritual convictions may spark strong affective reactions in the clinician (Kelly, 1995).

If therapy generally is an intimate experience, then addressing religious and spiritual issues in therapy intensifies this intimacy. Most clinicians recognize that they have religious sentiments, feelings, or commitments, but they do not address or integrate these issues. Clinicians need to confront such reticence and seriously attend to this material.

The task of assessing religion and spirituality involves an understanding of the implications of the patient's beliefs, with an eye toward clarifying how these beliefs may enhance or complicate the patient's well-being. By carefully monitoring countertransference, one is not embroiled in the rightness or wrongness of beliefs but achieves a deeper appreciation of often highly significant factors that affect the patient.

CONCLUSIONS

This chapter has emphasized the importance of assessing religious and spiritual material in psychotherapy in order to ascertain a fuller and deeper understanding of the patient. This discussion considered problems inherent in the assessment of religion and spirituality for the clinical setting. Although definitional, methodological, and measurement difficulties exist, religious issues should not be abandoned in psychotherapy given their significance for emotional well-being.

If we are to understand the effects of religion and spirituality on health, we will need to be sensitive to the inherently ambiguous, mysterious, and sometimes elusive aspects of these fields. Competent supervision and training in these issues are essential for clinicians. As psychology continues to explore the significance of religion and spirituality and as research defines which aspects of these dimensions constitute healthy and unhealthy experiences, with sensitivity to bias, assessment instruments will continue to be refined. It is important that these efforts maintain an appreciation for the complexity inherent in psychological work involving religion and spirituality; this significant dimension should never again suffer sweeping reductionism, be approached as unidimensional, or, worst of all, be discounted. A caveat is made regarding expectations of assessing religious and spiritual issues. Given the essential subject matter of religion and spirituality (i.e., concerns of faith, goodness, and holiness), while applying scientific methodology to understand better such phenomena, "humility" is needed regarding the extent and capability possible of the scientific methodology ever to measure thoroughly religion and spiritual experiences.

The RSHI has been presented to offer specific guidelines for inquiry regarding spirituality and religion. Additionally, recommendations have been offered to assist the clinician in the assessment and management of his or her countertransference regarding religious and spiritual material. Treatment begins when the therapist provides opportunities for the patient to explore and discover him- or herself through a relationship that is characterized by cohesion and trust. Discussion of religious and spiritual concerns, when approached with both openness and discretion, allows the patient and clinician to develop such a relationship. Through the process of assessing spiritual and religious concerns in psychotherapy, personal freedom—a goal shared by psychotherapy and by religion and spirituality—is within our grasp.

APPENDIX.
RELIGION AND SPIRITUAL HISTORY INVENTORY

This religious and spiritual history inventory presents an outline that incorporates basic lines of inquiry for ascertaining a patient's religious history. It is not intended as a standard questionnaire to be implemented verbatim as part of a psychological interview. On the basis of the interviewee's clinical needs, the clinician may select directions of inquiry suggested by this outline to explore specific aspects of religion and spirituality in the patient's life.

I. Current Information
  A. Patient:
    1. Age:
    2. Sex:
    3. Marital status:
    4. Religion:
    5. Cultural background:
    6. Education:
    7. Occupation:
  B. Parents (names):
    1. Ages:
    2. If deceased, dates of death and ages at death:
    3. Birthplaces:
    4. Marital status (married, separated, divorced, remarried):
    5. Religions:
    6. Cultural backgrounds:
    7. Educations:
    8. Occupations:
    9. Attitudes toward religion and spirituality:
    10. Commitments to religious or spiritual practice:
    11. Quality of relationship with your parents:
    12. Quality of relationship between parents:
  C. Siblings:
    1. Ages:
    2. Sexes:

    3. Marital statuses:
    4. Religions:
    5. Educations:
    6. Occupations:
    7. Attitudes toward religion and spirituality:
    8. Your feelings toward siblings:
  D. Marital partner (name):
    1. Age:
    2. Sex:
    3. Marital status:
    4. Religion:
    5. Education:
    6. Cultural background:
    7. Occupation:
    8. Attitudes toward religion and spirituality:
    9. Quality of relationship with marital partner:
    10. Spouse's attitudes and practices concerning religion and spirituality—
        e.g., does he or she share beliefs and practices?
  E. Children (names):
    1. Ages:
    2. Sexes:
    3. Marital statuses:
    4. Religions:
    5. Educations:
    6. Occupations:
    7. Attitudes toward religion and spirituality:
    8. Quality of your relationship with your children:
    9. Quality of your children's relationships among one another:

II. Childhood Religion and Spirituality
  A. Attitudes toward religion and spirituality in family of origin
    1. Quality of these attitudes: Positive   Neutral   Negative
    2. Frequency of discussion of religion in the home:
    3. Practices of religion (in community/home)—e.g., prayer at meals,
       church attendance:
    4. Do you think your parents believed in God? Explain.
  B. Experiences with religion and spirituality during childhood
    1. Significant sources for learning about religion:
    2. Significant impressions about religion—e.g., earliest memory:
    3. At what age:
    4. Degree of interest in religion and spirituality as a child:
    5. Relationship with God, the Transcendent, or Higher Power as a
       child:
    6. Experience with and frequency of prayer as a child:

C. Formal religious education
 1. Experience with organized religion and/or formal roles in religious traditions during childhood:
 2. Significance of religious traditions during childhood:
 (Go to IV, D if patient is a child.)

III. Adolescent Religion and Spirituality
 A. Changes in religious or spiritual convictions during adolescence
  1. Degree/nature of changes:
  2. Effect of these changes on family life:
  3. Effect of these changes on personal life:
  4. Effect of these changes on social life:
 B. Experience with religion and spirituality during adolescence
  1. Significant sources of learning about religion:
  2. At what age:
  3. Degree of interest in religion and spirituality as an adolescent:
  4. Relationship with God, the Transcendent, or a Higher Power as an adolescent:
  5. Experience with and frequency of prayer as an adolescent:
 C. Formal religious education
  1. Experience with organized religion and/or formal roles in religious traditions during adolescence:
  2. Significance of religious traditions during adolescence:
  3. Did religious thinking influence in any way your attitudes toward: dating, sexuality, identity, and intimacy?
  (Go to IV, D if patient is an adolescent.)

IV. Adulthood Religion and Spirituality
 A. Changes in religious or spiritual convictions during adulthood
  1. Degree/nature of changes:
  2. Effect of these changes on family life:
  3. Effect of these changes on personal life:
  4. Effect of these changes on social life:
 B. Experience with religion and spirituality during adulthood
  1. Significant sources of learning about religion:
  2. At what age(s):
  3. Do you believe in God?
  4. Degree of interest in religion and spirituality:
  5. Relationship with God, the Transcendent, or a Higher Power:
  6. Experience with and frequency of prayer:
 C. Formal religious education
  1. Experience with organized religion and/or formal roles with religious community during adulthood:
  2. Significance of religious traditions during adult life:

D. Why is spirituality/religion/God important to you or not important to you?

E. Current experience with religion and spirituality

   1. Do you consider yourself a religious person? Explain.

   2. Does religious ritual or symbolism play a part in your life? Fasting? Retreats? Confession? Meditation? Other spiritual activities:

   3. Do you pray? When do you pray? Does God or a Higher Power answer your prayers?

   4. What are your feelings about God or a Higher Power?

   5. How do you imagine, define, or picture God? (Option: illustrate)

   6. Do you believe in an afterlife? Why or why not?

   7. Are your current beliefs similar to those of your family? If so, how deeply have your parents' beliefs shaped and determined your own? If not, to what do you attribute your differing ideologies?

   8. What have your beliefs meant to you?

   9. Do religion and spirituality affect your daily life? Explain.

  10. What aspects of your religion and spirituality are most appealing?

  11. What aspects of your religion are least appealing? Are there any that you do not uphold? Explain.

  12. Describe any conversions or extraordinary religious experiences. What has been your most moving spiritual experience?

  13. What gives your life meaning? Explain.

  14. What do you feel is the purpose of life? Explain.

  15. What are the beliefs and values that guide your life? Explain.

  16. Do you believe that there is one true religion? Explain.

  17. When you feel despair, what renews your hope? Explain.

  18. Do you draw on your religion and spirituality during difficult or stressful times? Explain. Note:
(Behavioral, e.g., church attendance, specific details)
(Cognitive, e.g., seeking "answers")
(Affective, e.g., comfort enhancement)
(Existential, e.g., God's plan)

  19. To what extent does your religion and spirituality provide you with fellowship or connection to others? Explain.

  20. How do you understand the relationship between your religion and spirituality and the concerns and work of therapy? Explain.

  21. When you encounter problems, do you then turn them over to God ("Thy Will be done")? Do you handle them yourself, or do you work together with God?
Explain.

  22. Have you experienced the presence of holiness, sacredness, or awe? Explain.

V. Personal Comments

REFERENCES

Aguinis, H., & Aguinis, M. (1995). Integrating psychological science and religion. *American Psychologist, 50*(7), 541–542.

Allport, G. W., & Ross, J. M. (1967). Personal religious orientation and prejudice. *Journal of Personality and Social Psychology, 5*, 432–443.

American Psychiatric Association. (2000). *Diagnostic and statistical manual of mental disorders IV-TR* (DSM IV-TR). Washington, DC: Author.

American Psychological Association. (1992). Ethical principles of psychologists and code of conduct. *American Psychologist, 47*, 1597–1611.

Benson, J., & Stark, M. (1996). Reason to believe. *Natural Health, 26*(3), 72–78.

Bhugra, D. (1996). Religion and mental health. In D. Bhugra (Ed.), *Psychiatry and religion: Context, consensus and controversies* (pp. 1–4). London: Routledge.

Chirban, J. T. (1981). *Human growth and faith: Intrinsic and extrinsic motivation in human development.* Washington, DC: University Press of America.

Chirban, J. T. (1992, August). *B. F. Skinner's struggle with religion.* Invited address presented at the annual meeting of the American Psychological Association, Washington, DC.

Chirban, J. T. (1996a). *Interviewing in depth: The interactive–relational approach.* Thousand Oaks, CA: Sage.

Chirban, J. T. (1996b). Spiritual discernment and differential diagnosis: Interdisciplinary concerns. In J. T. Chirban (Ed.), *Personhood: Orthodox Christianity and the connection between body, mind, and soul* (pp. 35–43). Westport, CT: Bergin & Garvey.

Chirban, J. T. (2001). Introduction. In J. T. Chirban (Ed.), *Sickness or sin? Spiritual discernment and differential diagnosis* (pp. 1–9). Brookline, MA: Holy Cross Press.

Chirban, J. T. (in press). Enhancing the skills of mental health practitioners: Treating mind and body and spirit. In D. S. Satin (Ed.), *The twenty-second annual Erich Lindemann memorial lecture.* New York: Jason Aronson.

Fitchett, G., & Handzo, G. (1998). Spiritual assessment, screening, and intervention. In J. C. Holland (Ed.), *Psycho-oncology* (pp. 790–808). New York: Oxford University Press.

Fowler, J. W. (1981). *Stages of faith: The psychology of human development and the quest for meaning.* New York: Harper & Row.

Fowler, J. W. (1996). Pluralism and oneness in religious experiences: William James, faith development theory, and clinical practice. In E. P. Shafrankse (Ed.), *Religion and the clinical practice of psychology* (pp. 165–186). Washington, DC: American Psychological Association.

Fowler, J. W., & Keen, S. (1985). First presentation: Jim Fowler—Life patterns: Structure of trust and loyalty. In J. W. Bergman (Ed.), *Life maps: Conversations on the journey of faith* (pp. 14–101). Waco, TX: Word Books.

Frankl, V. E. (1963). *Man's search for meaning: An introduction to logotherapy* (I. Lasch, Trans.). Boston: Beacon Press.

Freud, S. (1961). Future of an illusion. In J. Strachey (Ed. and Trans.), *The standard edition of the complete works of Sigmund Freud* (Vol. 21, pp. 1–57). London: Hogarth Press. (Original work published 1927)

Goldbourt, U., Yaeri, S., & Madalie, J. H. (1993). Factors predictive of longterm coronary heart disease mortality among 10,059 male Israeli civil servants and municipal employees. *Cardiology, 82,* 100–121.

Gorsuch, R. (1994). Religious aspects of substance abuse and recovery. *Journal of Special Issues, 51,* 65–83.

Gorsuch, R. L., & Miller, W. R. (1999). Assessing spirituality. In W. R. Miller (Ed.), *Integrating spirituality into treatment: Resources for practitioners* (pp. 147–164). Washington, DC: American Psychological Association.

Hill, P. C., & Hood, R. W., Jr. (1999). *Measures of religiosity.* Birmingham, AL: Religious Education Press.

Hoshmond, L. T. (1995). Psychology's ethic of belief. *American Psychologist, 50*(7), 540.

Jung, C. G. (1933). *Modern man in search of a soul.* New York: Harcourt, Brace & World.

Kass, J. D., Friedman, R., & Lesserman, J., Lesserman, J., Zuttermeister, P. C., & Benson, H. (1991). Health outcomes and a new index of spiritual experience. *Journal for the Scientific Study of Religion, 30*(2), 203–211.

Kelly, E. W., Jr. (1995). *Spirituality and religion in counseling and psychotherapy: Diversity in theory and practice.* Alexandria, VA: American Counseling Association.

Kuhn, C. C. (1988). A spiritual inventory of the medically ill patient. *Psychiatric Medicine, 6*(2), 87–99.

Larson, A. D., & Milano, M. (1995). Are religion and spirituality clinically relevant in health care? *Mind/Body Medicine, 1*(3), 147–157.

Levin, J. S., & Chatters, L. M. (1998). Research on religion and mental health: An overview of empirical findings and theoretical issues. In H. G. Koenig, (Ed.), *Handbook of religion and mental health* (pp. 33–50). San Diego, CA: Academic Press.

Lowenthal, K. M. (1995). *Mental health and religion.* London: Chapman & Hall.

Lukoff, D., Francis, L., & Turner, R. (1992). Towards a more culturally sensitive DSM-IV: Psychoreligious and psychospiritual problems. *Journal of Nervous and Mental Diseases, 180,* 673–682.

Lukoff, D., Lu, D., & Turner, R. P. (1998). From spiritual emergence to spiritual problem: The transpersonal roots of the new DSM-IV category. *Journal of Humanistic Psychology, 38*(2), 21–50.

Maddi, S. R. (1970). The search for meaning. In W. S. Arnold & M. Page (Eds.), *Nebraska Symposium on Motivation* (Vol. 18, pp. 137–186). Lincoln, NB: University of Nebraska.

Maugans, T. A. (1996). The spiritual history. *Archives of Family Medicine, 5,* 11–16.

McCullough, M. E., & Larson, D. B. (1999). In W. R. Miller (Ed.), *Integrating spirituality into prayer treatment: Resources for practitioners* (pp. 85–110). Washington, DC: American Psychological Association.

Meissner, W. W. (1984). *Psychoanalysis and religious experience.* New Haven, CT: Yale University Press.

Merwick, C. (1995). Should physicians prescribe prayers for health? Spiritual aspects of well-being considered. *Journal of the American Medical Association, 273* (20), 1561–1562.

Miller, W. R. (Ed.). (1999). *Integrating spirituality into treatment: Prayer resources for practitioners.* Washington, DC: American Psychological Association.

Pargament, K. I. (1997). *The psychology of religion and coping: Theory, research, practice.* New York: Guilford Press.

Pargament, K. I., Kennell, J., Hathaway, W., Grevengoed, N., Newman, J., & Jones, W. (1988). Religion and the problem-solving process: Three styles of coping. *Journal for the Scientific Study of Religion, 27,* 90–104.

Richards, P. S., & Bergin, A. E. (1997). *A spiritual strategy for counseling and psychotherapy.* Washington, DC: American Psychological Association.

Richards, P. S., & Bergin, A. E. (Eds.). (2000). *Handbook of psychotherapy and religious diversity.* Washington, DC: American Psychological Association.

Rizzuto, A. (1979). *The birth of the living God: A psychoanalytic study.* Chicago: University of Chicago Press.

Rizzuto, A. (1992). Christian worshipping and psychoanalysis in spiritual truth. In J. T. Chirban (Ed.), *Personhood: Orthodox Christianity and the connection between body, mind, and soul* (pp. 51–60). Westport, CT: Bergin & Garvey.

Shafranske, E. P. (Ed.). (1996). *Religion and the clinical practice of psychology.* Washington, DC: American Psychological Association.

Shafranske, E. P. (2000). Religious involvement and professional practices of psychiatrists and other mental health professionals. *Psychiatric Annals, 30*(8), 1–8.

Shafranske, E. P., & Malony, N. H. (1990). Clinical psychologists: Religious and spiritual orientations and their practice of psychotherapy. *Psychotherapy, 27,* 72–78.

Skinner, B. F. (1953). *Science and human behavior.* New York: Macmillan.

Skinner, B. F. (1976). *Particulars of my life.* New York: Knopf.

Skinner, B. F. (1983). *A matter of consequences.* New York: Knopf.

Sloan, R. P., Bagiella, E., & Powell, T. (1999). Religion, spirituality, and medicine. *Lancet, 353,* 664–667.

Spero, M. H. (1981). Countertransference in religious therapists of religious patients. *American Journal of Psychotherapy, 35*(4), 565–576.

Stoddard, G. A. (1993). Chaplaincy by referral: An effective model for evaluating staffing needs. *Caregiver Journal, 10*(1), 37–52.

Stolorow, R. (1991). Chapter 2. In R. Curtis (Ed.), *The relational self: Theoretical convergences in psychoanalysis and social psychology.* New York: Guilford.

Tan, S.-Y. (1996). Religion in clinical practice: Implicit and explicit integration. In E. P. Shafranske (Ed.), *Religion and the clinical practice of psychology* (pp. 365–390). Washington, DC: American Psychological Association.

Vande Kemp, H. (1996). Historical perspective: Religion and clinical psychology in America. In E. P. Shafranske (Ed.), *Religion and the clinical practice of psychology* (pp. 71–112). Washington, DC: American Psychological Association.

Watzlawick, P. (1977). *How real is real? Confusion, disinformation, communication.* New York: Guilford Press.

Ward, L. C. (1995). Religion and science are mutually exclusive. *American Psychologist, 50*(7), 542–543.

12

-◄O►-

SPIRITUAL INTERVENTIONS IN HEALING AND WHOLENESS

SIANG-YANG TAN
NATALIE J. DONG

As demonstrated in previous chapters, the connection between faith and health has a growing empirical foundation. Positive correlations have been found to exist between religious factors and physical health (Caine & Kaufman, 1999; George, Larson, Koenig, & McCullough, 2000; King, 2000; Koenig, 1999; Larson & Larson, 1994; Larson, Swyers, & McCullough, 1998; Levin & Vanderpool, 1991). Although reviews of specific aspects of religiosity have yielded relatively consistent positive findings (Bergin, 1991; Payne, Bergin, Bielema, & Jenkins, 1991), the specific nature of the relationship between religious factors and health outcomes is unclear (Hill & Butter, 1995). It is clear, however, that the high population base rates of religiosity indicate that a large portion of patients presenting for medical or mental health care will have significant religious beliefs and practices (Rowan, 1996). With about 95% of the United States population declaring belief in God (Miller, 1999), health care providers must be sensitive to religious and spiritual concerns. We believe they should also be aware of ways in which they or others can intervene spiritually to help bring healing and wholeness.

HEALTH AND WHOLENESS

In this chapter, we take the approach that the state of health, or being healthy, is not simply the absence of disease or illness. Although the presence of a physical disease process contributes significantly to a lack of health, it is certainly possible for a person to be free of disease yet still not feel healthy. There is a subjective quality to health that may be more adequately incorporated by the terms "wholeness" or "wellness" (see also Diener, 2000; Myers, 2000a, 2000b). Miley (1999) utilizes the concept of well-being to address this more holistic, subjective approach to health and healing. He contends that how we deal with stress is central to the development and maintenance of well-being. He states that this is the focus of the area of health psychology that deals with the promotion of healthy behaviors and prevention of chronic diseases through behavioral and lifestyle changes. As such, we approach well-being as a broadly conceptualized term encompassing those facets of the individual that impinge on behavior and lifestyle—personality, spiritual beliefs, culture, social context, and cognitions, as well as physical abilities and limitations. A psychology of wholeness thereby precludes the isolation or treatment of one facet of the individual independently from other facets (see also Salovey, Rothman, Detweiler, & Steward, 2000; Taylor, Kemeny, Reed, Bower, & Gruenewald, 2000). We take the approach that the physical, spiritual, and psychological domains of the individual are interrelated and interactive. Therefore, comprehensive treatment of the whole person must be cognizant of, or sensitive to, each of these interactive domains.

Miller and Thoresen (1999) state that "health is better conceived of as a latent construct like personality, character, or happiness, a complex multidimensional construct underlying a broad array of observable phenomena" (p. 4). In Miller and Thoresen's proposed conceptualization, health includes three broad domains: suffering, functional ability, and subjective inner peace or coherence in life. These domains encompass cognitive, emotional, and spiritual aspects of the person, in addition to the physical.

Although the precise definition of the constructs of health and wholeness can be debated, it remains apparent that health is far more than the absence of disease. As stated by Miller and Thoresen (1999), "if health is more than the absence of disease, and broader than the single dimension of suffering, then a healer's task is larger than the detection and eradication of a specific disease state" (p. 5).

SPIRITUALITY

Various definitions of the terms "religion" and "spirituality" have been utilized (see Plante & Sherman, Chapter 1, this volume). Richards and Bergin (2000) define religion as a "subset of the spiritual" (p. 5). In their approach to understanding religion and spirituality, the spiritual refers to experiences, beliefs, and phenomena that touch on the transcendent and existential aspects of life. The religious is understood by Richards and Bergin as having to do with theistic beliefs, practices, and feelings.

In contrast to Richards and Bergin, Pargament (1997) defines religion "as a process, a search for significance in ways related to the sacred" (p. 32) and spirituality as a search for the sacred, so that spirituality is a core function of religion. In this approach, religion is the more broad-based term under which spirituality is subsumed. We have chosen to use this latter definition of religion.

A large majority of North Americans hold a belief in God, a supreme being or supernatural order, life after death, angels, or other supernatural beings. Many of these people consider their spiritual beliefs to be important to finding a source of strength and direction in life. Twelve-step groups are just one example of the pervasive belief in and reliance on some kind of higher supernatural power for strength and direction. Although "spiritual wellness" is itself a debated topic (Ingersoll, 1998), it nonetheless appears that spirituality is an important source of meaning and can be an important component to overall subjective wellness and quality of life (Clark, 1998).

Although spirituality and religion have been distinguished from each other in various ways, religious organizations remain an important resource for improving people's spiritual lives regardless of how "religion" and "spiritual" are defined. Religious organizations, such as churches, synagogues, temples, and mosques, can and do provide a structure and context within which individuals can have spiritual experiences in a corporate setting. Religious organizations can also provide a context in which there are shared experiences of searching for what is sacred, learning ways of entering into spiritual experiences (e.g., fasting, or prayer), transmitting meaning beyond the self, and growing or maintaining a relationship with God. It must also be recognized that some people have unhealthy or negative spiritual experiences within a religious organization or in their own individual spiritual experience. It may therefore be necessary to distinguish individual spiritual experiences from broader religious experiences, beliefs, and teachings.

The interaction between religion and spirituality, as well as the subjective nature of individual experiences, certainly points to the importance of clearly understanding the spiritual and religious beliefs of the individual client prior to utilizing a spiritual or religious intervention. The importance of understanding the client's perspective and world view is addressed by contemporary psychoanalytic subjectivity theories (e.g., Stolorow & Atwood, 1979) with their emphasis on recognizing the different sets of experienced realities held by the therapist and the client. Religious or spiritual beliefs, practices, and experiences must be understood from within the client's world in the same way in which we seek to understand cognitive barriers to treatment, personality variables, or other issues that can impinge on health promotion and maintenance.

CULTURAL CONTEXT IN FAITH AND HEALING

Although culture in itself is not predictive of faith and it's implications for healing and wholeness, culture does provide a broad context within which to understand religious faith and spiritual beliefs. An awareness of the world view and values within cultural groups and across religious beliefs is useful as health care professionals seek to facilitate healing and wholeness in the lives of their patients. In this section, we specifically discuss religious and spiritual themes among Asian Americans and their implications for healing. For information about diverse religious traditions and cultural approaches to faith, the reader is referred to Richards and Bergin (2000; see also Fukuyama & Sevig, 1999). Although awareness of broad cultural patterns is important, the individual patient must also be understood from the perspective of his or her unique beliefs, values, and traditions.

Asian American Culture and Faith Perspectives

To speak of *an* Asian American culture and faith perspective is something of a misnomer. Asian Americans are a diverse group, including people whose origins are Chinese, Japanese, Korean, Filipino, Asian Indian, Southeast Asian, and Pacific Islander. More than 50 groups speaking any of more than 30 different languages are included in this category (Sue, Nakamura, Chung, & Yee-Bradbury, 1994). We discuss traditional belief systems (e.g., Taoism, Buddhism, and Confucian philosophy), in addition to describing the faith perspectives of Christian Asian Americans (see Tan & Dong, 2000).

Traditional Culture, Values, and Beliefs

Traditional Asian ethnic groups often hold beliefs in the existence of the spirit world and a recognition of multiple gods who rule the universe (Hopfe, 1983). Deceased ancestors are often seen as links to the spirit world, and their assistance may be cultivated by maintaining a shrine or altar in the home at which ancestors are remembered and offerings may be made. Illness may be seen as resulting from neglect or offense to ancestors or as the result of malevolent spirits who must be appeased.

Confucian principles have had a widespread influence throughout Asia. A system of ethics focusing on proper or harmonious social order (Hopfe, 1983), Confucian principles influence communication patterns within the family, as well as between the patient and the health professional. Communication is often transmitted through the father or the eldest male in the family, and health professionals are treated with deference and respect. Traditional Asian American families may hesitate to question the authority or judgment of health care professionals and may hesitate to openly assert their wishes or treatment preferences directly to their health care providers.

Buddhist perspectives on fate and suffering may affect traditional Asian responses to illness and personal suffering. A passive acceptance of discomfort or pain may express an approach to suffering as something that must be quietly endured. Some schools of Buddhism assert that all existence is suffering and life is full of pain (Wenhao, Salomon, & Chay, 1993). Consequently, traditional Asian patients may hesitate to seek relief from pain or other discomfort.

Many Asian Americans follow the principles of feng shui, which is a Chinese system of beliefs focused on the proper arrangement of buildings, rooms, furniture, and other objects. According to feng shui, proper placement achieves harmony and balance and thus brings good fortune and good health to the practitioner. The individual who experiences poor health may seek to alter the placement of household objects to achieve the proper flow and balance of energy in the home.

Religious Traditions

Although reliable demographic information is not available, it is apparent that Asian Americans subscribe to a variety of religious belief systems. Whereas over 70% of Korean Americans are Protestant Christians, Filipinos are heavily Catholic (Kim, 1996; Santa Rita, 1996). Chinese Americans may follow Buddhism, ancestor worship, or Christianity; Japanese Americans may follow Shintoism, Buddhism, or Christianity; and Vietnamese Americans are likely to follow Buddhism or Christianity. Other people from Southeast Asia are likely to follow Hinduism, Buddhism, or animism.

Many Asian Christians hold a world view that incorporates the existence of the supernatural, including a belief in the demonic and in spiritual warfare (Tan, 1991a, 1999). Many Asian Christians, particularly in the evangelical and charismatic traditions, rely on intercessory prayer and the power of the Holy Spirit in day to day coping. They may also interpret difficulties or illnesses as the work of demonic forces or spiritual warfare.

APPROACHES TO INTERVENTION

In this section, we describe spiritual interventions that can be implemented by health care professionals at all levels. We also discuss the role of the church in holistic care. Many interventions, such as prayer and meditation, can be implemented by persons subscribing to a variety of spiritual and religious beliefs. We also provide information on spiritual interventions from our own perspective and experience within the Christian tradition.

In spiritual assessment (Hill & Hood, 1999; see also Chirban, Chapter 11, this volume) and intervention it is crucial that health care professionals address the patient from within his or her belief system. Patients should be encouraged to utilize spiritual resources that are consistent with their values and traditions, such as prayer and meditation, and to seek the assistance of spiritual leaders such as pastors, rabbis, and priests. Health care professionals who hold different religious beliefs from their patients can encourage them to seek out spiritual resources from within their faith community.

A substantial body of interdisciplinary literature has been forming to develop a spiritual orientation for psychotherapy and psychology (e.g., Becvar, 1997; Canda & Furman, 1999; Cornett, 1998; Fukuyama & Sevig, 1999; Genia, 1995; Hood, Spilka, Hunsberger, & Gorsuch, 1996; Kelly, 1995; Lovinger, 1990; Miller, 1999; Richards & Bergin, 1997, 2000; Shafranske, 1996; Steere, 1997; Walsh, 1999; West, 2000) and can serve as a basis for exploring spiritual interventions within other disciplines. For example, Richards and Bergin (1997) provide a helpful table summarizing definitions and examples of various religious and spiritual interventions (Harris, Thoresen, McCullough, & Larson, 1999; see also Thoresen, Harris, & Oman, Chapter 2, this volume).

GUIDELINES FOR IMPLEMENTING SPIRITUAL INTERVENTIONS

Spiritual interventions should always be implemented with clinical sensitivity, ethical wisdom, and careful balance to avoid under- or overusing spiritual resources (see Tan, 1996b). The health care provider must use discernment in assessing whether the client is ready to use spiritual resources, especially if the client is not religious or is struggling with his or her faith. When the health care provider differs from the patient on some topic of faith or religious belief, she or he should be careful to maintain a respectful attitude and refrain from imposing his or her opinion on the client. Health care providers should also assess their own competence with spiritual interventions (Tan, 1993, 1996b; Tan & Gregg, 1997; see also Chirban, Chapter 11, and Shafranske, Chapter 13, this volume). Providers who are not comfortable using spiritual interventions or who are not sufficiently trained to be able to do so competently should refer religiously committed patients to appropriate resources within their religious belief systems or to another, more appropriately trained or experienced provider (Tan, 1993).

Tan (1994) discusses a number of potential dangers in the use of religious psychotherapy that are also relevant to the use of spiritual interventions in health care (see also Moon, 1997). The major dangers cited in Tan are as follows:

1. Imposing therapist religious beliefs or values on the client, thus reducing client freedom to choose.

2. Failing to provide sufficient information regarding therapy to the client.
3. Violating the therapeutic contract by focusing mainly or only on religious goals rather than on therapeutic goals.
4. Lacking competence in the area of exploring client values ethically or conducting religious therapy appropriately.
5. Arguing over doctrinal issues rather than clarifying them.
6. Misusing or abusing spiritual resources such as prayer, thus avoiding dealing with painful issues.
7. Blurring important boundaries or parameters necessary for the therapeutic relationship to be maintained.
8. Assuming ecclesiastical authority and performing ecclesiastical functions inappropriately when referral to ecclesiastical leaders may be warranted.
9. Applying only religious interventions to problems that may require medication or other medical and/or psychological treatments.

In spite of its potential dangers, the appropriate use of spiritual interventions can also provide a unique resource to patients. Worthington (1986) identifies a number of concerns held by evangelical Christians that may also apply to other patients who hold strong religious beliefs. He points out that patients may fear that secular therapists will neglect religious concerns, deal with religious belief events as pathological or only psychological, fail to comprehend religious ideas or terminology, presume that religious patients share nonreligious cultural values or norms, promote therapeutic conduct that contradicts their morals, and negate revelation as a valid source of truth.

Even after a determination has been made that explicit spiritual interventions are appropriate and the patient is ready to use spiritual resources, this type of intervention should only be implemented after informed consent to do so has been obtained from the patient (Tan, 1996b; see also Tan, 1994; Richards & Bergin, 1997). Spiritual interventions that are implemented must be relevant to the patient and to his or her problems. Further, spiritual interventions should be tailored to the patient's particular needs and problems rather than using scripted or routine prayers and teaching.

INTERVENTIONS AT THE INDIVIDUAL LEVEL: FOR THE PRACTITIONER

This section focuses on specific approaches to spiritual intervention that can be implemented by the health care provider on behalf of his or her patients or that the health care provider can encourage his or her patients to imple-

ment themselves. Although these interventions can be used by persons subscribing to a variety of religious and spiritual beliefs, we also provide examples arising from our own experience and Christian religious perspective.

Prayer

Prayer is a widely used resource for people in the United States. A 1993 Gallup poll cited by McCullough and Larson (1999) found that 90% of North
Americans pray at least occasionally. Specific prayers for healing can be utilized by the person seeking health and wholeness, by friends or family members, by church or religious group members and leaders, and by members of
the health care profession. Beyond specific requests for physical healing,
prayer can provide the person who prays with greater hope, security, peace,
meaning, alleviation of depression, tension reduction, and increased subjective well-being (Hood et al., 1996; McCullough, 1995; Pargament, 1990).

Health care practitioners can encourage patients who have spiritual or
religious beliefs to pray about their concerns. Prayers can be for specific
requests for healing. However, prayer can also be a resource to facilitate
coping with illness or psychological distress (see Tan, 1996a). Patients who
pray can gain a greater measure of acceptance, peace, comfort, strength,
knowledge of God's will, or closeness to God. The many dimensions of
prayer include, but are not limited to, confession, adoration or praise,
thanksgiving, petition for oneself, and intercession for others (Tan, 1996a).
Prayer can also include being quiet in solitude and simply waiting and listening. Patients can be encouraged to utilize prayer in the form best suited to
them, to help them find strength, courage, hope, and peace.

In addition to encouraging patients to pray themselves or family members to pray for a loved one, health care professionals can pray with or for
their patients themselves. For patients with religious beliefs, prayer by or
with their provider can positively affect the provider–patient relationship.
Patients may feel a stronger alliance with their provider, feel cared for, and
feel a greater sense of being understood. A stronger provider–patient alliance
can facilitate the patient's trust and willingness to comply with treatment
regimens. Providers who offer to pray with or for their patients should carefully evaluate how they will word their offer, because some patients or families may interpret such an offer as a sign of doom or failure by the provider.

Empirical studies of the effects of intercessory prayer on health outcomes (e.g., Byrd, 1988; Sicher, Targ, Moore, & Smith, 1998) have yielded
equivocal results. These studies have been sharply criticized (Dossey, 1993;
see also Sloan, Bagiella, & Powell, Chapter 14, this volume) for a number of
methodological problems. Although research in this area has significant limits, it does provide a tantalizing suggestion that intercessory prayer may
result in tangible positive differences in outcome. However, the possible neg-

ative effects of prayer also need to be further investigated (Dossey, 1997). Care should therefore be taken in who we pray for, how we pray, and what we pray for.

Many religious traditions engage in different forms of prayer. One model of Christian healing prayer is described in detail in Blue (1987; see also Tan, 1996a). This model of prayer includes five steps: (1) interviewing, (2) choosing a prayer strategy, (3) praying for specific results, (4) assessing the results, and (5) giving postprayer direction. Blue states that this model is well suited for use by those who have little or no background in healing ministry to the sick. Caine and Kaufman (1999), also writing from a Christian perspective, suggest the following when using prayer and faith for healing: (1) expressing personal faith, (2) calling for elders to pray for and minister to us, (3) confession of sins, (4) laying on of hands, and (5) use of modern medicine as an avenue of God's healing.

Forgiveness

Harris et al. (1999) provide a useful discussion of the use of forgiveness interventions. Helping clients to learn how to forgive both themselves and others can be a major focus in psychotherapy. Forgiveness can be used with or without reference to religious beliefs (McCullough, Sandage, & Worthington, 1997; Richards & Bergin, 1997) and may be one of the most frequently used forms of spiritual intervention in psychotherapy (Richards & Bergin, 1997).

Patients who are sick or in pain may be experiencing anger toward themselves for past behaviors or choices made, especially if they have influenced the development, maintenance, or exacerbation of a medical condition. Patients may be angry toward others for past events or for medical decisions that they perceive as harmful. Family relationships may erupt in conflict over changing roles and adapting to a sick family member. Helping patients to forgive can reduce their level of hurt, anger, and perceived offense and improve their mood and emotional state (Harris et al., 1999). Forgiving oneself and others can increase subjective well-being in spite of ongoing medical problems.

Laying on of Hands

Touch is a powerful means of communicating caring and promoting healing (for an in-depth examination of the use of touch in psychotherapy, see Hunter & Struve, 1998). Touch has been a significant element of Christian healing, following numerous New Testament examples of Jesus healing the sick through the use of touch (e.g., Matthew 8:14–15). For patients comfortable with this approach, the laying on of hands is a way in which Christian health care providers can continue the healing ministry of Jesus. Other religious traditions may also have specific forms of healing prayer that can be implemented as appropriate.

As with other forms of spiritual intervention, providers must first carefully assess the appropriateness and the positive treatment potential of the intervention. For some patients, particularly those with histories of physical or sexual abuse, the use of touch may be strongly contraindicated. Additionally, caution should be exercised with patients who have difficulties with trust, paranoia, and social avoidance, as well as those for whom touch would be physically painful.

When using the laying on of hands in prayer for healing, Caine and Kaufman (1999) recommend: (1) ask permission first, (2) cultivate an open attitude and free yourself of negative feelings, (3) pray with a partner, (4) use simple but specific prayer requests, (5) visualize while praying, and (6) periodically check with the person being prayed for to see what he or she is experiencing. Health care providers who are not adequately equipped or whose religion does not have a tradition of healing prayer can encourage their patients to seek out spiritual leaders who can minister to them in this way. Many churches have special healing services in which the laying on of hands and intercessory prayer are utilized. Health care providers may find it helpful to identify local churches in which such services are held so that they can appropriately refer interested patients.

Meditation

In some Eastern traditions, meditation offers a means of transcending the illusions of daily life, becoming more conscious of one's immediate experience, or achieving a state of nonjudgmental detachment. Practitioners of meditation can become more attuned to their experiences in the present moment without preconceptions, judgments, and assumptions. By cultivating the practice of meditation, some patients may experience greater calmness, less emotional reactivity to uncomfortable symptoms, and greater appreciation for the present moment. For example, Eastern meditation practices have been used to help patients with chronic pain achieve detachment from their pain and increase their functional abilities (see Kabat-Zinn, 1993).

From a Christian perspective, meditation is a means of seeking attachment to God and entering into His presence (Foster, 1978). Through meditation, the individual may receive specific direction, a word of comfort, or increased peace from spending time with God. Meditation can enhance a patient's sense of God's care for him or her, decrease emotional distress, and enhance emotional resources for coping with pain or illness.

In some Eastern practices, meditation focuses on breathing or on a particular word or object. Meditation can also focus on achieving a state of passively observing one's own mind, simply noticing the thoughts or images, that arise. In this latter approach, practitioners seek to avoid judgment of the thoughts or images as well as to avoid focusing on the thoughts and images themselves. For example, patients who struggle with pain management might seek to passively observe their pain, then let it go and watch it float away like a cloud in the breeze.

One approach to Christian meditation is detailed by Foster (1978). Foster begins with preparing to meditate by seeking an appropriate place and finding a comfortable posture for meditation. Specific meditation exercises, including ones designed to facilitate "centering" (a time to become still), are included.

Tan (1996a) describes David Ray's suggested steps for Christian meditation. These steps include: (1) select a word for the day and a Bible verse to meditate on; (2) get in a comfortable and relaxed position; (3) repeat your meditation cue; (4) use conscious thought to think about your word for the day and your Bible verse; (5) close your eyes to communicate with God more personally; (6) use mental pictures or imagery to let the Bible verse come alive; (7) pray, conversing openly with God, and (8) open your eyes as you end your time of meditation. Meditation on Scripture can be helpful as a way to learn more of God's truth, to grow in trust, and to put one's life into proper perspective.

Solitude and Personal Retreats

In our contemporary society replete with pagers, cell phones, laptop computers, and fax machines, solitude is undervalued and underutilized. Periods of solitude alone with God or in personal retreats can be helpful to the religious or spiritual person who suffers from chronic pain or other illness. "The major thing a private retreat accomplishes is to create an open empty space in our lives" (Foster, cited in Tan, 1996a, p. 99) where we can "come to hear God's speech" (p. 99). Foster (1978) has numerous insights and suggestions regarding solitude and private retreats (see also Tan & Gregg, 1997).

Finding a time of silence and a "quiet place" are essential to solitude. This quiet place can range from a chair in the home to a bench in the park to a weekend mountain cabin. The key is to find or create a place in which the patient is free from distraction and where his or her silence is honored. It is also important to avoid overstructuring this time of solitude. "Sometimes nothing should be done—simply and intentionally 'waste' time for God" (Foster, cited in Tan, 1996a, p. 100).

Solitude and private retreats can help to deepen the patient's relationship with God and increase faith and hope, even during times when God seems distant or doesn't make sense. Periodic times of solitude open a space in which the patient can experience God's love and power, can see with God's perspective, and can know with more certainty that God desires to and will work things out for good (Foster, 1978; Tan, 1996a). A time of retreat and solitude may facilitate the patient's achieving greater acceptance of his or her illness and increase his or her willingness to comply with treatment regimens. Patients may find that their psychological distress is reduced and that they are able to better cope with their pain or illness. Some patients may find that periodic times of retreat enhance their overall quality of life and sense of well-being in spite of their pain or other difficulties.

Fellowship and Worship

As pointed out by Foster (1978), we need to seek a balance of solitude and fellowship in our lives. The support, encouragement, and help of others is crucial to patients who are ill or in pain. Taking time to meet with others, as well as time to be in solitude, is especially important for those who are sick or in pain because "pain not only isolates us from one another, but even from ourselves" (Hauerwas, 1986, p. 77).

In addition to providing support, encouragement, and prayer, meeting with others in times of fellowship can provide a distraction from pain or illness, thus bringing a respite for the patient (Tan, 1996a). Special small groups for those who are ill or suffering from chronic pain can also provide a forum for sharing coping strategies and resources, including praying for one another.

Some people with chronic pain or illness find that regular times of worship are helpful. These times of worship can be in quiet time alone with God or in corporate worship in a church service, fellowship, or small group, or perhaps with a spouse or family. Such worship times usually include singing or listening to worship music, giving prayers of thanks and praise to God, and periods of silence.

Health care providers can encourage their patients to seek out opportunities for meeting with others and for worship. Many patients may need referral assistance to help them break a pattern of loneliness and isolation that exacerbates their medical needs. Maintaining a referral listing of local community centers, cultural groups, and churches and religious groups is an important step to meeting the care needs of these patients.

Multidisciplinary Care Teams

We recognize that in the modern medical world of managed care and limited time spent with each patient, implementing the aforementioned interventions in a sensitive and ethical manner can be impractical, if not impossible. One approach that is particularly useful in private group practices of primary care physicians is to include a mental health professional and/or a pastor as a part of the practice group (Albers, 1989). This approach to holistic health care affords the patient the opportunity to address his or her emotional and spiritual needs as they arise in the health care environment. Immediate referral to an on-site mental health professional or religious leader allows the patient to have his or her needs addressed in a professional environment without the barrier of needing to establish a separate appointment at another location.

Alternatively, for the medical professional working independently or in a setting in which it is not possible to hire an allied health care professional, she or he can develop a referral network of mental health care professionals and religious/spiritual leaders. Especially in large, urban settings, in which patients may come from diverse religious and spiritual backgrounds, it is essential to develop a network of appropriate referrals.

INTERVENTIONS AT THE CORPORATE LEVEL: FOR RELIGIOUS ORGANIZATIONS

This section focuses on approaches to spiritual interventions that can be implemented by religious organizations and groups. Although churches, synagogues, temples, mosques, and other religious organizations from a variety of belief systems can implement these strategies, we also provide more specific examples from our own experience and Christian religious perspective.

Visitation Ministry

A powerful and visible way in which religious groups can minister to those who are ill or in pain is through the ministry of visitation. For example, visitation by a pastor, priest, rabbi, or other spiritual leader can offer comfort, encouragement, prayer, and relief from isolation. "A hallmark of a true, caring visitation ministry is being able to spend unlimited time to meet the needs of the patient" (Albers, 1989, p. 176).

Visitation ministry includes efforts to meet the material needs of the patient. This may involve organizing members of a religious group to provide meals, cleaning, or baby-sitting or to run errands. This may also include providing financial assistance, especially if the patient is the primary wage earner in the family. A program of visitation can help to reduce social isolation, decrease stress by providing for tangible needs, and facilitate increased subjective well-being in spite of ongoing illness or pain. Albers (1989) offers a number of specific suggestions for ways in which a comprehensive visitation ministry can be organized.

Lay Counseling Ministry

Many patients who are ill or in pain struggle emotionally and spiritually. Patients and their families can become isolated from others and have difficulty managing the stresses and changes in their families as they adapt to caring for an ill family member. Providing counseling to patients and their families through a lay counseling ministry can be an effective means of meeting the needs of individuals and families (see Tan, 1991b, 1997). Churches, synagogues, temples, and mosques can utilize nonprofessionals or paraprofessionals in either a formal or an informal counseling ministry. Such lay counseling services are usually provided free of charge and therefore will not add more financial burdens to patients and their families. Religious organizations should also maintain a referral network of appropriate professional counselors who can meet the needs of individuals whose problems are beyond the scope of lay counselors or pastoral care.

12-Step Groups

Religious organizations can provide sponsorship of 12-step groups for members of their group and the community (see Harris et al., 1999, for evidence regarding spiritual and religious features of 12-step groups). Twelve-step groups are explicitly based on transcendent religious principles and can help people who are struggling with the problems caused by excessive alcohol or drug use, as well as a broader range of dependency or addiction problems.

For patients suffering adverse medical consequences from their addictions, maintaining freedom from their addictions can be a critical element of treatment and prevention of further problems. Maintenance of sobriety is also an important component of reducing health risk factors (e.g., risk of HIV/AIDS among drug users).

Medical Needs and Referrals

Many members of religious groups may need medical care but be unable to afford to pay for such care. Religious leaders can develop a network of physicians in their church or religious group or in the local community who may be willing to provide needed care *pro bono* in such situations. Religious groups can also make arrangements with physicians to pay for some or all of the cost for a member to receive needed care.

A Community of Caring

Religious leaders of all faiths can work to create a community in which caring is embodied in the actions of a religious group as it cares for others in the group and in the larger community. As a community of faith, members can be present for one another in significant ways in the midst of illness, pain, and hurt. An important way in which religious organizations can be present is through ongoing small groups and prayer groups. These groups can provide support, prayer, and encouragement to those members who become ill, as well as to new members who join as a means of receiving support. Religious groups can also organize support groups, perhaps focused on specific areas of need, in which people can join together in their mutual need for support, encouragement, and prayer.

The Christian church is intended to be a community of caring and prayer for others in which there is prayer for the sick (e.g., James 5:16), care for widows and orphans, the poor, the homeless, and those who suffer injustice (e.g., Isaiah 1:17). As stated by Hauerwas (1986), the church is a group of people who are called together by God. Because of God's faithfulness, members are to learn how to be faithfully present for one another, "for what does God require of us other than our unfailing presence in the midst of the world's sin and pain?" (p. 80).

As we find ways to be faithfully present to one another, we serve not only the individual who is in need but also a larger purpose. Hauerwas (1986) states that "medicine needs the church not to supply a foundation for its moral commitments, but rather as a resource of the habits and practices necessary to sustain the care of those in pain over the long haul" (p. 81). In learning how to simply *be* with others in the midst of suffering, we offer a paradigm for healing professionals who work in the midst of pain, suffering, and death.

Religious groups provide an important forum in which to address the challenging questions of life and to respond to the frustrations of those who are ill or in pain. Many people who are struggling with illness or pain wonder where God is or whether He hears their prayers. When God does not make sense, the church can seek to provide an environment in which questions can safely be asked and can provide a context for understanding the perplexities of faith. Pain and illness might be a path to deeper faith, to greater reliance on God's grace, spiritual growth, or discipline, or to greater empathy for others (Tan, 1996a). Some religious traditions (e.g., Buddhist) might provide meaning in understanding suffering as integral to life. Regardless of the particular beliefs held by a religious tradition, it is important to recognize the individual nature of each person's suffering and each person's faith journey and to avoid making routine judgments about the religious meaning of an individual's suffering and illness.

CONCLUSIONS

The Swiss physician Paul Tournier (1965) wrote that "[humankind] . . . is a unity: body, mind, and spirit ... to treat a man is to treat him therefore, in his entirety" (p. 136). If indeed such is the case, as a growing body of research seems to indicate, our modern health care system with its emphasis on the biological independent of the psychological and the spiritual must be adapted to provide care for the whole person.

As health care providers seek to address the needs of the individual patient, we believe it is of crucial importance that they do so from within the religious paradigm of the patient. Ethical patient care demands respect for the beliefs of the patient and sensitivity to the needs and readiness of the patient for spiritual interventions. The health care professional must also address his or her own spiritual life to adequately and appropriately address the spiritual needs of patients. Knowledge of the patient's heritage, culture, and potential problems that may arise out of religious faith or cultural beliefs can equip the professional to sensitively and competently meet the needs of patients.

Affordability and lack of third-party reimbursement is a significant barrier to holistic health care. Additionally, in a managed care climate in which maintaining a high volume of patients is necessary, most physicians do not have the time to address the psychological and spiritual needs of their patients. Nevertheless, a growing body of evidence points to the indivisibility of physical, psychological, and spiritual health and well-being. Expanding mental health care coverage in health insurance plans may make needed services more affordable for those who need care. Community leaders in medicine, mental health, and religious communities can work together to find creative ways to provide integrated care that address the needs of the whole person. Community-based health care centers that can intervene medically, psychologically, and spiritually are one approach to meeting this challenge. Greater efforts at building collaborative interdisciplinary alliances will help to facilitate the creativity needed to provide holistic health care in a changing medical environment.

As health care providers implement religiously or spiritually oriented interventions, it is crucial that they do so with the utmost ethical caution and professional care. We believe that, as ethical interventions are implemented, it is also critically important to conduct high-quality studies to evaluate the interventions used in treatment. Further research is needed to evaluate the efficacy of religious interventions, who they are most appropriate for, and when and how they are to be implemented to achieve positive effects. Johnson (1993), Harris et al. (1999), and Thoresen et al. (Chapter 2, this volume) provide a set of helpful guidelines for future research. We believe that thoughtful, ethical interventions and high-quality, rigorous evaluation will yield information helpful to increasing overall well-being and health outcomes.

REFERENCES

Albers, G. R. (1989). *Counseling the sick and terminally ill.* Dallas, TX: Word.

Becvar, D. S. (1997). *Soul healing: A spiritual orientation in counseling and therapy.* New York: Basic Books.

Bergin, A. E. (1991). Values and religious issues in psychotherapy and mental health. *American Psychologist, 46,* 394–403.

Blue, K. (1987). *Authority to heal.* Downers Grove, IL: InterVarsity Press.

Byrd, R. C. (1988). The therapeutic effects of intercessory prayer in a coronary care unit. *Southern Medical Journal, 81,* 826–829.

Caine, K. W., & Kaufman, B. P. (1999). *Prayer, faith and healing.* Emmaus, PA: Rodale Press.

Canda, E. R., & Furman, L. D. (1999). *Spiritual diversity in social work practice.* New York: Free Press.

Clark, C. C. (1998). Wellness self-care by healthy older adults. *IMAGE: Journal of Nursing Scholarship, 30,* 351–355.

Cornett, C. (1998). *The soul of psychotherapy: Recapturing the spiritual dimension in the therapeutic encounter.* New York: Free Press.

Diener, E. (2000). Subjective well-being: The science of happiness and a proposal for a national index. *American Psychologist, 55,* 34–43.

Dossey, L. (1993). *Healing words: The power of prayer and the practice of medicine.* New York: HarperCollins.

Dossey, L. (1997). *Be careful what you pray for . . . you just might get it.* New York: HarperCollins.

Foster, R. J. (1978). *Celebration of discipline: The path to spiritual growth.* New York: Harper & Row.

Fukuyama, M. A., & Sevig, T. D. (1999). *Integrating spirituality into multicultural counseling.* Thousand Oaks, CA: Sage.

Genia, V. (1995). *Counseling and psychotherapy of religious clients.* Westport, CT: Praeger.

George, L. K., Larson, D. B., Koenig, H. G., & McCullough, M. E. (2000). Spirituality and health: What we know, what we need to know. *Journal of Social and Clinical Psychology, 19,* 102–116.

Harris, A. H. S., Thoresen, C. E., McCullough, M. E., & Larson, D. B. (1999). Spiritually and religiously oriented health interventions. *Journal of Health Psychology, 4,* 413–433.

Hauerwas, S. (1986). *Suffering presence: Theological reflections on medicine, the mentally handicapped, and the church.* Notre Dame, IN: University of Notre Dame Press.

Hill, P. C., & Butter, E. M. (1995). The role of religion in promoting physical health. *Journal of Psychology and Christianity, 14,* 141–155.

Hill, P. C., & Hood, R. W. (Eds.). (1999). *Measures of religiosity.* Birmingham, AL: Religious Education Press.

Hood, R. W., Jr., Spilka, B., Hunsberger, B., & Gorsuch, R. (1996). *The psychology of religion: An empirical approach* (2nd ed.). New York: Guilford Press.

Hopfe, L. M. (1983). *Religions of the world.* New York: MacMillan.

Hunter, M., & Struve, J. (1998). *The ethical use of touch in psychotherapy.* Thousand Oaks, CA: Sage.

Ingersoll, R. E. (1998). Refining dimensions of spiritual wellness: A cross-traditional approach. *Counseling and Values, 42,* 156–165.

Johnson, W. B. (1993). Outcome research and religious psychotherapies: Where are we and where are we going? *Journal of Psychology and Theology, 23,* 297–308.

Kabat-Zinn, J. (1993). Mindfulness meditation: Health benefits of an ancient Buddhist practice. In D. Goleman & J. Gurin (Eds.), *Mind–body medicine: How to use your mind for better health* (pp. 259–275). Yonkers, NY: Consumer Reports Books.

Kelly, E. W. (1995). *Religion and spirituality in counseling and psychotherapy.* Alexandria, VA: American Counseling Association.

Kim, B.-L. C. (1996). Korean families. In M. McGoldrick, J. Giordano, & J. K. Pearce (Eds.), *Ethnicity and family therapy* (2nd ed., pp. 281–294). New York: Guilford Press.

King, D. E. (2000). *Faith, spirituality, and medicine: Toward the making of the healing practitioner.* New York: Haworth Pastoral Press.

Koenig, H. G. (1999). *The healing power of faith: Science explores medicine's last great frontier.* New York: Simon and Shuster.

Larson, D. B., & Larson, S. (1994). *The forgotten factor in physical and mental health.* Rockville, MD: National Institute of Healthcare Research.

Larson, D. B., Swyers, J. P., & McCullough, M. E. (Eds.). (1998). *Scientific research on spirituality and health: A consensus report.* Rockville, MD: National Institute for Healthcare Research.

Levin, J. S., & Vanderpool, H. Y. (1991). Religious factors in physical health and the prevention of illness. *Prevention in Human Services, 9,* 41–64.

Lovinger, R. J. (1990). *Religion and counseling.* New York: Continuum.

McCullough, M. E. (1995). Prayer and health: Conceptual issues, research review, and research agenda. *Journal of Psychology and Theology, 23,* 15–29.

McCullough, M. E., & Larson, D. B. (1999). Prayer. In W. R. Miller (Ed.), *Integrating spirituality into treatment: Resources for practitioners* (pp. 85–110). Washington, DC: American Psychological Association.

McCullough, M. E., Sandage, S. J., & Worthington, E. L. (1997). *To forgive is human.* Downers Grove, IL: InterVarsity Press.

Miley, W. M. (1999). *The psychology of well being.* Westport, CT: Praeger.

Miller, W. R. (Ed.). (1999). *Integrating spirituality into treatment: Resources for practitioners.* Washington, DC: American Psychological Association.

Miller, W. R., & Thoresen, C. E. (1999). Spirituality and health. In W. R. Miller (Ed.), *Integrating spirituality into treatment: Resources for practitioners* (pp. 3–18). Washington, DC: American Psychological Association.

Moon, G. W. (1997). Training tomorrow's integrators in today's busy intersection: Better look four ways before crossing. *Journal of Psychology and Theology, 25,* 284–293.

Myers, D. G. (2000a). *The American paradox: Spiritual hunger in an age of plenty.* New Haven, CT: Yale University Press.

Myers, D. G. (2000b). The funds, friends, and faith of happy people. *American Psychologist, 55,* 56–67.

Pargament, K. I. (1990). God help me: Toward a theoretical framework of coping for the psychology of religion. *Research in the Social Scientific Study of Religion, 2,* 195–224.

Pargament, K. I. (1997). *The psychology of religion and coping: Theory, research, practice.* New York: Guilford Press.

Payne, I. R., Bergin, A. E., Bielema, K. A., & Jenkins, P. H. (1991). Review of religion and mental health: Prevention and the enhancement of psychosocial functioning. *Prevention in Human Services, 9,* 11–40.

Richards, P. S., & Bergin, A. E. (1997). *A spiritual strategy for counseling and psychotherapy.* Washington, DC: American Psychological Association.

Richards, P. S., & Bergin, A. E. (Eds.). (2000). *Handbook of psychotherapy and religious diversity.* Washington, DC: American Psychological Association.

Rowan, A. B. (1996). Religious beliefs and health psychology: Empirical foundations. *Health Psychologist, 18,* 16–17.

Salovey, P., Rothman, A. J., Detweiler, J. B., & Steward, W. T. (2000). Emotional states and physical health. *American Psychologist, 55,* 110–121.

Santa Rita, E. (1996). Filipino families. In M. McGoldrick, J. Giordano, & J. K. Pearce (Eds.), *Ethnicity and family therapy* (2nd ed., pp. 324–330). New York: Guilford Press.

Shafranske, E. P. (Ed.). (1996). *Religion and the clinical practice of psychology.* Washington, DC: American Psychological Association.

Sicher, F., Targ, E., Moore, D., & Smith, H. S. (1998). A randomized, double-blind study of the effect of distant healing in a population with advanced AIDS. *Western Journal of Medicine, 169,* 356–363.

Steere, D. A. (1997). *Spiritual presence in psychotherapy: A guide for caregivers.* Bristol, PA: Brunner/Mazel.

Stolorow, R., & Atwood, G. (1979). *Faces in a cloud.* Northvale, NJ: Aronson.

Sue, S., Nakamura, C. Y., Chung, R. C., & Yee-Bradbury, C. (1994). Mental health research on Asian Americans. *Journal of Community Psychology, 22,* 61–67.

Tan, S. Y. (1991a). Counseling Asians. *Urban Missions, 9,* 42–50.

Tan, S. Y. (1991b). *Lay counseling: Equipping Christians for a helping ministry.* Grand Rapids, MI: Zondervan.

Tan, S. Y. (1993, January). *Training in professional psychology: Diversity includes religion.* Paper presented at the Midwinter Conference of the National Council of Schools of Professional Psychology (NCSPP), La Jolla, CA.

Tan, S. Y. (1994). Ethical considerations in religious psychotherapy: Potential pitfalls and unique resources. *Journal of Psychology and Theology, 22,* 389–394.

Tan, S. Y. (1996a). *Managing chronic pain.* Downers Grove, IL: InterVarsity Press.

Tan, S. Y. (1996b). Religion in clinical practice: Implicit and explicit integration. In E. P. Shafranske (Ed.), *Religion and the clinical practice of psychology* (pp. 365–387). Washington, DC: American Psychological Association.

Tan, S. Y. (1997). The role of the psychologist in paraprofessional helping. *Professional Psychology: Research and Practice, 28,* 368–372.

Tan, S. Y. (1999). Cultural issues in Spirit-filled psychotherapy. *Journal of Psychology and Christianity, 18,* 164–176.

Tan, S. Y., & Dong, N. J. (2000). Psychotherapy with members of Asian American churches and spiritual traditions. In P. S. Richards & A. E. Bergin (Eds.), *Hand-*

book of psychotherapy and religious diversity (pp. 421–444). Washington, DC: American Psychological Association.

Tan, S. Y., & Gregg, D. (1997). Disciplines of the Holy Spirit. Grand Rapids, MI: Zondervan.

Taylor, S. E., Kemeny, M. E., Reed, G. M., Bower, J. E., & Gruenewald, T. L. (2000). Psychological resources, positive illusions, and health. American Psychologist, 55, 99–109.

Tournier, P. (1965). The healing of persons. San Francisco: Harper & Row.

Walsh, F. (Ed.). (1999). Spiritual resources in family therapy. New York: Guilford Press.

Wenhao, J., Salomon, H. B., & Chay, D. M. (1993). Transcultural counseling and people of Asian origin: A developmental and therapeutic perspective. In J. McFadden (Ed.), Transcultural counseling: Bilateral and international perspectives (pp. 239–259). Alexandria, VA: American Counseling Association.

West, W. (2000). Psychotherapy and spirituality: Crossing the line between therapy and religion. London: Sage.

Worthington, E. L., Jr. (1986). Religious counseling: A review of published empirical research. Journal of Counseling and Development, 64, 421–431.

13

―◁○▷―

THE RELIGIOUS DIMENSION OF PATIENT CARE WITHIN REHABILITATION MEDICINE

The Role of Religious Attitudes, Beliefs, and Personal and Professional Practices

EDWARD P. SHAFRANSKE

Fifty-four million Americans are living with disabilities (McNeill, 1997). This represents approximately one-fifth of the U.S. population. If we include those whose lives are touched by persons with physical and mental disabilities (e.g., family members and significant others), this number begins to approximate the universe of Americans. This finding punctuates the importance of providing psychological care that is sensitive to the inclusive range of individual patient differences, as well as of summoning all available resources. Also, in light of the high incidence of disabilities, it is expected that general features of American culture are broadly expressed within this clinical population and that of their caregivers. Therefore, features of cultural diversity, including religious and spiritual orientation, should be brought into any discussion of psychological treatment. Further, resources that are naturally occurring and available within the environment may be solicited by psychologists and integrated into their approaches to intervention. This is particularly relevant in providing services that aim to establish or reinforce strategies for psychological coping that will assist both in the immediacy of medical treatment and in rehabilitation, as well as provide a foundation for a meaningful future.

This chapter proposes that the provision of religious and spiritual resources is integral to a holistic model of patient care within rehabilitation medicine. It considers the role of religious and spiritual belief, affiliation, and practice as potential contributors to coping and introduces exemplars of religious observance that may be employed within an inclusive and culturally sensitive model of psychological care. The discussion begins with a brief overview of religion and the psychology of coping, presents models integrating religious resources within patient care, includes a review of current practice in rehabilitation by presenting the findings of surveys of physicians and psychologists, and concludes with recommendations for practice, research, and training.

RELIGION AND THE PSYCHOLOGY OF COPING

Coping emerges out of the backdrop of cultural forces (Pargament, 1997). The nature of one's appraisals, emotional reactions, and behavioral responses is shaped by attributions, which to a great extent is socially mediated. The individual coconstructs meaning within the social contexts of family, neighborhood, and community and determines forms of response and coping. It is useful, therefore, to identify sources of coping within the wide landscape of American culture.

One distinctive feature of American culture and consciousness is found in religiosity. Recent surveys have found that over 95% of the U.S. population believe in God (Gallup, 1994), that over 50% pray at least once a day (National Opinion Research Center [NORC], 1973), that 93% identify with a religious group (Kosmin & Lachman, 1993), and that over 80% report that religion is "fairly" or "very" important in their lives (Gallup, 1994). Kosmin and Lachman (1993) suggest that religious affiliation may be a more important source of group identification than features of diversity such as race or ethnicity. Gallup (1995), following a review of 50 years of survey data, concluded: "the depth of religious commitment often has more to do with how Americans think and act than do other key background characteristics, such as level of education, age, and political affiliation." A review of the demographics of religiosity consistently portrays America throughout its history and into the present as a nation of religious believers. In this light, religiosity appears to be a distinctive feature that requires consideration in all aspects of applied psychology, including the psychology of coping and psychological treatment.

Beyond demographics, an argument can be made that facing changes in health status, engaging in the process of rehabilitation, and living with disabilities necessarily involves ontological issues and demands the development of coping strategies. Belief and faith commitments contribute to forming attributions about the causes and meanings of physical and mental illness and disability and provide a platform for sustaining, constructing, and transforming personal significance. Religious and spiritual beliefs and practices contribute to an orienting system that determines, in part, an individual's method of coping. An orienting system can be seen as the sum of influences, individual and collective, conscious and unconscious, located within the individual and positioned outside as social forces that shape personal meaning and behavior. Lazarus (2000), concerning stress and coping, commented, "The conceptual bottom line . . . is the *relational meaning* that an individual constructs from the person–environment relationship. That relationship is the result of appraisals of the confluence of the social and physical environment and personal goals, beliefs about the self and world, and resources" (p. 665).

Pargament (1997) proposed that religion and coping converge because religion is a *relatively available* part of the orienting system and because it is a *relatively compelling* way of coping. As a culturally sanctioned source of meaning, religion plays a significant role in an individual's orienting system. Religious beliefs, transmitted within the family system and reinforced by the local community, encourage the development of consciously held systems of attribution, as well as unconscious representations and organizing principles (Shafranske, 1992). The religious dimension within an orienting system not only provides answers to life's explicitly religious questions but also, more fundamentally, shapes perceptions, attributions, and affects in its construction of subjective experience. Aspects of transcendent, spiritual orientations are implicitly expressed within popular culture and produce a world view in which secular and sacred perspectives are seamlessly woven to provide coherence to broad categories of meaning. Orienting systems that are socially and individually constructed precede and are available to meet the challenges inherent in life. When an individual faces a life-altering event, such as catastrophic injury, disability, or illness, the existing orienting system is elicited to bring comprehension and to conserve and sustain coherence of personal meaning.

The salience of religion within an orienting system varies among individuals. The importance an individual places on religious and spiritual meanings is determined by a host of factors, including availability of alternative sources of orientation, functions within the familial and community culture, and effectiveness in furnishing coping resources in previous challenges. Contributing as well to salience is religion's ability to provide a compelling solution to the crisis at hand. The crisis to which religion is most attuned concerns the maintenance of personal meaning and supplying hope in the face of disillusionment. Changes in health status by injury or illness often prompt crises in an individual's sense of self and self-efficacy and may challenge basic assumptions and personal faith. Disability may shake an individual's psychological and ontological foundations. That bad things happen to good people is no trivial matter. Rather, such events call into question one's fundamental understanding of the nature of existence and one's life within Being. Ordinary means of adjustment may be inadequate to address the ontological underpinnings of illness. Religion is compelling because it provides a means to grapple with the ineffable and provides solutions to what Clifford Geertz (1966) has named "crises of interpretability." Disability and catastrophic illness often challenge individuals' commonplace understandings of meaning and the nature of existence, however ordained. Religion provides a context in which to assimilate the profound experiences of human limitation and to accommodate beliefs about the meaning of life and its pleasures and challenges.

Religion contributes to coping by either conserving or transforming an individual's significance in the face of challenge or disillusionment (Pargament, 1997). In addition to providing a belief response to crises of interpretability, religion provides rituals, observances, a community of faithful, and forms of direct community support and intervention to assist an individual to cope with the challenges he or she is facing. Pargament (1997) in the most thorough assessment of religion and the psychology of coping, concluded:

> The seemingly straight-forward question, "Does religion work," could not be answered with a simple "yes" or "no." Instead, the answer depends on the kind of religion one is talking about, who is doing the religious coping, and the situation that the person is coping with. Depending on the interplay among these variables, religion can be helpful, harmful, or irrelevant to the coping process. . . . Several other conclusions are warranted: (1) Religious coping seems especially helpful to more religious people, (2) religion can moderate or deter the effects of life stress, or both, and (3) religious coping adds a unique dimension to the coping process. (p. 312)

In addition to the role of religion in the psychology of coping, there is accumulating empirical evidence identifying religion to be an important variable in health. Systematic reviews of empirical research and survey data suggest a positive correlation between religious commitment and participation and health status (Ellison & Levin, 1998; Matthews, Larson, & Barry, 1993; Levin & Chatters, 1998; see also Thoresen, Harris, & Oman, Chapter 2, this volume). Religious involvement has been shown to be associated with quality of life (see Sherman & Simonton, Chapter 7, and Remle & Koenig, Chapter 8, this volume) and mental health (Plante & Sharma, Chapter 10, this volume) and serves as an epidemiological protective factor (McCullough, Chapter 3, this volume). In sum, religious involvement appears to be a salient variable in the psychology of coping, has been found to be associated with mental and physical health, and may offer resources, particularly to religious patients, in the provision of medical and psychological care to persons living with disabilities or in rehabilitation.

In light of the demographics of religious commitment in America, of the theoretically and empirically established role of religious coping, and of the relationship between religion and health status in general, it is necessary to ask, How might religious and spiritual resources be integrated into medical and psychological treatment? and How do providers address religious and spiritual dimensions in rehabilitation medicine and in providing services to persons living with disability? These questions are important in light of past research that found that clinicians in psychiatry and in the specialties of clinical and counseling psychology employed religious interventions primarily based on personal rather than professional factors. These mental health practitioners differed significantly from the general population in respect to personal religious beliefs, affiliations, and practices and, although they appeared to be sensitive to spirituality and respectful of others' religious commitments, had little or no training respective of religious issues (Bergin & Jensen, 1990; Shafranske & Gorsuch, 1985; Shafranske & Malony, 1990a, 1990b; Shafranske, 1996b, 2000a, 2000b).

MODELS FOR INTEGRATION OF RELIGIOUS RESOURCES IN MEDICAL TREATMENT

Values permeate the offering of medical treatment; this is particularly the case in interventions directed at the psychological sequelae associated with physical illness and disability. Jerome Frank (Frank & Frank, 1961/1991) suggested that psychotherapy, an exemplar of psychological treatment, at its heart counters demoralization through the transformation of meanings. Within all forms of psychological care exist implicit belief systems that shape clinical interventions and ultimately influence the attributions patients use to construct their subjective experiences. Psychology shares with religion the focus on the personal heuristics that people use to make sense of their lives. These heuristics derive from beliefs concerning the fundamental nature of human existence. From this perspective, it may be found that psychological treatment inevitably involves religious sentiment as broadly defined.

Further, it may be argued that psychological treatment cannot be divorced from the individual who is providing the care. The individual characteristics of the clinician, including, for example, features of personality, gender, ethnicity, culture, and religious faith and values, are necessarily conjoined with attitudes, knowledge, and skills obtained through professional training. Religious sentiment (or its obverse, the belief in the absence of a transcendent perspective) informs the treatment process in both seen and unseen ways. Also, physicians and psychologists are called to be responsive to the meanings that their patients bring to treatment concerning their physical and psychological difficulties. Whether or not care providers are personally invested in religious discourse, they often become engaged in dialogue involving religious language and meaning as they are entrusted to listen to the meanings constructed by their clients. Psychological intervention, to the extent to which it intends to influence a person's orienting approach, involves the religious or spiritual dimension.

Once I have argued that religious issues are necessarily involved in psychological treatment, a technical issue emerges concerning the clinical approach to be taken in respect to religious issues in practice. Tan (1996; see also Tan & Dong, Chapter 12, this volume) suggested two broadly defined models to address religious and spiritual issues in applied clinical practice: implicit and explicit integration. Implicit integration involves a respectful acceptance of the client's religious beliefs and values and may include consideration of the role of faith in daily life. There is no initiative, however, on the part of the clinician to bring spiritual issues to the foreground of the clinical discourse nor to employ religious resources in the service of the treatment. Within this model religiosity remains a background feature that, although acknowledged and respected, is not actively elicited nor explicitly integrated into treatment.

Explicit integration of religion in clinical practice "directly and systematically deals with spiritual or religious issues in therapy, and uses spiritual resources like prayer, Scripture or sacred texts, referrals to church or other religious groups or lay counselors, and other religious practices" (Tan, 1996, p. 368). In this model, the client's religious or spiritual orientation is explicitly integrated into psychological treatment. Spiritual practices rooted in a person's religious tradition—for example, prayer—may be brought directly into the therapeutic process. Although religiosity is not a requirement, clinicians employing an explicit integration approach are often personally religious and may hold faith perspectives congruent with those of their clients.

The specific form of integration in a given case is established by a number of factors, including therapeutic relationship, treatment goals and orientation, salience of religion or spirituality, participation in spiritual practices by the patient, and personal and professional orientation and training of the clinician. Integration is located on the continuum between purely implicit and explicit models and takes into consideration features of culture and the ongoing collaboration of the patient and clinician in their intersubjective construction of the therapeutic relationship. For a patient for whom religion appears primarily to be a background element, an implicit approach to integration may be taken in which a gradual exploration of the role of religious beliefs on attributions concerning illness, for example, might be undertaken. On the other hand, for a patient for whom religion holds a central position in daily life and who presents a history in which religious beliefs and observances have been readily utilized as sources of support, religious resources, such as prayer or collaboration with a chaplain, might be readily incorporated into a holistic treatment plan through explicit integration.

If medical and psychological treatment is viewed as inevitably involving personal religious or spiritual issues, and further, if religious coping is potentially a potent resource for medical rehabilitation, then programmatic studies need to be undertaken to establish the legitimacy of integration within the scope of professional practice. An assessment of the present status of religious resources in rehabilitation medicine and psychology is a necessary first step. The following presents a summary of such an assessment. It includes an examination of religious beliefs, affiliations, and practices of physicians and psychologists and their attitudes and practices, respective of religious resources. Religious resources are defined as general approaches, as well as specific interventions, that are derived from or include aspects of religious and spiritual beliefs and practices, for example, meditation or religious attributions.

METHOD

A survey approach was selected that allowed descriptive and correlational procedures to be performed. Four survey instruments were developed that included items taken from previous studies of psychologists and from national polls (Gallup, 1994; NORC, 1993) and items developed by the National Institute on Aging and the Fetzer Institute Working Group. Items from the Brief Multidimensional Measure of Religiousness/Spirituality were selected to contribute to collaborative research sponsored by the Fetzer Institute/National Institute on Aging (1999). Two questionnaires containing different item formats were developed for each of the physician and psychologist samples. A personal cover letter, survey, prepaid return envelope, nonparticipant response form, and request for results form were included; a follow-up postcard was sent approximately 2 weeks after the initial mailing.

A sample of 620 members, fellows, and associates of the American Psychological Association (APA) Division 22: Rehabilitation Psychology and a random sample of 1,000 physician members of the American Medical Association who specialize in rehabilitation medicine were randomly selected.

These sample sizes were chosen to insure that a response rate at or above 30% would yield results with a sampling error of no greater than ± 10%. A nonparticipant form was sent with the survey to assess the representativeness of the data and potential nonrandom response bias.

Three hundred twenty-eight rehabilitation physicians completed and returned questionnaires; 130 surveys were undeliverable. A return rate of 37.8% was obtained. The participants were 67.1% male and 32.9% female; average age was 44 (SD=10.4). Sixty-five percent reported that all of their professional time was dedicated to this specialty area.

Two hundred and forty completed questionnaires and 54 nonparticipant forms were returned by the psychologists; 47 protocols were returned as undeliverable. This reflects a response of 51.4% of the psychologist sample. The completed questionnaires reflect a response rate of 41.9%. The participants were 63% male and 37% female; average age was 49 (SD = 9). Greater than half of the psychologists reported that 100% of their professional time was dedicated to this specialty area.

The return rate for the psychologists was evaluated to be acceptable, taking into consideration usual rates of return for this professional group. The physician response rate, although lower than obtained in some national surveys, was evaluated as adequate for the purposes of an initial investigation (Thran & Berk, 1993). The findings should be interpreted conservatively, taking into consideration a likely bias of the respondents toward valuing the religious or spiritual dimension in professional practice. It was assumed that participants holding religion or spirituality as personally important would be more likely to complete a questionnaire in which religion and spirituality were the subject of study. This assumption was tested in a comparison analysis between participants and nonparticipants.

Although a significant difference was not found between the participants and nonparticipants concerning the importance of religion (t (212) = .809, $p < .49$) due to low rates of salience in both groups, significant differences were found in the other three comparison items. The following differences were identified between participant and nonparticipant psychologists. Nonparticipants dedicated less professional time to rehabilitation psychology (M = 38.20, SD = 36.71, compared with M = 73.81, SD = 30.96; t (213) = 5.73, $p < = .001$). Participants rated spirituality as more important (M = 1.68, SD = .77) in comparison with the nonparticipants (M = 2.07, SD = .62; t = (211) 2.52, $p < .05$) and reported religious and spiritual issues to be more involved in treatment (t = (210) 2.94, $p < .005$). (Note: These variables were treated as interval data based on $N > 100$.) This suggests that involvement and salience in the study's areas of interest, that is, religion, spirituality, and rehabilitation psychology, influenced a participant's behavior in completing the questionnaire. Further, this comparison indicated, as in previous studies (Shafranske, 1996b), that questionnaire respondents were more likely to be interested in religious and spiritual issues in psychological treatment and were also likely to be positively biased toward the spiritual dimension. Findings based on their responses are skewed to reflect a more positive orientation of the relevance of religious and spiritual issues in psychological treatment than may actually exist.

RESULTS

Religious Belief, Affiliation, and Practice

A number of items assessed the religious beliefs, affiliations, and practices of physicians and psychologists. Physicians' involvement in religion and spirituality was questioned through a self-description item and an assessment of salience (see Tables 13.1, 13.2, and 13.3). These data show that the majority of physicians consider themselves to be religious and that over 90% of the respondents rated spirituality to be fairly important or very important. Their ratings of salience of religion were not significantly dissimilar to those of the general population when matched by education.

TABLE 13.1. Importance of Religion Reported by Physicians and Psychologists and the Public at Large (Percentages)

	Very important	Fairly important	Not very important	No opinion
For total sample				
National sample[a]	58.0	30.0	11.0	1.0
National sample[b]	59.0	29.0	12.0	< 1.0
By education[b]				
Postgraduate	50.0	35.0	15.0	< 1.0
College graduate	51.0	35.0	15.0	< 1.0
College incomplete	56.0	33.0	11.0	< 1.0
No college	64.0	29.0	7.0	< 1.0
Physicians/rehabilitation medicine[c]	46.7	29.7	22.4	1.2
Physicians/psychiatry[d]	38.2	18.5	41.7	1.9
Psychologists/rehabilitation[e]	40.6	29.3	29.3	0.8
Psychologists/clinical–counseling[f]	26.0	22.0	51.0	0.0

[a]Gallup Poll (April 30–May 2, 1999).
[b]1993 Gallup Poll, Gallup (1994).
[c]Random sample of physicians specializing in rehabilitation medicine (N = 328) (Shafranske, 1998).
[d]Random sample of members of the American Psychiatric Association (N = 105) (Shafranske, 2000).
[e]Random sample of American Psychological Association Division 22 (Rehabilitation Psychology) members (N = 242) (Shafranske, 1998).
[f]Random sample of American Psychological Association members listing degrees in Clinical Psychology or Counseling Psychology (N = 253) (Shafranske, 1996b).

TABLE 13.2. Comparison of the Importance of Religion and Spirituality (Percentages)

	Very important	Fairly important	Not very important	No opinion
Physicians/rehabilitation medicine[a]				
Salience of religion	46.7	29.7	22.4	1.2
Salience of spirituality	57.6	34.8	7.6	0.0
Physicians/psychiatry[b]				
Salience of religion	38.2	18.5	41.7	1.9
Salience of spirituality	56.4	24.8	17.8	1.0
Rehabilitation psychologists[c]				
Salience of religion	27.0	28.0	43.0	2.0
Salience of spirituality	50.0	30.0	19.0	1.0
Clinical and counseling psychologists[d]				
Salience of religion	26.0	22.0	51.0	0.0
Salience of spirituality	48.0	25.0	26.0	0.0

Note. [a]Random sample of physicians specializing in rehabilitation medicine (N = 328) (Shafranske, 1998). [b]Random sample of members of the American Psychiatric Association (N = 105) (Shafranske, 2000). [c]Random sample of American Psychological Association Division 22 (Rehabilitation Psychology) members (N = 242) (Shafranske, 1998). [d]Random sample of American Psychological Association members listing degrees in Clinical Psychology or Counseling Psychology (N = 253) (Shafranske, 1995).

TABLE 13.3. Comparison of Self-Description of Religiosity and Spirituality (Percentages)

	Physicians[a] (N = 158)	Psychologists[b] (N = 121)
To what extent do you consider yourself a religious person?		
Very religious	18.4	15.7
Moderately religious	42.3	34.7
Slightly religious	29.8	27.3
Not religious at all	9.5	22.3
To what extent do you consider yourself a spiritual person?		
Very spiritual	27.3	37.2
Moderately spiritual	48.3	43.8
Slightly spiritual	20.3	10.7
Not spiritual at all	4.2	8.2

[a]Random sample of physicians specializing in rehabilitation medicine (N = 328) (Shafranske, 1998). [b]Random sample of American Psychological Association Division 22 (Rehabilitation Psychology) members (N = 242) (Shafranske, 1998).

The psychologists were similar to their physician colleagues in their ratings of salience. Forty-one percent rated religion as very important and 29% as fairly important. This sample differed in some regards from previous samples of counseling and clinical psychologists. It is interesting to note that both physicians and psychologists specializing in rehabilitation rate salience of religion higher than their counterparts in psychiatry and clinical and counseling psychology (Shafranske, 2000b). Consistent with other surveys of psychologists is the finding that spirituality, which may connote a more individual than institutional expression of religious sentiment, receives higher ratings of salience.

As in previous studies (Shafranske, 1996b), differences were found in certain features of religiosity between psychologists and the general population. Psychologists differ significantly in their report of the salience of religion (t (198) = 6.01, p < .0001) and appear to hold different religious beliefs. An examination of ideological positions that psychologists endorse suggests that greater than one-third believe in a personal God (see Table 13.4). Although this scale has not been used in national polls, an inspection of the available data supports the conclusion that the vast majority of Americans believe in a personal God. Ninety-five percent believe in God (Hoge, 1996), 90% pray to God, and almost half report that they have occasionally or regularly "received a definite answer to a specific request" (Princeton Religion Research Center, 1993, p. 49). In contrast, the majority of psychologists do not believe in a God who is immanently involved in the events of the world. Greater than 15% believe that notions of God are illusions, although no one indicated that such faith positions are irrelevant.

Less than 50% of the psychologists actively or regularly participate in religion, and less than one-third agreed with the statement, "My whole approach to life is based upon my religion." A decline in religious involvement exists in comparing current to family of origin assessments of affiliation (see Figure 13.1). This may suggest that psychologists as a group may be unique in their orientation to religious sentiment and may be significantly different from the general population in terms of involvement in organized religion. However, this finding may not necessarily indicate a distinct perspective by psychologists but rather may be reflective of a more general trend that finds salience of religious commitment inversely related to education. Relatively low religious affiliation has been found generally within the professorate, particularly among psychology faculty (Politics of the Professorate, 1991; Shafranske, 1996b). Further, survey research of the general public suggests that even though 7 in 10 Americans report belonging to a church or synagogue, a more modest number regularly participate. About 40% of the U.S. population and about 33% of the psychologist respondents reported that they had attended church or synagogue in the previous 7 days. Over 20% of the psychologists reported that they attended religious services

TABLE 13.4. Ideological Orientations

	Percentage of agreement		
Ideological statement	Rehabilitation psychologists[a]	Clinical psychologists[b]	Clinical and counseling psychologists[c]
There is a personal God of transcendent existence and power whose purposes will ultimately be worked out in human history.	36.4	29.6	23.9
There is a transcendent aspect of human experience which some persons call God but who is not imminently involved in the events of the world and human history.	10.7	10.3	13.6
There is a transcendent or divine dimension which is unique and specific to the human self.	9.9	9.3	6.8
There is a transcendent or divine dimension found in all manifestations of nature.	27.3	20.8	31.1
The notions of God or the transcendent are illusory products of human imagination; however, they are meaningful aspects of human existence.	15.7	25.9	23.5
The notions of God or the transcendent are illusory products of human imagination; therefore, they are irrelevant to the real world.	0	2.0	1.2
No response	0	2.2	0

[a]Random sample of APA Division 22 (Rehabilitation Psychology) members ($N = 121$) (Shafranske, 1998).
[b]Random sample of APA Division 12 (Clinical Psychology) members ($N = 409$) (Shafranske & Malony, 1990).

every week or more; 55%, approximately once a month, and about 16% once or twice a year. This reflects a common pattern in church involvement in which there is a highly devout and active core membership, a large group of persons who identify themselves as members of a church and who sometimes participate, and a smaller group who hold a religious preference, maintain church affiliation, yet rarely participate. It is likely, taking into account the bias in the respondents, that psychologists are less involved in institutional religion than the general public; however, this difference appears to be modest. It was also found that psychologists, when involved in religion, are intrinsic (religion as endowing personal meaning) and extrinsic-personal (means to gain personal comfort and security) rather than extrinsic-social (means to social gains) in their religious orientation as measured by single-item scales (Gorsuch & McPherson, 1989; see also Sherman & Simonton, Chapter 6, this volume).

The assessment of psychologists' sensitivity to the religious dimension changes character when one asks about spirituality. As presented in Table 13.2, importance increases to 80%, with 50% indicating spirituality as "very important." About 80% of the sample considers themselves to be "moderately" or "very" spiritual in contrast to 50% being "moderately" or "very" religious (Table 13.3). This finding suggests that psychologists are not antithetical to the spiritual dimension. Rather, their expression or form appears to be more private, idiographic, and less institutionally derived. Forty-three percent reported that they had had a religious or spiritual experience that changed their lives with 84% indicating that these experiences resulted in a gain in faith. These data suggest that rehabilitation psychologists are different from the general population in terms of the specific form that their spiritual orientation takes; however, that difference may be modest.

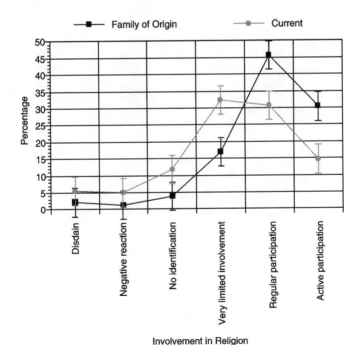

FIGURE 13.1. Comparison of the family of origin and current religious involvement of rehabilitation psychologists.

Clinical Practice

Clinical practice was assessed by survey items focusing on attitudes, experiences, and behaviors. Embedded as a research assumption is the premise that professional practice is informed by personal beliefs and attitudes, as well as by formal graduate education and clinical training. Further, such attitudes and beliefs are influenced by experiences extant of professional training. The discussion of clinical practice begins with a look into the personal experiences and attitudes of clinicians.

Psychologists were asked whether religion was involved in how they understood or dealt with stressful situations in their own lives (See Figure 13.2). Over 65% reported that their religion was either somewhat or very involved, although less than one-quarter reported that "what religion offers them most is comfort in times of trouble and sorrow." Fifty-two percent of the psychologists and the physicians reported that involvement in rehabilitation had influenced their faith. A review of narrative responses of the psychologists suggested that the majority experienced a strengthening in their religious convictions and an increased sensitivity to the human condition and respect for life through their work in rehabilitation. The personal reli-

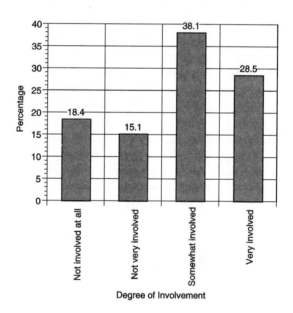

FIGURE 13.2. Rehabilitation psychologists' ratings on the extent to which religion is involved in understanding or dealing with stressful situations in their own lives.

gious convictions of the psychologists were found to influence their attitudes and behaviors regarding the use of religious or spiritual interventions. However, clinicians in general appear to be sensitive to the appearance of religious, spiritual, and ontological issues in rehabilitation.

Greater than 50% of the physicians reported that religious or spiritual issues or "loss of meaning" were involved "a great deal of the time" or "often" in treatment; 38.2% stated this as "sometimes" and 10.9% as "rarely." Psychologists were posed three items focusing on different aspects of religious or spiritual content in rehabilitation treatment (see Figure 13.3). In their view, more broadly stated ontological issues involving "the loss of purpose or meaning in life" were most often seen. Over 80% of the respondents indicated that religious or spiritual issues were involved in treatment and that patients attribute a religious meaning to their medical condition at least some of the time. These findings suggest that clinicians encounter, to varying degrees, patients for whom religious or spiritual issues influence the treatment process. This raises the question, How do psychologists address the religious or spiritual issues of their patients in the course of treatment?

This question was answered through an assessment of attitudes and

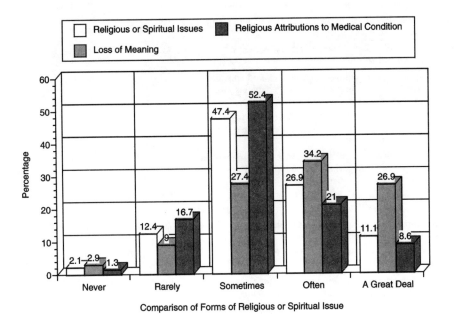

FIGURE 13.3. Rehabilitation psychologists' ratings of the extent to which religious and spiritual issues, "loss of meaning," and religious attributions for medical conditions are discussed during therapy with patients with disabilities.

behaviors. A number of items addressing professional attitudes were posed that focused on parameters of practice and self-perception of comfort and competence in addressing religious or spiritual issues in clinical practice. These statements are presented in Table 13.5. Although the majority believe that psychologists are ill prepared to offer religious and spiritual resources, less than 20% stated that they were "not comfortable addressing patient's religious and spiritual needs." This is striking in light of the fact that few report any attention to these issues within clinical training. This may suggest that confidence in one's own ability to respond competently is greater than that extended to one's peers. Even when clergy are available to furnish religious or spiritual resources, the majority of psychologists would not decline to offer these resources themselves. From these responses, it appears that most of the psychologists in this sample are personally comfortable in offer-

TABLE 13.5. Attitudes among Rehabilitation Psychologists Concerning the Use of Religious Resources

	Percentage of agreement[a]				
	SD	D	UD	A	SA
Psychologists are ill prepared to offer religious and spiritual resources.	3.1	27.8	15.5	45.3	10.3
I do not feel comfortable addressing patient's religious and spiritual concerns.	29.2	43.8	10.4	10.4	6.3
Psychologists should not use religious and spiritual resources in treating patients when chaplains and other local ministers and rabbis are available.	25.7	44.3	11.3	11.3	7.2
A psychologist must personally have religious or spiritual faith in order to use a religious or spiritual resource in treatment.	29.9	41.2	9.3	17.5	2.06
A psychologist should disclose their faith orientation prior to any examination of religiosity and spirituality with a patient.	20.6	44.3	15.5	14.4	5.15
Psychologists should not provide religious or spiritual resources unless the patient initiates.	3.1	13.4	20.6	35.1	27.8
Attempting to change a patient's religious outlook or attributions is unethical.	6.25	12.5	12.5	34.4	34.4
If a patient asked me to pray with them I would decline.	15.6	40.6	17.7	15.6	10.4
If it were empirically demonstrated that the use of a specific religious intervention was efficacious then psychologists should offer that intervention regardless of their personal religious beliefs.	12.4	25.8	17.5	32.0	12.4

[a]SD, strongly disagree; D, disagree; UD, undecided; A, agree; SA, strongly agree. Random sample of American Psychological Association Division 22 (Rehabilitation Psychology) members (N = 190) (Shafranske, 1998).

ing religious and spiritual resources, although, curiously, they believe that their colleagues, most likely similarly trained as themselves, are in general not adequately prepared to do so. This may more accurately reflect an endorsement of their personal openness to addressing spiritual issues than a claim of competence over their colleagues.

The majority would not initiate religious or spiritual interventions absent the request of the patient and appear to respect the autonomy of a patient's faith perspective, viewing it to be unethical to attempt to change a patient's religious outlook or attributions. This statement is of interest in light of the observation that psychotherapists implicitly and explicitly attempt to change the attributions and world views of their clients, for example, through cognitive reframing, psychoanalytic interpretation, and so forth.

Psychologists appear to be reluctant to disclose their personal faith orientations. This hesitation may reflect the assumption of clinical neutrality and may be related to the view that religious or spiritual resources should be offered as psychological treatment interventions in which the personal beliefs of the clinician are not essential features. In other words, the personal attributes and commitments of the clinician are not relevant to offering a particular therapeutic, no matter its religious or spiritual origin. Indeed, over 70% disagreed that faith commitment was necessary to offer a religious or spiritual resource. An inference could be drawn, therefore, that most believe that such resources could be offered as technical, clinical interventions. In this regard, Propst, Ostrom, Watkins, Dean, and Mashburn (1992) found that nonreligious cognitive therapists were more effective in offering religious cognitive–behavioral therapy than in offering nonreligious cognitive therapy to religious clients. However, if the argument is raised that religious or spiritual resources can be offered in a neutral fashion as technical interventions, then it is surprising that there was a mixed response to an item concerning the use of empirically supported interventions. The question was posed, "If it were empirically demonstrated that the use of a specific religious intervention was efficacious then psychologists should offer that intervention regardless of their personal religious beliefs." Thirty-six percent agreed, 38% percent disagreed, and 18% were undecided. This finding may suggest that personal factors are viewed as playing a role in the selection of a therapeutic intervention or may reflect a more general reticence to adhering to rote application of empirically supported forms of treatment. Physicians were asked whether they would pray for a patient if requested by the patient. Ninety percent indicated they would pray for the patient; 55% of the psychologists would pray with him or her. Interestingly, if it were presented to psychologists that a spiritual intervention such as prayer were scientifically demonstrated to improve patient progress, only 55% would perform the intervention, and 41.2% would refer the patient to a member of clergy. Although the items were not equivalent, it appears that factors beyond the empirical and scientific influence the possible use of religious or spiritual interventions.

A further assessment of clinician attitudes and behaviors was conducted through an inventory of the use of religious resources. Psychologists were asked to indicate which interventions they have performed, would recommend, would approve, or would disapprove. A general finding as illustrated in Figure 13.4 is that, as the intervention becomes more active and requires direct clinician involvement or personal commitment and participation, the endorsement and performance decreases. For example, 78% recommend or perform "knowing patients' religious backgrounds," but just over 10% recommend prayer to or pray with a patient. This may also be an artifact of training and experience; psychologists typically conduct an intake interview in which a wide array of demographic information is solicited, including religion. This is in distinction to a unique intervention such as prayer, which emanates from an explicit religious context. Inspection of the data suggests a relatively narrow range of the use of interventions, despite a relatively high approval rating. Fifty-three percent approve "recommending religious jour-

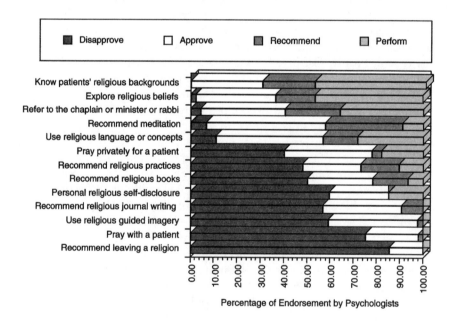

FIGURE 13.4. Attitudes toward and use of religious and spiritual interventions by rehabilitation psychologists.

nal writing," and yet only 6% report having performed that intervention. It may be that clinicians find such interventions to be acceptable in the abstract yet the interventions may not come to mind due to the minimal exposure to these interventions within formal clinical training.

An analysis of variance was conducted to investigate the role of personal faith commitment in the performance of specifically religious interventions. The extent to which one considers oneself religious was found to be significantly related to the performance of religious interventions F (1, 89) = 7.01, $p < .001$. This supports previous studies in which personal religiosity was related to the performance of religious interventions (Shafranske, 1996b; Shafranske, 2000b).

A review of the data provides the conclusion that issues of religiousness and spirituality, broadly defined, often emerge within treatment of persons living with disabilities and that psychologists to varying degrees respond through the use of religious resources. Attitudes toward the use of explicit religious resources suggest a degree of openness, although few perform these interventions. Those who hold a personal religious orientation are more likely to use more explicitly religious or spiritual resources in treatment.

Clinical Training

As previously reported, the majority of the rehabilitation psychologists disagreed with the statement that they felt uncomfortable in addressing religious and spiritual concerns. One might wonder where that degree of confidence comes from in light of the majority's opinion that psychologists are ill prepared to respond to these issues. The answer may be found in formal clinical training, which is the appropriate venue for developing competence. Eighty-two percent of the sample reported, however, that religious and spiritual issues were rarely or never presented and discussed (See Figure 13.5). This finding is consistent over a number of national and regional studies (see Shafranske, 1996b, for a summary.) Less than 5% reported that these issues were presented often or a great deal of the time. In addition, the majority assessed their training respective of these issues to be inadequate (see Figure 13.6). In light of the lack of exposure and training in the use of religious and spiritual resources in treatment, psychologists may be forced to primarily rely on personal beliefs and experiences in forming clinical strategies. It appears that they have not been provided adequate education, training, and supervision to incorporate a program of religious coping within rehabilitation. This finding is striking when a comparison is drawn between the frequency with which religious or spiritual issues occur in psychological treatment in rehabilitation and the frequency with which these issues are presented in clinical training.

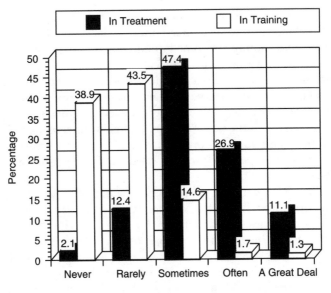

FIGURE 13.5. Rehabilitation psychologists' ratings of the extent to which religious or spiritual issues were part of their training and of the extent to which these issues are encountered in treatment.

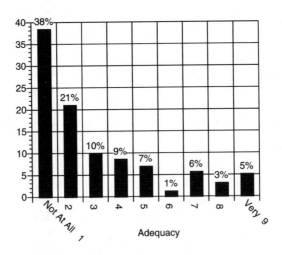

FIGURE 13.6. Self-report by rehabilitation psychologists of adequacy of training in religious and spiritual issues.

DISCUSSION

This study adds further support to the observation that psychologists differ from the general population to a moderate extent in terms of their religious beliefs, affiliations, and practices. It appears, however, that psychologists are respectful of the beliefs of others and, in fact, value personal spirituality. Training respective of religious and spiritual issues in rehabilitation psychology mirrors that in other applied specialty areas—it is minimal and is assessed by the majority to be inadequate. The lack of education and clinical training is troubling in light of the frequency with which religious or spiritual issues are presented in rehabilitation and in consideration of the potential benefits that religious and spiritual resources may offer in the psychology of coping. Although religious issues were rarely, if ever, discussed in graduate education and clinical training, few clinicians report discomfort in addressing the religious and spiritual concerns of their patients. Psychologists appear to be receptive to the incorporation of religious and spiritual interventions within rehabilitation. Both physicians and psychologists appear to be willing to pray with a patient if requested; however, they would not initiate such a behavior regardless of whether such an intervention were demonstrated to be efficacious. Those who integrate religious and spiritual resources or approve in principle of offering religiously oriented interventions appear to be strongly influenced by personal rather than professional commitments. This is understood as the logical default position in light of the paucity of training in this regard and reconfirms the position that personal values inevitably influence the treatment process. It appears that a gap exists in the training of psychologists respective of religious and spiritual issues. Although the training experiences of physicians in rehabilitation medicine were not specifically assessed in this study, it is likely that they also receive minimal exposure. This was found to be the case in a survey of physicians specializing in psychiatry (Shafranske, 2000b).

A remedy is required to insure adequate preparation to address the religious and spiritual issues of patients as they directly affect treatment. Further, in light of the theoretical and empirical evidence of the role of religion in the psychology of coping, research and clinical training is required to bring all resources to the assistance of patients. This effort will be enhanced through the publication of theoretical, empirical, and applied scholarship by professional organizations and academic presses (Shafranske, 1996a; Richards & Bergin, 1997; Miller, 1999; Richards & Bergin, 2000; Koenig, 1998), funded collaborative research programs (Fetzer Institute, 1997), and the development of curricula (Larson, Lu, & Swyers, 1996). Further, psychologists are ethically compelled to consider issues of diversity, including religiosity, in providing psychological treatment (American Psychological Association, 1992). Graduate education and clinical training should include discussion of religious and spiritual commitments and practices as components of diversity. National accrediting bodies relevant to rehabilitation have specified that the spiritual needs of patients be addressed (Commission on the Accreditation of Rehabilitation Facilities, 1993; Joint Commission on Accreditation of Healthcare Associations, 1993).

Advances in treatment occur through systematic empirical research based on the foundation of multidisciplinary and theoretical scholarship. Institutional support should be directed to investigate the constituents of religious coping, both as naturally occurring processes within the community and as specific clinical procedures. Clinical interventions, as they become empirically supported, should be introduced systematically within graduate education and training with requisite supervision. An ongoing dialogue is required between the professions of rehabilitation psychology and allied professions, including professionals in pastoral care and chaplains, to better articulate the appropriate collaborative model for integrating religious coping into treatment. Efforts should be made to establish protocols for referral to and collaboration with religious professionals, for example, rabbis and ministers, as well as for the direct provision of religious and spiritual resources. It should be emphasized that any form of integration of religious and spiritual resources in treatment should be offered in an ethical and culturally sensitive manner (Tan, 1994; Yarhouse & VanOrman, 1999). For example, should psychologists be encouraged to individually initiate a specific intervention protocol, or should the guidelines encourage the development of collaborative treatment arrangements? Minimally, clinicians should be encouraged to consider clergy to be religious professionals who may serve an essential role as consultants and coparticipants in treatment provision (Weaver et al., 1997). Further, any initiatives in this arena should be undertaken with respect for the diversity that exists among clinicians and patients and with the acknowledgment that such intervention protocols should be uniquely tailored to the individual client and clinical context. This requires the development of assessment procedures that will reliably assess the nature of an individual's religious and spiritual life and his or her use of religious modes of coping. It should always be kept in mind that a wide diversity exists within what appears to be a homogeneous religious population; one may believe in God, but that hardly indicates the dynamic role of faith within one's life. Further, investigators and clinicians should be mindful of the increasing diversity of religious expression in America and the interaction of religiosity with other features of diversity, that is, race, ethnicity, and gender.

In conclusion, religious coping offers an additional resource to persons in rehabilitation and to those living with disabilities. Further investigation is required to establish treatment efficacy and to develop comprehensive training in the use of treatment regimens that incorporate religious and spiritual resources. At minimum, efforts need to be made within the profession to address what is consistently reported to be minimal attention to religious and spiritual issues within graduate education and clinical training.

ACKNOWLEDGMENT

This study was supported by a research contract awarded by the Fetzer Institute, Kalamazoo, Michigan.

REFERENCES

American Psychological Association. (1992). Ethical principles of psychologists and code of conduct. *American Psychologist, 47*, 1597–1611.

Bergin, A. E., & Jensen, J. P. (1990). Religiosity of psychologists: A national survey. *Psychotherapy, 27*, 3–7.

Commission on the Accreditation of Rehabilitation Facilities. (1993). *1993 standards manual for organizations serving people with disabilities.* Tucson, AZ: Author.

Ellison, C. G., & Levin, J. S. (1998). The religion–health connection: Evidence, theory and future directions. *Health Education and Behavior, 25*, 700–720.

Fetzer Institute. (1997). *Roles of religiousness and spirituality in medical rehabilitation and the lives of persons with disabilities research program.* Kalamazoo, MI: Author.

Fetzer Institute/National Institute on Aging. (1999). *Multidimensional measurement of religiousness/spirituality for use in health research.* Kalamazoo, MI: John E. Fetzer Institute.

Frank, J. D., & Frank, J. B. (1991). *Persuasion and healing* (3rd ed.). Baltimore: Johns Hopkins University Press. (Original work published 1961)

Gallup, G., Jr. (1994). *The Gallup poll: Public opinion 1993.* Wilmington, DE: Scholarly Resources.

Gallup, G., Jr. (1995). Fifty years of Gallup surveys on religion. *The Gallup Report No. 36.* Princeton, NJ: The Gallup Organization.

Geertz, C. (1966). Religion as a cultural system. In C. Geertz (Ed.), *Anthropological approaches to the study of religion* (pp. 87–125). London: Tavistock.

Gorsuch, R. L., & McPherson, S. E. (1989). Intrinsic/Extrinsic measurement: I/E-Revised and single-item scales. *Journal for the Scientific Study of Religion, 28*(3), 348–354.

Hoge, D. (1996). Religion in America: The demographics of belief and affiliation. In E. Shafranske (Ed.), *Religion and the clinical practice of psychology* (pp. 21–41). Washington, DC: American Psychological Association.

Joint Commission on Accreditation of Healthcare Associations. (1993). *The joint commission accreditation manual for hospitals. 1993.* Chicago: Author.

Koenig, H. G. (Ed.). (1998). *Handbook of religion and mental health.* San Diego, CA: Academic Press.

Kosmin, B., & Lachman, S. (1993). *One nation under God: Religion in contemporary American society.* New York: Crown.

Lazarus, R. S. (2000). Toward better research on stress and coping. *American Psychologist*, 55(6), 665–673.

Larson, D. B., Lu, F. G., & Swyers, J. P. (1996). *Model curriculum for psychiatry residency training programs: Religion and spirituality in clinical practice*. Rockville, MD: National Institute for Healthcare Research.

Levin, J. S., & Chatters, L. M. (1998). Religion, health, and psychological well-being in older adults: Findings from three national surveys. *Journal of Aging and Health*, 10(4), 504–531.

Matthews, D. A., Larson, D. B., & Barry, C. P. (1993). *The faith factor: An annotated bibliography of clinical research on spiritual subjects*. Bethesda, MD: National Institute for Healthcare Research.

McNeill, J. M. (1997). Americans with disabilities: 1994–95. *Current Population Reports* (Report No. C3.186:P-70/2/61). Washington, DC: U.S. Department of Commerce.

Miller, W. R. (1999). *Integrating spirituality into treatment: Resources for practitioners*. Washington: American Psychological Association.

National Opinion Research Center (1973). *General social survey*. Chicago: University of Chicago.

Pargament, K. I. (1997). *The psychology of religion and coping: Theory, research, practice*. New York: Guilford Press.

Politics of the Professorate. (1991, July–August). *The Public Perspective*, pp. 86–87.

Princeton Religion Research Center. (1993). *Religion in America*. Princeton, NJ: Author.

Propst, L. R., Ostrom, R., Watkins, P., Dean, T., & Mashburn, D. (1992). Comparative efficacy of religious and non-religious cognitive–behavioral therapy for the treatment of clinical depression in religious individuals. *Journal of Consulting and Clinical Psychology*, 60, 94–103.

Richards, I. S., & Bergin, A. E. (1997). *A spiritual strategy for counseling and psychotherapy*. Washington, DC: American Psychological Association.

Richards, I. S., & Bergin, A. E. (2000). *Handbook of psychotherapy and religious diversity*. Washington, DC: American Psychological Association.

Shafranske, E., & Gorsuch, R. (1985). Factors associated with the perception of spirituality in psychotherapy. *Journal of Transpersonal Psychology*, 16, 231–241.

Shafranske, E. P. (1992). God-representation as the transformational object. In M. Finn & J. Gartner (Eds.), *Object relations theory and religion* (pp. 57–72). Westport, CT: Praeger.

Shafranske, E. P. (Ed.). (1996a). *Religion and the clinical practice of psychology*. Washington, DC: American Psychological Association.

Shafranske, E. P. (1996b). Religious beliefs, affiliations, and practices of clinical psychologists. In E. Shafranske (Ed.), *Religion and the clinical practice of psychology* (pp. 149–162). Washington, DC: American Psychological Association.

Shafranske, E. P. (2000a). Religion and psychology: Psychologists' personal and professional beliefs, practices, and training. In A. Kazdin (Ed.), *Encyclopedia of psychology* (pp. 46–47). New York: American Psychological Association and Oxford University Press.

Shafranske, E. P. (2000b). Religious involvement and professional practices of psychiatrists and other mental health professionals. *Psychiatric Annals*, 30(8), 1–8.

Shafranske, E. P., & Malony, H. N. (1990a). Clinical Psychologists' religious and spiritual orientations and their practice of psychotherapy. *Psychotherapy*, 27(1), 72–78.

Shafranske, E. P., & Malony, H. N. (1990b). California psychologists' religiosity and psychotherapy. *Journal of Religion and Health*, 29(3), 219–231.

Tan, S.-Y. (1994). Ethical considerations in religious psychotherapy: Potential pitfalls and unique resources. *Journal of Psychology and Theology*, 22, 389–394.

Tan, S.-Y. (1996). Religion in clinical practice: Implicit and explicit integration. In E. Shafranske (Ed.), *Religion and the clinical practice of psychology* (pp. 365–387). Washington, DC: American Psychological Association.

Thran, S. L., & Berk, M. L. (1993). Surveys of physicians. In *Proceedings of the international conference on establishment surveys* (pp. 83–92). Alexandria, VA: American Statistical Association.

Weaver, A. J., Samford, J. A., Kline, A. E., Lucas, L. A., Larson, D. B., & Koenig, H. G. (1997). What do psychologists know about working with the clergy? An analysis of eight APA journals: 1991–1994. *Professional Psychology: Research and Practice*, 28(5), 471–474.

Yarhouse, M. A., & VanOrman, B. T. (1999). When psychologists work with religious clients: Applications of the general principles of ethical conduct. *Professional Psychology: Research and Practice*, 30(6), 557–562.

PART IV

⊷◦⊶

COMMENTARIES ON RESEARCH CONCERNING FAITH AND HEALTH

14

◄O►

WITHOUT A PRAYER

Methodological Problems, Ethical Challenges, and Misrepresentations in the Study of Religion, Spirituality, and Medicine

RICHARD P. SLOAN
EMILIA BAGIELLA
TIA POWELL

Claims about religion, spirituality, and health appear with increasing frequency today, both in the popular media and in professional journals. This trend is based in part on evidence that patients want to consider broad alternatives to conventional medical practice and on published studies linking religion and health outcomes. Correspondingly, there are increasing calls to incorporate religious and spiritual activities into clinical practice. We recently demonstrated that much of the empirical literature purported to show that religious activity is associated with beneficial health outcomes suffers from methodological shortcomings and, as a result, is weak and inconclusive (Sloan, Bagiella, & Powell, 1999). Moreover, attempts to connect religion and medicine raise significant ethical concerns. Despite the publication of several recent methodologically sounder studies, the evidence still is weak and, for many reasons, provides no justification for breaking down the walls between religion and medicine, as Matthews and Larson recommend (Matthews & Larson, 1997). In this chapter, we cover the methodological and ethical problems raised by attempts to make religious activities adjunctive medical treatments.

METHODOLOGICAL PROBLEMS

Failure to Control for Multiple Comparisons

When we test a hypothesis that a given risk factor is significantly associated with some outcome, we measure a degree of uncertainty. This uncertainty is quantified as the probability of incorrectly rejecting the null hypothesis of no association and falsely declaring that such an association exists, that is, committing a Type I error. The probability of committing a Type I error should not exceed 5%, the standard significance level used in statistical testing. Thus we are willing to tolerate falsely declaring an association between a risk factor and an outcome no more than 5 times out of 100. For every statistical test of an association between a risk factor and an outcome, the probability of a false positive is fixed. However, when conducting multiple tests, we increase the likelihood of a Type I error. For example, if we conduct as many as six tests, each at the 5% significance level, the chance of having at least one false positive will be about 26%. That is, we will have 26% probability of declaring an association between one of the risk factors and the outcome to be true when in fact it is false and merely the product of chance.

Conducting repeated tests is not wrong in itself if we recognize that we are increasing the chance of committing a Type I error and adjust the significance level accordingly. There are numerous ways to control for multiple comparisons, and most of the computerized statistical packages have incorporated these methods.

Many studies in the literature on religion and health fail to make adjustments for the greater likelihood of finding a statistically significant result when conducting multiple statistical tests. A paper examining the relationship between religious activities and blood pressure (Koenig et al., 1998) provides a particularly instructive example. In this paper, at least 126 statistical tests are conducted with no control at all for multiple comparisons. Using a simple Bonferroni correction for multiple comparisons, that is, dividing the standard 5% level by the number of comparisons, yields a critical significance level of .0004. None of the comparisons in this paper achieved this level of statistical significance.

In a retrospective study (Levin, Lyons, & Larson, 1993), the relationships between frequency of prayer and six items measuring subjective health were examined. Analyses of variance were conducted on each of these six perceptions of health, and three revealed effects of frequency of prayer at the .05 level of statistical significance. Another recently published study reported that religious attendance was inversely associated with levels of interleukin-6 (IL-6), a component of the immune system, in the elderly (Koenig et al., 1997). However, IL-6 was one of eight outcome variables, and there was no attempt to control for multiple comparisons, as the authors themselves reported. In such studies, adjustment of alpha levels to control for multiple comparisons would render these findings nonsignificant.

Similar problems arise in the famous study by Byrd (Byrd, 1988). In this double-blind study, patients in a coronary care unit (CCU) were assigned randomly either to standard care or to receiving daily intercessory prayer by three to seven born-again Christians. Patients and their doctors did not know which patients were receiving prayer. Twenty-nine outcome variables were measured, and on six of them, the prayer group had fewer newly diagnosed problems; but there was no control for multiple comparisons. Moreover, the six significant outcomes were not independent: The prayer group had less newly diagnosed heart failure and fewer newly prescribed diuretics, two outcomes directly related to each other. The prayer group also had less newly diagnosed pneumonia and fewer newly prescribed antibiotics, outcomes also related to each other.

This failure to control for multiple comparisons characterizes much of the literature that examines relationships between religious activities and health outcomes.

Covariates: Confounders and Mechanisms

Confounders such as behavioral and genetic differences and stratification variables such as age, gender, education, ethnicity, socioeconomic status, and health status may play an important role in the relationship between religion and health. Failure to control for these factors can lead to biased estimation of this relationship, a particularly acute problem in the nonexperimental research that characterizes this literature. How do confounders lead researchers to make mistakes about an association between a risk factor and an outcome? Consider the following example: Systolic blood pressure increases linearly with the number of times one votes in presidential elections. Should we conclude that voting is a risk factor for hypertension and advise people not to vote?

If we probe only slightly, we discover that after controlling for age, the relationship between systolic blood pressure and frequency of voting disappears. In this example, age is a confounding variable. The relationship between high systolic pressure and voting exists only because age is directly associated with both.

Multivariate methods address this problem, permitting estimation of the magnitude of the association between religious variables and health outcomes while controlling for the effects of other variables. However, use of these methods requires complete presentation of the results, that is, at least the regression coefficients and the corresponding confidence intervals for all of the variables in the statistical model. Reports that fail to do this are incomplete and may be misleading.

Attempts to assess the effect of religiosity on health outcomes illustrate this problem. Increased religious devotion, operationalized as service as a Roman Catholic priest (Michalek, Mettlin, & Priore, 1981) or nun (Timio et al., 1997), a Mormon priest (Gardner & Lyon, 1982), or a Trappist or Benedictine monk (de Gouw, Westendorp, Kunst, Mackenbach, & Vandenbroucke, 1995), is associated with reductions in morbidity and mortality. In fact, these findings are attributable almost entirely to confounding: These groups differ from the general population in codes of conduct that proscribe behaviors associated with risk, including some or all of the following: smoking, alcohol consumption, sexual activity, psychosocial stress, and in some cases, consumption of meat. In fact, most of these cases were selected for study precisely because of these codes of conduct.

In a series of studies from Israel (Friedlander, Kark, & Stein, 1986; Goldbourt, Yaari, & Medalie, 1993; Kark et al., 1996), religiosity, measured as religious orthodoxy, also was shown to confer health benefits. However, one of these (Friedlander et al., 1986) was a case-control study, the deficiencies of which—recall bias and difficulty in establishing causality—are widely known. In another (Goldbourt et al., 1993), a multivariate model (presented in their Table 6) predicting coronary heart disease mortality included standard risk factors but omitted religion, and no information on risk ratio or confidence intervals or even level of statistical significance was provided. Finally, in a study matching secular and religious kibbutzim on geographic locale (Kark et al., 1996), use of the same regional hospital, and similar number of members over 40 years of age, all-cause mortality was significantly greater among members of the secular kibbutzim. However, the strategy of matching insures equivalence of groups only on the matched variables. As a consequence, the groups differed on dietary habits, smoking, cholesterol, and marital status, with the secular group having greater risk, as the authors themselves report. The multivariate analysis of mortality did not control for these factors.

The problem of confounding and other covariates also affects studies that claim that religious behaviors influence health outcomes. In some studies using large data bases, this problem can be addressed. Both the Alameda County Study and the Tecumseh Community Health Study found that frequency of attendance at religious services was inversely associated with mortality (House, Robbins & Metzner, 1982; Strawbridge, Cohen, Shema & Kaplan, 1997). However, after control for all relevant covariates, this relationship held only for women, not for men. In another large study, attendance at religious services was associated with increased functional capacity in the elderly (Idler & Kasl, 1997), but after control for appropriate covariates, this relationship held for only 3 of the 7 years in which outcome data were collected. There was no effect on mortality (Idler & Kasl, 1992). In a smaller study, religiosity predicted mortality in the elderly poor but only among those in poor health (Zuckerman, Kasl, & Ostfeld, 1984).

In many other studies, failure to control adequately for important covariates results in the assertion of significant findings when none may exist. For example, Pressman, Lyons, Larson, and Strain (1990) reported that among elderly women after surgical repair of broken hips, religiousness was associated with better ambulation status, measured as the amount of assistance required and distance walked, at discharge (Pressman et al., 1990). Although the analysis controlled for severity of health condition, it failed to control for age, a critical variable when studying functional capacity in the elderly.

Similar problems characterize a report claiming that religious attendance and importance of religion interacted such that those high in both had lower diastolic (but not systolic) blood pressure than those low in both (Larson et al., 1989). The report contained no statistics on this interaction; and although potential covariates, such as socioeconomic status, age, smoking status, and body mass index, were measured, the absence of the statistical model makes it difficult to evaluate the findings. In another report, based on the same data set, frequency of church attendance was positively related to systolic (but not diastolic) blood pressure after control for Quetelet Index, smoking, and socioeconomic status (Graham et al., 1978). Neither data, the multivariate model, nor the amount of variance accounted for by the religious variable was presented. Moreover, there was no measure of health status, which can influence the capacity to attend church.

In some cases, problems of interpretation arise not so much in the original research but rather in secondary sources. A case in point is a report by Comstock and Partridge (1972), frequently cited as a demonstration of a positive association between church attendance and health. However, as Comstock himself later reported, this finding was most likely due to failure to control for the important covariate of functional capacity; that is, those with reduced capacity (and poorer health) were less likely to go to church (Comstock & Tonascia, 1977). This latter study rarely is cited. Similarly, Koenig reports that a study by Colantonio et al. (Colantonio, Kask, & Ostfeld, 1992) "found lower rates of stroke in persons who attended religious services at least once per week" (Koenig, 1997, p. 85). However, this was only the case for the univariate analysis; the effect disappeared altogether after covariates such as levels of physical function were added to the analysis. Levin, in a review of a review, reported that 22 of 27 studies of religious attendance and health showed a significant positive relationship (Levin, 1994), despite his own previous assertion that associations between attendance and health are highly questionable because this literature is characterized by numerous methodological problems, including the failure to adjust for confounders and covariates (Levin & Vanderpool, 1987).

Although, as we discuss subsequently, more recent studies have addressed this problem using multivariate analyses, this is not always the case. In a widely cited paper, Koenig, Hays, et al. (1999) report that church attendance was associated with longer survival in a cohort of elderly participants, even after control for relevant covariates and confounders. However, in the analysis, as the authors report, a subscale measuring social interaction "was dropped because it included membership in church-related groups that would confound the analysis" (p. 372). Thus this analysis is unable to distinguish social interactions taking place in church from social interactions more generally. Given a recent finding that social and productive activities predicted survival in a similar cohort (Glass, Mendes de Leon, Marottoli, & Berkman, 1999), it is entirely conceivable that the effect that Koenig, Hays, et al. (1999) report reflects social activity in general.

An important distinction should be made between confounding factors and mechanisms. A confounding factor is a variable associated with both the risk factor of interest and the outcome but is not in the causal pathway between the two. Thus a confounder induces a spurious relationship between a risk factor and an outcome. Accounting for the effect of the confounder eliminates the relationship.

A mechanism, on the other hand, is in the causal path that connects the risk factor to the outcome. For example, the association between smoking and lung cancer is explained by high levels of nicotine and carbon monoxide. In this case, the covariates (carbon monoxide and nicotine levels) not only are related to both the risk factor (smoking) and the outcome (lung cancer) but also are in the causal path between the two. High levels of nicotine and carbon monoxide represent a mechanism by which smoking increases the risk of lung cancer. When a covariate truly is a mechanism and not a confounder, statistically controlling for it will eliminate a true relationship between the risk factor of interest and the outcome.

A further complication in considering whether a factor is a confounder or a mechanism arises from the ambiguity of causal direction inherent in a correlation. It may be, for example, that attendance at religious services and social support are significantly correlated. However, we cannot be certain about the causal direction of this relationship. Church attendance may lead to increased social support, but it is equally plausible that it may result from social support, that is, people with extensive social interactions may have acquaintances who attend religious services and, because of this, they decide to attend for themselves. In this case, it is social support that leads to church attendance, not the other way around. And of course, a significant correlation between attendance and support may be explained by a common factor associated with both variables.

Until the causal direction of associations between religious activities and other variables is unambiguous, there is no reason to believe that those variables represent the mechanism by which religious attendance leads to better health. Thus proper adjustment for their possible confounding effect should be made.

Bad Science: Misinterpretation of Data and Fishing for Findings

Even when studies are carefully conducted and show associations between religious activities and health outcomes, problems arise in interpretation of these findings. Thus, for example, well-conducted epidemiological studies showing that attendance at religious services was associated with reduced mortality (Hummer, Rogers, Nam, & Ellison, 1999; Oman & Reed, 1998) reflect only associations at the population level; they provide no evidence that making recommendations to patients to attend religious services actually will lead to increased attendance, let alone to better health (Sloan et al., 2000). Evidence from epidemiological studies must be confirmed by clinical trials before it can be converted into clinical recommendations.

One common problem with observational studies such as the ones often reported in this literature is that individuals assign themselves to the risk category. This phenomenon can lead to biased associations resulting from self-selection. Individuals choose to attend religious services; they are not assigned randomly to attend. This self-selection may represent a prototype of risk factors, that is, attending religious services may be only one of several related factors that predispose people or to protect them from specific events. This possibility cannot be dismissed without a trial in which participants are assigned at random to different experimental conditions.

Although epidemiological results generally are confirmed by clinical trials, this is not always the case. For example, recent results from randomized clinical trials suggest that, contrary to the evidence from epidemiological studies, a low-fat, high-fiber diet does not protect from colorectal cancer (Alberts et al., 2000; Schatzkin et al., 2000). Only a clinical trial, in which patients are randomly assigned either to receive or not receive a recommendation to attend religious services, could help to determine whether such a recommendation will lead to increased church attendance and ultimately to better health. Because there are likely to be significant differences between the health effects of attending religious services on one's own and those of attending because one's physician recommends it, a trial such as this would be problematic, difficult to conduct, and yield meaningless results.

Further misinterpretation of data is found in the recently published meta-analysis of studies of religious involvement and mortality, in which the association between religious attendance and mortality is described as robust (McCullough, Hoyt, Larson, Koenig, & Thoresen, 2000). Studies such as these are used to justify recommending that physicians encourage patients to engage in a wide range of religious activities.

Of course, the studies reviewed by McCullough et al. (2000) are epidemiological in nature and therefore cannot shed light on interventions to promote religious activities. In addition to this problem, however, the authors simply misread their own findings. In their meta-analysis, McCullough et al. calculated an unadjusted odds ratio of 1.29 for this association. As the authors themselves noted, "odds ratios near 1.0 indicate weak or nonexistent associations between variables, whereas odds ratios greater than 3.0 represent strong associations between variables" (p. 212). Moreover, after adjustment for important covariates, for example, gender, race, income, education, functional status, and so forth, the odds ratio (OR) dropped to 1.23, with a p value = 0.306. Nonetheless, the authors report that the relationship between religious activity and mortality was real and "robust." As the p value for the OR after adjustment for covariates indicates, this OR is not real. Moreover, an OR of 1.23 or 1.29 is anything but robust.

Consider, by comparison, the ORs typically seen in biomedicine: The OR for the association of lipoprotein(a) with coronary heart disease in young women, after adjustment for age, smoking, education, body mass index, systolic blood pressure, total cholesterol, triglycerides, and HDL, was 2.90 (95% CI, 1.6 to 5.0; Orth-Gomer et al., 1997). Odds ratios for the association of leisure time activities and cardiac arrest were of a similar magnitude, for example, 2.94 for participants who did not perform gardening activities more than 60 min/week in contrast to those who did, 3.70 for participants who did not walk more than 60 min/week compared with to those who did, and 2.94 for participants who did not engage in high-intensity activities compared with those who did, after adjustment for standard covariates (Lemaitre et al., 1999). Exposure to environmental tobacco smoke was associated with lung cancer (OR = 3.90) after adjustment (Rapiti, Jindal, Gupta, & Boffetta, 1999).

Even for psychosocial factors, the ORs typically are far greater. Everson et al. (Everson, Kaplan, Goldberg, & Salonen, 2000) recently reported that hopelessness conferred a greater than three-fold increased risk for becoming hypertensive (OR = 3.22, after adjustment for standard risk factors). Frasure-Smith, Lespérance, and Talajic (1995) showed that depressive symptomatology following myocardial infarction conferred a substantially elevated risk of mortality (OR = 6.64, after adjustment for risk factors). In a meta-analysis of intervention trials, Linden, Stossel, and Maurice (1996) demonstrated that patients with coronary artery disease who did not receive psychosocial treatments had greater mortality and cardiac recurrence rates during 2-year follow-up, with ORs of 1.70 for mortality and 1.84 for recurrence, after adjustment for risk factors. Each of these ORs is significant and substantial, in contrast to the miniscule and nonsignificant OR of 1.23 reported by McCullough et al. (2000).

Another illustration of bad science is provided by a recently published paper from Koenig's group (Helm, Hays, Flint, Koenig, & Blazer, 2000) that examined associations between private religious behavior (e.g., prayer, reading the Bible) and mortality. In the overall analysis, they found no association. However, after dichotomizing participants by functional status (those with and those without impairments), the authors reported that among the unimpaired, private religious behavior was associated with a significant survival advantage, even after control for relevant confounders. They justify this analytic strategy by suggesting that "praying in a foxhole", that is, offering prayers when already impaired and presumably in times of need at the end of life, may be different from a "long-term habit of private devotionals" (p. M402). This represents breathtaking post hoc hypothesizing. First, it is axiomatic that in survival analyses, variables known to influence survival, for example, functional status, are entered prior to variables under investigation, in this case private religious behavior. When in the overall analysis, the authors followed this approach, they found no effect of religious behavior, and this is where the analysis should have ended. Second, how do the authors know that those with impairments do not have a lifetime history of private devotionals? Third, and most important, the authors' strategy violates all standards of scientific methodology: Cutting the sample into enough pieces and analyzing each one separately eventually will produce a significant p value by chance alone. Why stop with functional status? Why not look separately at men and women, blacks and whites, younger versus older elderly, those living alone versus those living with others? This simply is bad science.

With physicians increasingly called on to practice evidence-based medicine, it simply is unacceptable to recommend practices whose efficacy has not been demonstrated and that, as we indicate in the next section, raise substantial ethical concerns. The argument that the empirical literature justifies engaging in religious activity as adjunctive medical treatments is unsupported.

ETHICAL ISSUES

In addition to questions about the empirical studies of purported relationships between religious activity and health outcomes, there are significant ethical concerns. Here we address four such concerns: coercion, privacy, doing harm, and discrimination.

Coercion

Health professionals, even in these days of consumer advocacy, retain influence over their patients by virtue of their medical expertise. When doctors depart from areas of established expertise to promote a nonmedical agenda, they abuse their status as professionals. Thus we question making inquiries into the patient's spiritual life in the service of making recommendations that link religious practice with better health outcomes. In *The Healing Power of Faith*, Koenig (1999) provides recommendations to enhance the health of those who are not religious (pp. 280–281):

- Consider attending a church or synagogue.
- Consider reading religious scriptures.
- Try to emulate the behavior of truly religious/spiritual persons at your place of work.

He even provides advice for patients who already are religious (pp. 277–278):

- Consider attending services more frequently.
- Attend a prayer or Scripture study group weekly.
- Get up 30 minutes earlier and spend that time in prayer.
- Take a few minutes each day to pray with your family.

Advice such as this may be perfectly appropriate from the clergy, but in the context of a physician–patient interaction, it is inappropriate and potentially coercive. Do we really want physicians dispensing advice about our religious lives? And if doctors are to make coercive recommendations to patients, should they not select those interventions with the greatest likelihood of benefit? Because more than one-half of Americans are obese and approximately 25% still smoke, a conscientious doctor ought to address these problems before asking a patient to spend that time in prayer. Particularly in this era of 8-minute patient visits any minute of discussion on one subject, such as religion, means not discussing something else, such as hypertension. Any recommendation to do one thing, such as pray, decreases the likelihood of a patient following another recommendation, such as smoking cessation or dieting. Thus, when doctors take on the work of the clergy, they become both bad clergy and bad doctors.

Privacy

A second ethical consideration involves the limits of medical intervention. For many patients, religious pursuits are a private matter, even if the evidence were to show a solid link between religious activity and health. Socio-economic status and marital status, for example, are associated with health outcomes (Adler et al., 1994; Ebrahim, Wannamethee, McCallum, Walker, & Shaper, 1995), but physicians do not dispense advice that presumes to enhance them. Evidence also suggests that for women, early rather than late childbearing may reduce the risk of various cancers (Lambe, Thorn, Sparen, Bergstrom, & Adami, 1996; Ramon et al., 1996), but we would recoil at a physician recommending to a young woman, either married or single, that she have a child to reduce this risk. These matters are personal and private, even if they are related to health. Many patients regard their religious faith as even more personal and private.

Doing Harm

A third ethical problem concerns the possibility of actually doing harm. Linking religious activities and better health outcomes can be actively harmful to patients, who already must confront age-old folk wisdom that illness is due to their own moral failure (Gould, 1981; Groopman, 2000). Within any individual religion, are the more devout adherents "better" people, more deserving of health than others? If evidence showed health advantages of some religious denominations over others, should physicians be guided by this evidence to counsel conversion? Attempts to link religious and spiritual activities to health are reminiscent of the now discredited research suggesting that different ethnic groups show differing levels of moral probity, intelligence, or other measures of social worth (Gould, 1981). Because all humans, devout or profane, ultimately will succumb to illness, we wish to avoid the additional burden of guilt for moral failure for those whose physical health fails before our own.

Discrimination

A fourth ethical concern is discrimination. Proponents of making religious activity an adjunctive medical treatment assert that there is substantial evidence that religious activity is associated with beneficial health outcomes. "We have recently completed a systematic review of over 1200 studies on the religion/health relationship. . . . The vast majority of these studies show a relationship between greater religious involvement and better mental health, better physical health, or lower use of health services" (Koenig, Idler, et al., 1999, p. 124). These same proponents recommend that physicians probe patients' spiritual history to determine if religion and spirituality are important in treating their medical condition. Matthews et al. (1998) recommend that clinicians ask, "What can I do to support your faith or religious commitment?" to patients who respond favorably to questions about whether religion or faith are "helpful in handling your illness" (p. 123). Thus recommendations to encourage religious activity are to be made only to those patients who affirm their importance and not to those who do not. This creates an interesting and difficult ethical dilemma: Given their assertion of the overwhelming evidence that religious activity confers health benefits, how can they in good conscience withhold this recommendation from patients for whom religion is not important? This is like determining patients' views on antibiotics before recommending them to treat pneumonia. It creates two classes of patients: one for whom an effective and life-extending treatment is recommended and another for whom it is not. To do this surely is unethical, given the purported strength of the evidence. Their hesitation suggests that these health practitioners do not really believe their own recommendations are based in fact. They know they have strayed into the problematic area of individual choice and personal values. Suspecting that the weight of medical science fails to support them, they cannot make their recommendations with a clear conscience.

CONCLUSIONS

Serious methodological and empirical issues continue to plague the literature on religion and health. Even well-conducted studies demonstrate only a weak or nonexistent association, and these associations exist only at the epidemiological level. Without compelling evidence from intervention studies to demonstrate that promoting religious activity actually leads to improved health outcomes, no empirical basis exists for making religious activity adjunctive medical treatments.

Beyond the empirical literature, there are important ethical concerns surrounding associations between religion and health that have barely been addressed, let alone resolved. In a country of growing religious heterogeneity, the possibility of serious ethical conflicts from unwarranted medical intrusions into religious life is real.

These conclusions are relevant to the issue of bringing religious activity into medical practice. Concerns of patients about religion and health are best addressed by clergy, to whom referrals can readily be made. Professional clergy, whether they are health care chaplains or not, do not have conflicting roles in these matters, as physicians do. They are not bound by the limits of science. Neither are their relationships with patients troubled by role asymmetry with regard to health. Matters of religion and health may indeed be important to patients, but they are not the business of doctors.

REFERENCES

Adler, N. E., Boyce, T., Chesney, M. A., Cohen, S., Folkman, S., Kahn, R. L., & Syme, S. L. (1994). Socioeconomic status and health: The challenge of the gradient. *American Psychologist, 49,* 15–24.

Alberts, D. S., Martinez, M. E., Roe, D. J., Guillen-Rodriguez, J. M., Marshall, J. R., van Leeuwen, J. B., Reid, M. E., Ritenbaugh, C., Vargas, P. A., Bhattacharyya, A. B., Earnest, D. L., Sampliner, R. E., Parish, D., Koonce, K., & Fales, L. (2000). Lack of effect of a high-fiber cereal supplement on the recurrence of colorectal adenomas. *New England Journal of Medicine, 342,* 1156–1162.

Byrd, R. C. (1988). Positive therapeutic effects of intercessory prayer in a coronary care unit population. *Southern Medical Journal, 81,* 826–829.

Colantonio, A., Kask, S. V., & Ostfeld, A. M. (1992). Depressive symptoms and other psychosocial factors as predictors of stroke in the elderly. *American Journal of Epidemiology, 136,* 884–894.

Comstock, G. W., & Partridge, K. B. (1972). Church attendance and health. *Journal of Chronic Disease, 225,* 665–672.

Comstock, G. W., & Tonascia, J. A. (1977). Education and mortality in Washington County, Maryland. *Journal of Health and Social Behavior, 18,* 54–61.

de Gouw, H. W. F. M., Westendorp, R. G. J., Kunst, A. E., Mackenbach, J. P., & Vandenbroucke, J. P. (1995). Decreased mortality among contemplative monks in the Netherlands. *American Journal of Epidemiology, 141,* 771–775.

Ebrahim, S., Wannamethee, G., McCallum, A., Walker, M., & Shaper, A. (1995). Marital status, change in marital status, and mortality in middle aged British men. *American Journal of Epidemiology, 142,* 834–842.

Everson, S. A., Kaplan, G. A., Goldberg, D. E., & Salonen, J. T. (2000). Hypertension incidence is predicted by high levels of hopelessness in Finnish men. *Hypertension, 35,* 561–567.

Frasure-Smith, N., Lespérance, G., & Talajic, M. (1995). Depression and 18–month prognosis after myocardial infarction. *Circulation, 91,* 999–1005.

Friedlander, Y., Kark, J. D., & Stein, Y. (1986). Religious orthodoxy and myocardial infarction in Jerusalem: A case control study. *International Journal of Cardiology, 10,* 33–41.

Gardner, J. W., & Lyon, J. L. (1982). Cancer in Utah Mormon men by lay priesthood level. *American Journal of Epidemiology, 116,* 243–257.

Glass, T. A., Mendes de Leon, C., Marottoli, R. A., & Berkman, L. F. (1999). Population based study of social and productive activities as predictors of survival among elderly Americans. *British Medical Journal, 319,* 478–483.

Goldbourt, U., Yaari, S., & Medalie, J. H. (1993). Factors predictive of long-term coronary heart disease mortality among 10,059 male Israeli civil servants and municipal employees. *Cardiology, 82,* 100–121.

Gould, S. J. (1981). *The mismeasure of man.* New York: Norton.

Graham, T. W., Kaplan, B. H., Cornoni-Huntley, J., James, S. A., Becker, C., Hames, C. G., & Heyden, S. (1978). Frequency of church attendance and blood pressure elevation. *Journal of Behavioral Medicine, 1,* 37–43.

Groopman, J. (2000, April 21). Your cancer isn't your fault. *New York Times*, p. A23.

Helm, H. M., Hays, J. C., Flint, E. P., Koenig, H. G., & Blazer, D. G. (2000). Does private religion activity prolong survival? A six-year follow-up study of 3,851 older adults. *Journal of Gerontology, 55A*, M400–M406.

House, J. S., Robbins, C., & Metzner, H. L. (1982). The association of social relationships and activities with mortality: Prospective evidence from the Tecumseh Community Health Study. *American Journal of Epidemiology, 116*, 123–140.

Hummer, R. A., Rogers, R. G., Nam, C. B., & Ellison, C. G. (1999). Religious involvement and U.S. adult mortality. *Demography, 36*, 273–285.

Idler, E. L., & Kasl, S. V. (1992). Religion, disability, depression, and the timing of death. *American Journal of Sociology, 97*, 1052–1079.

Idler, E. L., & Kasl, S. V. (1997). Religion among disabled and nondisabled persons: II. Attendance at religious services as a predictor of the course of disability. *Journal of Gerontology, 52B*, S306–S316.

Kark, J. D., Shemi, G., Friedlander, Y., Martin, O., Manor, O., & Blondheim, S. H. (1996). Does religious observance promote health? Mortality in secular and religious kibbutzim in Israel. *American Journal of Public Health, 86*, 341–346.

Koenig, H. G. (1997). *Is religion good for your health?* Binghamton, NY: Haworth Pastoral Press.

Koenig, H. G. (1999). *The healing power of faith*. New York: Simon & Schuster.

Koenig, H. G., Cohen, H. J., George, L. K., Hays, J. C., Larson, D. B., & Blazer, D. G. (1997). Attendance at religious services, interleukin-6, and other biological parameters of immune function in older adults. *International Journal of Psychiatry in Medicine, 27*, 233–250.

Koenig, H. G., George, L. K., Hays, J. C., Larson, D. B., Cohen, H. J., & Blazer, D. G. (1998). The relationship between religious activities and blood pressure in older adults. *International Journal of Psychiatry in Medicine, 28*, 189–213.

Koenig, H. G., Hays, J. C., Larson, D. B., George, L. K., Cohen, H. J., McCullough, M. E., Meador, K. G., & Blazer, D. G. (1999). Does religious attendance prolong survival? A six-year follow-up study of 3,968 older adults. *Journal of Gerontology, 54*, 370–376.

Koenig, H. G., Idler, E., Kasl, S., Hays, J. C., George, L. K., Musick, M., Larson, D. B., Collins, T. R., & Benson, H. (1999). Religion, spirituality, and medicine: A rebuttal to skeptics. *International Journal of Psychiatry in Medicine, 19*, 123–131.

Lambe, M., Thorn, M., Sparen, P., Bergstrom, R., & Adami, H. O. (1996). Malignant melanoma: Reduced risk associated with early childbearing and multiparity. *Melanoma Research, 6*, 147–153.

Larson, D. B., Koenig, H. G., Kaplan, B. H., Greenberg, R. S., Logue, E., & Tyroler, H. A. (1989). The impact of religion on men's blood pressure. *Journal of Religion and Health, 28*, 265–278.

Lemaitre, R. N., Siscovick, D. S., Raghunathan, T. E., Weinmann, S., Arborgast, P., & Lin, D. Y. (1999). Leisure-time physical activity and the risk of primary cardiac arrest. *Archives of Internal Medicine, 159*, 686–690.

Levin, J. S. (1994). Religion and health: Is there an association, is it valid, and is it causal? *Social Science and Medicine, 38*, 1475–1482.

Levin, J. S., Lyons, J. S., & Larson, D. B. (1993). Prayer and health during pregnancy: Findings from the Galveston Low birthweight survey. *Southern Medical Journal, 86*, 1022–1027.

Levin, J. S., & Vanderpool, H. Y. (1987). Is frequent religious attendance *really* conducive to better health? Toward an epidemiology of religion. *Social Science and Medicine, 24*, 589–600.

Linden, W., Stossel, C., & Maurice, J. (1996). Psychosocial interventions for patients with coronary artery disease. *Archives of Internal Medicine, 156*, 745–752.

Matthews, D. A., & Larson, D. B. (1997). Faith and medicine: Reconciling the twin traditions of healing. *Mind/Body Medicine, 2*, 3–6.

Matthews, D. A., McCullough, M. E., Larson, D. B., Koenig, H. G., Swyers, J. P., & Milano, M. G. (1998). Religious commitment and health status. *Archives of Family Medicine, 7*, 118–124.

McCullough, M. E., Hoyt, W. T., Larson, D. B., Koenig, H. G., & Thoresen, C. (2000).Religious involvement and mortality: A meta-analytic review. *Health Psychology, 19*(3), 211–222.

Michalek, A. M., Mettlin, C., & Priore, R. L. (1981). Prostate cancer mortality among Catholic priests. *Journal of Surgical Oncology, 17*, 129–133.

Oman, D., & Reed, D. (1998). Religion and mortality among the community-dwelling elderly. *American Journal of Public Health, 88*, 1469–1475.

Orth-Gomer, K., Mittleman, M. A., Schenck-Gustafsson, K., Wamala, S. P., Eriksson, M., Belkic, K., Kirkeeide, R., Svane, B., & Ryden, L. (1997). Lipoprotein(a) as a determinant of coronary heart disease in young women. *Circulation, 95*, 329–334.

Pressman, P., Lyons, J. S., Larson, D. B., & Strain, J. J. (1990). Religious belief, depression and ambulation status in elderly women with broken hips. *American Journal of Psychiatry, 147*, 758–760.

Ramon, J. M., Escriba, J. M., Casas, I., Benet, J., Iglesias, C., Gavalda, L., Torras, G., & Oromi, J. (1996). Age at first full-term pregnancy, lactation and parity and risk of breast cancer: A case-control study in Spain. *European Journal of Epidemiology, 12*, 449–453.

Rapiti, E., Jindal, S. K., Gupta, D., & Boffetta, P. (1999). Passive smoking and lung cancer in Chandigarh, India. *Lung Cancer, 23*, 183–189.

Schatzkin, A., Lanza, E., Corle, D., Lance, P., Iber, F., Caan, B., Shike, M., Weissfeld, J., Burt, R., Cooper, M. R., Kikendall, J. W., Cahill, J., Freedman, L., Marshall, J., Schoen, R. E., & Slattery, M. (2000). Lack of effect of a low-fat, high-fiber diet on the recurrence of colorectal adenomas. *New England Journal of Medicine, 342*, 1149–1156.

Sloan, R., Bagiella, E., & Powell, T. (1999). Religion, spirituality, and medicine. *Lancet, 353*, 664–667.

Sloan, R. P., Bagiella, E., VandeCreek, L., Hover, M., Casalone, C., Hirsch, T. J., Hasan, Y., Kreger, R., & Poulos, P. (2000). Should physicians prescribe religious activities? *New England Journal of Medicine, 342*, 1913–1916.

Strawbridge, W. J., Cohen, R. D., Shema, S. J., & Kaplan, G. A. (1997). Frequent attendance at religious services and mortality over 28 years. *American Journal of Public Health, 87,* 957–961.

Timio, M., Lippi, G., Venanzi, S., Gentili, S., Quintaliani, G., Verdura, C., Monarca, C., Saronio, P., & Timio, F. (1997). Blood pressure trend and cardiovascular events in nuns in a secluded order: A 30-year follow-up study. *Blood Pressure, 6,* 81–87.

Zuckerman, D. M., Kasl, S. V., & Ostfeld, A. M. (1984). Psychosocial predictors of mortality among the elderly poor. *American Journal of Epidemiology, 119,* 410–423.

15

◄❍►

RELIGION AND SPIRITUALITY IN THE SCIENCE AND PRACTICE OF HEALTH PSYCHOLOGY

Openness, Skepticism, and the Agnosticism of Methodology

TIMOTHY W. SMITH

In a remarkably brief period of time, health psychology has become a central element of the behavioral and biomedical sciences. Since its formal emergence in the 1970s, the field has made rapid advances in the study of psychological influences on and impact of physical health and illness. This research now guides an impressive array of applications in the prevention and management of illness, ranging from psychological interventions with individuals to organizational interventions and even to the design of public policy. The field has made an active effort to be inclusive and comprehensive by examining how issues of health and behavior vary with age, gender, ethnicity, sexual orientation, and socioeconomic status. Until recently, the topic of religion and spirituality has been relatively overlooked in health psychology. This volume makes clear that throughout the field's history there have been efforts to examine the role of these psychosocial constructs in the development, course, and impact of illness. However, given the level of religious involvement and the importance of spiritual concerns among many of the people that health psychologists study and treat, research on the topic seems notable in its scarcity. We know surprisingly little about the impact of religion and spirituality on health. Most health psychologists would readily agree that issues of diversity and sensitivity regarding ethnicity, age, sex, and sexual orientation are important considerations in the science and practice of health psychology. Yet this concern has not been applied to issues of religion and spirituality with the same enthusiasm and thoroughness.

Paralleling a renewed public interest in religion and spirituality, the scientific study of religion and health has grown in recent years, as has interest in matters of religion and spirituality in health care services. Yet, with seemingly equal energy, skeptical voices have also arisen in response, challenging the conclusions and even legitimacy of the field's recent attention to matters of faith. Common social wisdom encourages us to avoid discussions of religion in many settings for fear of the deeply held differences of opinion that may emerge. In polite company, we should stick to safer topics. In the case of the study of faith and health, it is too late to heed such advice. The disagreement is open and active.

Some of the conflicts are clear and substantive. Others seem misperceived. The competing misperceptions could be captured by two cartoons that appeared previously in the pages of *Science*. In the first, a chalkboard dense with seemingly scientific equations contains an open space in the middle, with the words "a miracle happens here." In some cases with justification (W. S. Harris et al., 1999), the current generation of skeptics might feel that this image reflects the inherent nature of "scientific" inquiry in faith and health. In the second, two lab-coated scientists stand before another chalkboard, similarly full of equations. One has drawn a huge "X" across the entire board, and the other asks, "That's it? That's peer review?" Researchers involved in the study of faith and health might understandably feel that their work is met with this automatic and unwelcoming response. Of course, the ideal scientific climate is one of equal shares of openness and skepticism, in which even unfamiliar and potentially provocative questions are posed but in which no conclusions are spared from critical analysis.

In this chapter, I discuss the status of research on faith and health from the perspective of health psychology research. I examine the representation of matters of religion and spirituality in each of the three major topics in health psychology, with an emphasis on conceptual and methodological issues in each area. Elsewhere (Smith & Ruiz, 1999), I have argued that the field can be segmented into the topics of (1) health behavior and prevention, (2) stress and disease, and (3) psychosocial aspects of medical illness and care. Religion and spirituality are relevant to each area, as noted by Plante and Sherman (Chapter 1, this volume), though future research must attend to recurring methodological and conceptual challenges in each of them. I then turn briefly to issues concerning the use of research on religion and spirituality as a guide to clinical services. There is much smoke but certainly some fire in the current debate about the role of religion and spirituality in the practice of clinical health psychology. However, these disagreements have parallels in other debates about the art and science of clinical practice. Finally, I suggest that the understandable tension at the core of the debate— if managed constructively—could stimulate many valuable contributions.

HEALTH BEHAVIOR AND PREVENTION THROUGH RISK REDUCTION

One of the central topics in health psychology is the role of health behaviors or "lifestyle factors" in the development of illness and premature mortality, as well as the effectiveness of risk-reducing preventive interventions. Smoking, inactivity, high fat diets, obesity, alcohol and drug abuse, unprotected sexual activity, and preventive practices (e.g., use of sunscreen and seat belts, participation in medical screenings, etc.) are examples of behaviors, or conditions heavily influenced by behaviors, that have an important impact on major public health threats. Indeed, many important causes of serious illness and premature death (e.g., cardiovascular disease, cancer, HIV/AIDS) are influenced to a considerable degree by such behaviors. Hence, understanding the influences on health behavior, the process of change in health behavior, and the effectiveness of related interventions represents an essential part of the research and applied agenda in health psychology and behavioral medicine.

Testing Models of Health Behavior

It is clear that matters of faith and health are relevant to this topic. For example, participation in some religious faiths involves reduced exposure to behavioral risks; because of prohibitions on tobacco and alcohol use, some religious groups have reduced risks for some illnesses and some causes of death. However, few would take the further step of recommending participation in any religious group solely for this reason. Aside from membership in specific religious denominations in which some behavioral risks are proscribed, are matters of faith related to health behavior? Willis, Wallston, and Johnson (Chapter 9, this volume) provide evidence that this is the case for one very important age group. They review evidence and report new findings that among adolescents, religious beliefs and religious coping are indeed associated with a more positive profile of health behaviors. Use of tobacco and alcohol in adolescence is a key predictor of exposure to these behavioral risks in adulthood and ultimately of the resulting risk of cancer, cardiovascular disease, and other sources of morbidity. Use of alcohol and engagement in risky sexual behavior also pose more immediate threats to health in ado-lescence. Hence, correlational evidence suggests that religious involvement may have beneficial effects on health behaviors.

The research reported by Willis et al. illustrates both the potential strengths and the challenges in health behavior research. In addition to their encouraging findings, Willis et al. demonstrate a commendable level of attention to conceptual clarity and psychometric properties of measures when discussing and assessing religious constructs. Clear conceptual defini-tions and conceptual models, as well as compelling evidence of the construct validity of psychosocial predictors of health behaviors, are essential in this area of research (Smith & Ruiz, 1999; Weinstein, 1993; Weinstein, Rothman, & Sutton, 1998). Further, the construct validity of measures of spiritual and religious concepts must include evidence of convergent *and* dis-criminant or divergent validity. In many areas of health behavior research, explication of what constructs specific measures do and do not assess is an essential but regrettably overlooked component in the accumulation of a systematic, cumulative body of knowledge (Smith & Rhodewalt, 1992; Smith & Ruiz, 1999). All too often, the "little theories" about the links between concepts and research operations receive short shrift in research programs primarily concerned with the "big theories" about how constructs are related. Inadequate attention to these issues has a variety of negative consequences. For example, religious, spiritual, or health behavior con-structs with very different names and definitions may be assessed with mea-sures that are psychometrically indistinguishable. This practice results in essentially tautological associations between what are interpreted as distinct constructs, as well as in the rediscovery of established relationships through the use of severely overlapping scales with different names. This problem is hardly unique to the assessment of spiritual and religious constructs, as it has been a problem in many areas of health psychology research. Yet, as health psychology expands into this area, attention to this issue can help avoid the limitations of other research areas. As suggested by Thoresen, Harris, and Oman (Chapter 2, this volume) and Sherman and Simonton (Chapters 6 and 7, this volume), investigators of religion and health recog-nize this fundamental methodological concern.

Previous theory and research on religion will be invaluable assets in the delineation and assessment of key constructs. Yet rigorous attention to psy-chometric concerns could be inconsistent with the often complex and subtle features of spirituality and religious activities. Chirban (Chapter 11, this vol-ume) presents the richness and nuance of this conceptual domain, and con-siderable care must be taken in applying the often blunt tools of psychomet-rics to capture it adequately. Perhaps a scoring system could be derived to accompany the semistructured clinical protocol he describes. This assess-ment could, in turn, be used as a common validation framework for comparing and contrasting less expensive self-report measures of these constructs. Elsewhere (Plante & Sherman, Chapter 1 and Sherman & Simonton, Chapter 6, this volume), the conceptual landscape in this area and the related assessment instruments are reviewed. A critical understanding of the strengths and weakness of these procedures is important in the design and interpretation of research on religious and spiritual influences on health behaviors.

Of course, it is also essential to use reliable and valid measures of health behaviors. Individual health behaviors are not closely correlated with each other, nor are they very stable over time (Norris, 1997). People who consume a high-fat diet may or may not exercise regularly, and their diet is likely to fluctuate considerably over time. Hence, rather than on a notion of a broadly and consistently healthy or unhealthy "lifestyle," research in this area must be based on a model of specific and changing health behaviors. Therefore, prospective designs are not valuable just through their increased informativeness about the possible direction of causality underlying relations among psychosocial variables and health behaviors; such designs are also valuable in providing information about the stability of effects over time.

There is widespread public knowledge and appreciation of the role of behavior in health. Virtually everyone "knows" that smoking, high dietary intake of saturated fat, inactivity, and excessive alcohol use are unhealthy. This fact renders the assessment of health behaviors through self-report potentially worrisome. Self-reports of behaviors widely recognized to be unhealthy and potentially undesirable create the possibility that such scales tap an unknown mixture of actual health behavior and socially desirable responding. In the context of research on religion and spirituality, this methodological concern is compounded by the possibility that measures of those constructs are also contaminated with similar response biases or artifacts (Sherman & Simonton, Chapter 6, this volume). Hence, correlations between self-reports of religious or spiritual beliefs and practices and self-reports of health behavior could be inflated by shared method artifacts, reflecting wholly or in part the impact of the "third variable" of socially desirable responding. Especially in large population studies, it may not be feasible to include more compelling measures of health behaviors. Nonetheless, measures that do not rely solely on self-reports permit stronger tests of research hypotheses. Further, evidence based on self-reports must be interpreted with caution.

Valid assessments of the inputs and outcomes in studies of religious and spiritual influences on health behavior are essential, but they are not the only critical features of strong research in this area. Conceptual models in this area typically specify mechanisms through which distal variables such as religion and spirituality might affect health behavior. These constructs (e.g., health values, coping behaviors, etc.) must also be assessed effectively, with attention to common artifacts and unintended overlap with measures of other constructs. Further, the statistical approaches used to evaluate these models must be matched to the conceptual hypotheses, as in discussions of the evaluation of mediating and moderating variables (Baron & Kenney, 1986; Holmbeck, 1997). Occasionally, models specify time-linked processes, such as stages of change in health behaviors. These models pose additional challenges in design and analysis (Weinstein et al., 1998). There are clear temporal aspects to many health behavior changes, as in the case of the poor stability of some changes (e.g., smoking cessation, weight loss). Tests of religious and spiritual predictors of initial changes may or may not provide information on the much more important issue of their stability. The potentially fluctuating nature of religious activity complicates further the challenges posed by temporal aspects of research design.

Although statistically significant associations, regardless of their magnitude, often have theoretical importance, research on health behavior is essentially driven by a practical concern. The overarching goal of reducing unhealthy behavior and thereby improving the public health makes effect sizes (i.e., estimates of the strength of association) important. The ultimate importance of health behavior research is actually reflected in the product of multiple effect sizes in the various links in the chain from determinants of health behavior and the often limited effectiveness of interventions in changing behavior to the magnitude of the impact of health behavior on what are typically multiply determined diseases (R. M. Kaplan, 1984). Finally, the relative importance and determinants of various health behaviors are likely to vary across the lifespan and as a function of sex, race, and socioeconomic status. Thus evaluations of the role of religious and spiritual factors in health behavior should attend to issues of external validity or generalizability across these dimensions. Further, the impact of religious and spiritual factors may itself vary as a function of the specific religious context or denomination.

Evaluating Risk-Reducing Interventions

Eventually, a systematic and cumulative body of evidence describing whether or not—and if so, how—religious and spiritual factors affect health behavior could guide the development, evaluation, and practical implementation of risk-reducing preventive interventions. It is clear that the evidence regarding the impact of religious factors on health behavior is suggestive and even encouraging but far from definitive. The research evidence regarding the mechanisms through which these factors influence health behavior is even less well developed. Hence, the research base has not matured to the point at which it provides a clear foundation for interventions.

Yet such interventions have been proposed, and some have been subjected to at least preliminary evaluation (A. H. Harris, Thoresen, McCullough, & Larson, 1999). Further, some segments of the population are eager for health behavior change approaches that are based on or are at least consistent with their religious and spiritual beliefs (Miller, 1999). In some organizations, such as Alcoholics Anonymous or 12-step programs for substance abuse, such interventions have a long history and a large if not definitive research literature. Yet clinical use of interventions lacking in empirical support is potentially problematic, as discussed later in this chapter. Further, empirical evaluation of religious and spiritual interventions for health behavior change that are not based on supported models of the role of these factors poses an additional risk. Interventions lacking a preliminary foundation in research on the religious and spiritual determinants of health behavior and the mechanisms of these effects could be found ineffective simply because they focus on the wrong factors. Evidence of the ineffectiveness of misdirected religious or spiritual health behavior change programs could potentially lead to a premature and far-reaching rejection of these approaches. More carefully and systematically derived interventions, in contrast, might be more likely to be found effective. Hence, a "rush to application" by proponents could have the paradoxical effect of reducing funding for further trials, support from health care providers, and acceptance by patients and health care professionals alike.

Whether or not they are based on supportive research on the determinants of health behavior and the process or mechanisms of health behavior change, research on the effectiveness of religiously and spiritually oriented interventions should incorporate common methodological features of intervention studies on health promotion. Some of the issues described herein are obviously relevant, such as the adequate assessment of behavioral outcomes and attention to the generalizability of results across important demographic variables. Other issues common to all clinical intervention studies are relevant as well, such as the selection of appropriate comparison groups (Chambless & Hollon, 1998), the integrity of intervention protocols (Waltz, Addis, Koerner, & Jacobson, 1993), the maintenance of behavior changes, the clinical or practical significance of intervention effects, and the quantitative management of attrition (Kendall, Flannery-Schroeder, & Ford, 1999).

Intervention studies also provide unique opportunities for experimental tests of models of health behavior. In order to capitalize on this opportunity, the relevant mediating (or explanatory) variables specified in the underlying conceptual model must be assessed and appropriate mediational analyses of intervention effects performed. Also, in addition to the clinical or practical significance of interventions, research on health behavior change increasingly addresses the complex issue of cost-effectiveness, especially in light of limited health care resources (Freidman, Subel, Meyers, Caudill, & Benson, 1995; R. M. Kaplan, 2000; Yates, 1994). In this case, the question is simply put: Are the benefits of spiritual or religious interventions for health behavior change sufficient to justify their costs, relative to current practices? Given the maturity of some of these research areas, the methodological "bar" is set quite high for many topics in health behavior change research (Compas, Haaga, Keefe, Leitenberg, & Williams, 1998), and proponents of the inclusion of religious and spiritual matters must take care to incorporate the critical features of design and analysis.

In health behavior change research, interventions are sometimes directed toward very large groups, such as the workplace or even whole communities (Hancock, Sanson-Fisher, & Redman, 1997). The evaluation of such approaches represents a complex problem of the planning and analysis of what are often quasi-experimental designs (Cook & Campbell, 1979). The social organization of religious practices lends itself to this form of intervention. Indeed, religious organizations provide an important public health resource for prevention and health behavior change, often with the additional benefit of inherent tailoring to specific demographic groups (e.g., obesity interventions for African American women). If such interventions are to go beyond service delivery to serve a research mission as well, they must address the daunting challenges of this type of research design and analysis (Hancock et al., 1997).

STRESS AND DISEASE

Certainly, one of the most provocative findings of recent research on religion and spirituality in health psychology and behavioral medicine comes from epidemiological studies; even when controlling for health behaviors (e.g., smoking, alcohol consumption), participation in religious activities seems to be associated with increased longevity and decreased risk of serious illness (McCullough, Hoyt, Larson, Koenig, & Thoresen, 2000; Thoresen et al., Chapter 2, and see also McCullough, Chapter 3, this volume). This finding is an example of the second major topic in health psychology—the effects of stress, emotions, and related psychosocial factors on the development of illness. Stressful life circumstances, personality characteristics, coping behavior, and features of the social environment affect physical health directly rather than through the intervening effects of health behaviors, presumably through the psychobiological correlates of stress and negative emotion (Lovallo, 1997). This topic has been a central feature of health psychology and behavioral medicine since the inception of these fields and accounts for a large portion of the public's interest in them. The basic model underlying this area of research begins with the premise that an individual's cognitive appraisal of the environment as posing a significant threat or demand evokes physiological changes in the individual. If sufficiently prolonged, severe, and repeated, these physiological changes can promote disease. Further, personality characteristics (e.g., chronic anger or hostility) and social circumstances (e.g., social support) render some individuals at greater or lesser risk of stress-induced illness by altering the frequency or magnitude of physiological responses. These effects of stress and related psychosocial processes have been extensively studied and are best understood in the case of two general areas—the effects of stress on the cardiovascular system (Rozanski, Blumenthal, & Kaplan, 1999) and on the immune system (Rabin, 1999).

Currently, four general research strategies are employed in this area. In the least informative, *human cross-sectional, case–control research*, the psychosocial characteristics of individuals with and without a specific illness are compared. This methodological approach is limited because psychosocial variables can be influenced by the development of illness, rendering this design quite susceptible to ambiguity about the direction of causality and other threats to internal validity (Cohen & Rodriguez, 1995). In the second approach—*human epidemiological research*—psychosocial variables are assessed in groups of individuals, and after a follow-up period the association of these factors with subsequent health is examined. It is important to note that many prospective studies of psychosocial constructs and health are based on small and select samples. Hence they are not epidemiological studies in the typical sense of this term. In the preliminary stage of some research areas, however, even small studies of convenience samples can be useful. *Animal research* permits a level of experimental manipulation of environmental stress and invasive assessments of disease processes that are clearly unethical in human research and therefore is an important complement to human research. Finally, *human mechanism research* examines the impact of stress and associated personality or social factors on the physiological changes believed to link them with disease.

For research concerning the potential impact of religious and spiritual factors on disease processes, two of these general strategies are clearly inappropriate. For obvious reasons it is unlikely that useful animal models of religion will be developed, and the impact of serious illness on religious and spiritual processes is so common that the cross-sectional comparison of clinical groups is uninformative. That is, higher levels of religious involvement in patients with serious illness compared with healthy controls is at least as likely to reflect a consequence of illness as it is a cause. For the other approaches, there are clear methodological challenges for research on the health consequences of faith.

Epidemiological Studies of Religion, Spirituality, and Health

Epidemiological research can be seen as essentially descriptive. The identification of reliable psychosocial predictors of morbidity and mortality is useful, even if it is not guided by conceptual models of how such factors influence health. However, in current health psychology and behavioral medicine, such models are increasingly seen as a requirement. At the simplest level, the potential pathways or mechanisms linking psychosocial risk factors and health must be at least generally described, and they must be medically plausible. Further, given that most diseases of interest have multifactorial pathophysiologies that change over time, the models of psychosocial influences on disease must attend to the natural history of disease processes. To date, epidemiological research on the effects of religious and spiritual involvement on health is not adequately grounded in such models. Arguably, simple statistical associations between these constructs and subsequent health are sufficiently important and novel that more complete models are not required at this point. However, such analyses must be structured so as to rule out obvious artifactual influences on the association between faith and health (see Sloan, Bagiella, & Powell, 1999, and Chapter 14, this volume). Once the current debate about whether or not the basic epidemiological association is robust and valid is settled (see Thoresen et al., Chapter 2; McCullough, Chapter 3; and Sloan et al., Chapter 14, this volume), further progress in the study of health consequences of religion and spirituality will require more complete models. The example put forth by Thoresen, Harris, and Oman (Chapter 2, this volume) is a valuable beginning in this regard.

The previous discussion about the absolute necessity in health behavior research of clear conceptual definitions of the religious and spiritual predictor variables and compelling evidence of the reliability and validity (i.e., convergent and divergent) of related measures is central to epidemiological studies of the health consequences of these constructs. The history of research on psychosocial predictors of health contains several instances in which incomplete attention to conceptual definitions and to the validity of assessment devices have impeded systematic progress (e.g., Funk, 1992; Rhodewalt & Smith, 1991). Confidence in the interpretation of statistical associations between measures of religious and spiritual variables and subsequent health is directly related to the validity of the assessments of these psychosocial constructs. The reviews of prospective studies included in this volume provide intriguing suggestions of the importance of this issue, such as the possibility that public religious participation is a more robust predictor of subsequent health than is more private religious activity. In such instances, clarity and precision in assessment have the potential to refine models of the mechanisms linking these predictors to health.

Religious and spiritual variables are likely to overlap with two widely studied classes of psychosocial risk factors—personality characteristics and social relationships. Therefore, in the process of measurement evaluation, it seems important to examine the association of religious and spiritual measures with established measures of these domains. Research of this type could alert investigators to possible instances in which the effects of personality, social relations, religion, and spirituality overlap, thereby facilitating an integrated rather than unintentionally redundant literature on psychosocial predictors of health. In the domain of personality, the growing acceptance of the Five Factor taxonomy of personality traits (Digman, 1990) provides a valuable tool for these types of integrative comparisons and contrasts. The well-validated Five Factor assessment devices provide the opportunity to identify the unique and distinguishing aspects of health-relevant individual differences in a known conceptual space (Smith & Williams, 1992; Gallo & Smith, 1998). In studies of the social correlates of religious and spiritual variables, care must be taken to include valid measures of both positive (e.g., social support) and negative (e.g., social conflict) features of the social environment, as both are related to health and both could be important correlates of religious and spiritual involvement. Examination of these potential associations helps sharpen our understanding of the measures and provides information about how religious and spiritual processes might influence health.

Equally important is the nature of the health outcome assessment. Studies of mortality have outcomes of obvious validity and importance, though analyses of all-cause mortality (i.e., all causes of death combined) can complicate the process of developing conceptual models because of the likely heterogeneity of mechanisms through which psychosocial factors influence general mortality. Similarly, medically documented outcomes (e.g., verified diagnosis of myocardial infarction or cancer) are also typically quite valid, and most research areas have general standards for the quantification or classification of such outcomes. More troublesome is the use of self-reports of health or other measures reflecting illness behavior rather than illness itself (e.g., visits to physicians, sick days). Measures of illness behavior certainly do reflect actual health. For example, self-reports of health predict subsequent mortality, even when physician ratings of health are controlled (e.g., G. A. Kaplan & Camacho, 1983). However, the correspondence between measures of illness behavior and actual illness is far from perfect, and the lack of overlap appears to be related to a variety of psychological constructs. For example, self-reports of physical symptoms in excess of actual illness are reliably correlated with the personality construct of neuroticism or negative affectivity (Costa & McCrae, 1987; Watson & Pennebaker, 1989). If religious or spiritual measures are similarly correlated with negative emotions, then what appears to be an association between religious or spiritual involvement and physical health could actually reflect the effects of neuroticism on unfounded somatic complaints. The importance of this concern is underscored by research reviewed by Plante and Sharma (Chapter 10, this volume), which demonstrates that religious measures are consistently related to measures of negative emotionality. Of course, subjective health is an important element of quality of life and therefore an outcome worth studying in its own right. Nonetheless, it is essential to make appropriately cautious interpretations when self-reported health is used as an outcome.

Even when valid indicators of psychosocial predictors and health outcomes are employed in prospective studies with large and well-defined samples, the inherently correlational design of these studies raises additional interpretive cautions. Positive effects suggest only that something captured by or correlated with the psychosocial measure predicts subsequent health. How much additional inference is scientifically appropriate depends on other features of the design and analysis, but strong causal conclusions of the sort that would support clinical recommendations for specific interventions are never appropriate. There are simply far too many third variables that can potentially account for the apparent effects of religious processes on health. It is methodologically indefensible to leap from correlational epidemiological findings across the expanse of causal ambiguity to clinical recommendations. Those who do so (e.g., Koenig, 1997) understandably meet with severe criticism (Sloan et al., Chapter 14, this volume).

The range of third variables that can potentially account for the apparent association between religious and spiritual factors and health not only necessitates interpretive caution but also identifies a valuable research agenda. It is clear that health behaviors, personality characteristics, and aspects of the social environment are candidates for research of this type. Traditionally, the analytic strategy in epidemiological research is directed toward identifying "independent" risk factors. For example, given that many smokers are physically inactive, is the statistical association of smoking with subsequent cardiovascular disease independent of the third variable of physical activity? In the case of psychosocial epidemiology, such issues are more appropriately framed as model testing. Can shared variance with health behavior account for the association of religious participation with mortality? If so, this does *not* indicate that religious participation is not important for health. Instead, it suggests a mechanism for the effects of religious variables on health. If statistical control of health behavior fails to eliminate the otherwise significant effect of religious participation on mortality, one might be tempted to conclude that health behaviors are not an important mechanism. However, confidence in this conclusion must be tempered by the possibility that limitations in the assessment of health behavior resulted in incomplete statistical control of this mechanism and therefore that the intervening impact of health behavior was "undercorrected."

Nonetheless, a comparative theory-testing approach to the problem of correlated risk factors is likely to advance our understanding of the health consequences of religion. For example, it would be useful to test the hypothesis that religious involvement affects health because it is more common among people who are high in Agreeableness and Conscientiousness and that these personality traits confer reduced risk of serious illness (Smith & Gallo, 2000). Alternatively, perhaps religious activity fosters social support, and this well-established protective factor accounts for its effects. Finally, recent developments in psychosocial epidemiology have demonstrated "place" effects on health. For example, when neighborhood and individual socioeconomic status are quantified, both have a prospective association with health outcomes (e.g., Waitzman & Smith, 1998). That is, the places we inhabit seem to influence our health independently of our personal qualities. Perhaps religious participation is a marker for such a "place" effect by which it is not the individual's characteristics but regular exposure to a safe, less threatening community that fosters health. Assessments of individual and local levels of religious participation, coupled with hierarchical data analyses, could distinguish individual versus community effects of religiousness.

Finally, psychosocial epidemiological research must take care to examine how risk factors may vary across key demographic groups and across the time course of disease. Obviously, it is essential to determine if the effects of such demographic factors account for the association between religious or spiritual factors and subsequent health in order to rule out artifacts. However, demographic factors could also delimit (i.e., moderate) the association of religious and spiritual involvement with health. For example, the effects of religious participation on mortality appear to differ for men and women (McCullough, Chapter 3, this volume), and may also vary across ethnicity, age, socioeconomic status, and level of initial health.

Mechanism Research

To date, reviews of the epidemiological research on religion, spirituality, and health offer the tentative conclusion that health behaviors do not provide a complete account of the association. Instead, some sort of stress-reducing or stress-buffering effect is hypothesized. If this is indeed a general class of mechanisms linking religious and spiritual processes to health, then associations of religious and spiritual factors with physiological processes must be documented. As outlined by Thoresen, Harris, and Oman (Chapter 2, this volume), as yet there is precious little evidence of such an association. Yet there is a wide range of conceptual and methodological approaches to the study of such links. Hence this relative gap in the literature on faith and health is also an important and feasible focus for future research. Sophisticated methodologies are available to examine the impact of religious and spiritual variables on the psychobiological mechanisms that could link them to health.

Laboratory-based studies typically involve the experimental manipulation of stressful tasks or challenges and assessment of hypothesized physiological mechanisms. The psychosocial risk factor the relationship of which with disease mechanisms is to be modeled is either measured or itself manipulated, depending on the specific research question. Cardiovascular, neuroendocrine, and even acute immune system changes are assessed in this paradigm. In such studies, care must be taken to select appropriate stressors so as to create a reasonable laboratory model of the stress process. Further, methodological issues are paramount in the collection and analysis of both the physiological and associated psychological (e.g., affective reactions, task appraisals, etc.) responses (for reviews, see Schneiderman, Weiss, & Kaufmann, 1989; Smith & Ruiz, 1999).

Laboratory studies of acute stress mechanisms afford advantages in experimental control and precision of measurement but can be criticized for their lack of realism and potentially limited generalizability to stress responses in the natural environment. Ambulatory studies of physiological responses (e.g., blood pressure, heart rate, cortisol level) provide a valuable supplement to laboratory methods. For example, the association of religious participation or forgiveness with ambulatory levels of blood pressure could be examined. Ambulatory physiological assessments can be combined with parallel self-report assessments of daily experiences. In this way, the effects of religious factors on both exposure to stressful events and physiological reactions to those events can be examined.

Chronic stress can also have deleterious physiological effects, and a variety of paradigms are available for examining the association of psychosocial factors with such responses. For example, the chronic stress of caregiving is associated with negative effects on immune activity (Kiecolt-Glaser & Glaser, 1995) and health (Schulz & Beach, 1999). The moderation of these effects by religious or spiritual factors could easily be examined. In short, many paradigms are available to test the hypothesis that faith affects health through the pathway of altered physiology. Even initial support for this sort of plausible mechanism would strengthen the research base considerably.

Associations between religious and spiritual variables and physiological stress responses would be consistent with the hypothesis that these psychosocial factors affect health through the pathway of altered stress. However, such associations provide only initial support. It must be established that these physiological responses are of sufficient type, magnitude, and frequency to be involved in the development of disease (Cohen & Rabin, 1998). Ultimately, the mediational models underpinning this research area could be tested in studies in which religious and spiritual variables are assessed along with the hypothesized physiological mechanisms, and appropriate analyses could indicate whether or not such mechanisms account statistically for the effects of these psychosocial factors on subsequent health. To be fair, such grand theory testing is extraordinarily rare in health psychology and behavioral medicine, but the design and analysis of large epidemiological studies could be directed in such a way as to make investigations possible.

PSYCHOSOCIAL ASPECTS
OF MEDICAL ILLNESS AND CARE

The final major topic in health psychology involves psychosocial aspects of acute and chronic medical illness. Included in this topic are studies of adjustment to acute and chronic diseases, the psychological impact of medical and surgical care, and the effects of adjunctive psychosocial treatments for illness. The chapters in this volume indicate that this third broad topic has been a major focus of the work on faith and health, including religiousness in adjustment to cancer (Sherman & Simonton, Chapter 7) and HIV/AIDS (Remle & Koening, Chapter 8) and spirituality-based interventions for medical conditions (Tan & Dong, Chapter 12). The future prospects for research on the role of religion and spirituality in adaptation to illness seem bright, though methodological issues inherent in this area of research must guide future studies.

Adjustment to Illness and Stressful Health Care

In order for researchers to identify predictors of adjustment to medical conditions and care, they must appreciate the specific symptoms, underlying pathophysiology, prognosis, and standard diagnostic and intervention procedures for a given condition. Only with this type of understanding of medical contexts will they design optimal studies of psychosocial influences on adaptation, as the illness and treatment context is a far-reaching determinant of the patient's experience. Further, these features of the medical context will suggest important outcomes and predictors. The work by Sherman and Simonton (Chapter 7, this volume) provides a good example of the necessary thoroughness. For most specific medical conditions, the conceptual domain has been well described and assessment devices developed and subjected to psychometric evaluation. Researchers embarking on studies of the role of religion and spirituality in adjustment to medical illness and care should examine this literature closely in order to select the best assessment devices and procedures. As with the previous two topics, clear conceptual definitions of religious and spiritual constructs, related variables, and a model of their hypothesized interrelations are important for systematic research. And again, well-validated measures of these constructs are essential.

Beyond these homilies on models and measures, several specific methodological issues must be addressed. For example, emotional adjustment is a frequent focus of research of this type. In many cases, measures of adjustment developed for medically healthy populations are employed, and they can produce misleading findings when used with medically ill persons. This is particularly the case when measures of depression are used with the medically ill. The somatic symptoms of depression (e.g., fatigue, disturbances in appetite, etc.) are typically highly diagnostic in medically healthy populations but can reflect symptoms of physical illness rather than emotional functioning in medical populations (Clark, Cook, & Snow, 1998; Peck, Smith, Ward, & Milano, 1989). Further, the implicit pathology model that underlies the selection of such measures must be questioned. Depressive reactions are common among the medically ill and have implications not only for quality of life but also for medical prognoses. However, the level of depressive symptoms among medical patients does not capture the full range of the potential effects of chronic illness on emotional adjustment. Most patients do not experience diagnosable depressive reactions, and normal emotional functions are better captured by a two-dimensional model of varying degrees of negative affect and independently varying degrees of positive affect (Watson & Tellegen, 1985). Measures of depressive symptoms collapse these dimensions (Watson et al., 1995), such that depression is a combination of high negative and low positive affect. Hence, a specific and comprehensive assessment of the impact of religious factors on emotional adjustment in the medically ill requires the use of measures of emotional adjustment that extend beyond the typical choices of depressive symptoms or other negative affects.

A great deal of research on adjustment to medical illness relies on self-report methods to assess emotional adjustment, physical activity levels, pain, and other consequences of illness. In addition to the typical artifacts involving social desirability, a common problem in research of this type involves overlap in item wording. In some cases, measures of distinct constructs include similarly worded items. Care must be taken, for example, to insure that measures of religious coping and related constructs do not contain item content reflecting emotional responses or activity levels (Sherman & Simonton, Chapters 6 and 7, this volume). Otherwise, such overlap can lead to inflated estimates of the role of these factors in adaptation to illness. When severe, this overlap produces "thinly veiled tautologies" (Coyne &

Gotlib, 1983) in which the contaminating emotional or functional content of religious predictor scales understandably correlates with the similar content on outcome measures.

In many areas of research, individual predictors and social-environment predictors of adjustment are examined separately. Yet individually oriented constructs (e.g., religious practices or spiritual values) are likely to be related to the patient's social context (e.g., availability of care and support). Hence studies that include both these categories of influence on adjustment to illness (e.g., Coyne & Smith, 1994; Manne & Zautra, 1989) may provide a more complete analysis of the effects of religion and spirituality. An often underemphasized social context influencing adaptation is the relationship between the patient and health care professionals. Adequacy of communication, interlocking perceptions and expectations, and interactions in this context are important influences on seeking care and on its quality and effectiveness (Duffy, Hammerman, & Cohen, 1988). In this regard, Shafranske (Chapter 13, this volume) identifies a critical area for continued research—the religious and spiritual views of health care providers.

Adjustment to medical illness is a dynamic process with a variety of potential patterns of change over time. When combined with the likely impact of health on religious and spiritual processes, it is clear that prospective designs have much to offer. However, selection of the time frame for sampling these changing processes must be guided by a thorough understanding of the specific medical condition and its treatment. In some medical conditions, relatively infrequent assessments may be adequate. In others, in which important outcomes fluctuate more rapidly, much more frequent assessments are necessary. In such cases, recent advances in the use of daily experience sampling and momentary assessments in health psychology (Affleck, Zautra, Tennen, & Armeli, 1999) could be useful in explicating the role of religion and spirituality in the everyday life of the medically ill. Much of the research on religious and spiritual influences on adjustment to illness examines the role of religiously oriented coping (Pargament, 1997) and is grounded in the general coping model of Lazarus and Folkman (1984). Research of this type should certainly attend to issues raised herein, especially the possible contamination of coping items with distress or disability and the likely social context of coping. However, the recent, broader critiques of coping assessment (e.g., Coyne & Gottlieb, 1996; Stone et al., 1998) suggest that patients do not provide accurate assessments of actual coping activities when they complete retrospective coping inventories. Inaccurate retrospective general summaries of coping behavior can produce misleading evidence about the role of religious coping in adaptation. Hence future research on religious coping should examine the newer methodologies that have been developed as supplements to standard approaches (e.g., Stone et al., 1998).

Evaluating Adjunctive Religious
and Spiritual Treatments

One of the major contributions of health psychology and behavioral medicine has been the design and empirical evaluation of psychosocial interventions for medical problems. The range of applications is impressive—from the management of acute pain and distress associated with surgery and aversive medical procedures to interventions to reduce chronic pain and disability to treatments to enhance adherence to essential medical regimens and interventions to reduce the negative impact of stress and negative emotions on the course of disease (Compas et al., 1998; Linden, Stossel, & Maurice, 1996). The work reviewed in this volume and elsewhere (A. H. Harris et al., 1999) raises the possibility that established standard psychosocial interventions could be enhanced by the addition of religious and spiritual approaches. Tan and Dong (Chapter 12, this volume) and Thoresen and his colleagues (Chapter 2, this volume) review some of the available approaches and the limited evidence of their effectiveness. It is fair to say that in no case is a religious or spiritual intervention approach in clinical health psychology or behavioral medicine supported by the same degree of empirical evidence of effectiveness as is available for traditional psychosocial interventions. Hence there is a clear need for clinical intervention research. As described previously, ideally such research would be guided by the yet-to-be-accumulated evidence of how religious and spiritual processes affect the development and course of illness through the pathway of stress or by similar evidence of the ways in which these factors affect the patient's adaptation to illness and care. Further, research of this type should be guided by established research guidelines in clinical health psychology and behavioral medicine, as reviewed here.

Outcome measures should be selected following careful consideration of the specific medical condition and a review of related assessment research. Multimethod assessments of outcomes are clearly preferred, especially in light of the fact that placebo and expectancy effects are well documented in health psychology and behavioral medicine (e.g., Turner, Deyo, & Loweser, 1994). Exacerbating this issue is the fact that religious and spiritual interventions are likely to convey transparent and perhaps compelling expectancies for improvement. Hence, in addition to using at least some outcome measures that are less susceptible to self-report artifacts and biases, researchers should select comparison groups in such a way as to control this effect (Schwartz, Chesney, Irvine, & Keefe, 1997). It is the unique rather than the nonspecific effects of religious and spiritual interventions that require evaluation.

The optimal timing of assessments and length of follow-up depend on the specific population and intervention under study. However, whereas brief, immediate effects are quite important in the case of adjustment to surgery or other stressful medical procedures (Auerbach, 1989), in most other cases the stability of effects over time is a critical concern (Compas et al., 1998). Further, unless the research question is quite novel, comparison of religious interventions with no-treatment or waiting-list comparison groups is not likely to provide meaningful increments in clinical knowledge, given the likely impact of nonspecific factors as discussed previously. In most cases, religious and spiritually oriented approaches could be usefully compared with traditional psychosocial interventions. One would anticipate that the relative effectiveness of such groups in a comparative trial would be influenced by the spiritual preferences of the patient. Hence questions of the moderation of religious and spiritual treatment effects are obviously important. Finally, once significant treatment effects are demonstrated, the issues of clinical significance (Kendall et al., 1999) and cost-effectiveness (Friedman et al., 1995) become relevant. Clearly, the research agenda in the evaluation of religious and spiritual interventions as adjuncts to standard medical care is extensive.

FAITH, ART, AND SCIENCE IN THE CLINICAL PRACTICE OF HEALTH PSYCHOLOGY

Health psychology is more than a field of inquiry; it is also intended to promote well-being. Applied endeavors in health psychology are grounded in the scientist–practitioner model in which health care services are guided by the results of empirical research. There is a growing emphasis on empirically supported therapies in clinical psychology in general (Chambless & Hollon, 1998) and behavioral medicine and health psychology as well (Compas et al., 1998). However, the immediate need for clinical services often outstrips the definitiveness and specificity of evidence about the optimal treatment of a particular condition presented by an individual client or patient. Even the most robust findings of clinically significant effects of well-defined interventions for equally well-defined conditions have varying impact at the level of individual clients. Hence generalizing from the empirical literature to individual clinical activities is always a complex, probabilistic process. In the best of circumstances, empirical evidence guides practice rather than guarantees its effectiveness. Further, individuals often have pressing health problems for which compelling evidence of effective treatment is lacking. In other instances, evidence derived from carefully controlled studies of groups of homogeneous individuals cannot be generalized conclusively to specific individuals with complex or multiple problems. Hence the art of application in any area of professional psychology always requires going beyond the available evidence. When critics of the clinical application of research on religion emphasize that such practices go well beyond the empirical support, we must remember that this is essentially always the case and varies only in the extent to which practice goes beyond evidence. Of necessity, practice with only limited empirical support is the typical case for quite a lot of clinical activities, even those of proponents of empirically supported therapies. Incalculable human suffering would accumulate in the wait for truly definitive evidence.

Yet the preceding review makes clear that the research base relevant to decisions about clinical assessment and interventions involving religious and spiritual issues is in many respects quite limited, especially in comparison with many areas in clinical health psychology and behavioral medicine. We know much more about the valid assessment and effective treatment of a variety of health risks (e.g., smoking, diet, alcohol abuse), specific conditions in which psychological issues are relevant (e.g., hypertension, coronary disease, cancer, HIV/AIDS, headache, arthritis, diabetes), and general clinical problems (e.g., adherence to medical regimens, adjustment to invasive medical procedures) than we know about the role of religious and spiritual matters in health and health care. Hence, bold clinical recommendations to pursue religious and spiritual activities in efforts to improve health and manage illness are suspect.

This does not mean that such issues should be actively avoided in clinical care. Rather, it means that tentativeness, caution, and sensitivity are required. Critics of the inclusion of religious and spiritual issues in health care are understandably and appropriately concerned with practices and recommendations that go beyond the available evidence. Even though it likely reflects the best of intentions, advice about religion or spirituality from a physician or psychologist that clearly goes beyond the legitimate conclusions supported by clinical science is just as inappropriate as unsupported advice about vitamins, diet, magnets, or any other type of intervention. However, the potential intrusion of medical and psychological authorities and experts into private matters of religion creates additional potential abuses. Religious or spiritual prescriptions could be seen as a coercive and potentially judgmental or distressing intrusion into private matters, cloaked in the veneer of scientific and medical authority. Sloan and his colleagues (Chapter 14, this volume) provide a brief review of some of the potential ethical and professional pitfalls in faith-based recommendations and interventions. Yet even the clear and compelling possibility of bad clinical practice does not necessarily preclude the inclusion of religious and spiritual concerns in clinical health psychology. Recent work has tried to articulate these ethical issues and establish appropriate professional guidelines for including religion and spirituality in the science and practice of psychotherapy (Miller, 1999; Richards & Bergin, 1997; Shafranske, 1996; see also Chirban, Chapter 11 and Tan & Dong, Chapter 12, this volume).

It may also be the case that psychologists are more informed about professional and ethical considerations at the interface of clinical care and faith than are some other members of the health care team. Psychologists presumably understand the essential nature of awareness, sensitivity, and respect in dealing with the patient's personal beliefs and practices. If attention to matters of faith grows in medicine, psychologists, like pastoral care counselors, may have a critical consultation–liaison role in guiding other members of the health care team in the appropriate, sensitive incorporation of these issues in assessment and care.

CONCLUSIONS: LIONS AND LAMBS WORKING TOGETHER

From this review, it is clear that matters of religion and spirituality are relevant to each of the foci of health psychology. When combined with the prevalence and importance of religious and spiritual concerns in the population, the emergence of this topic seems long overdue. However, the research findings are in many instances preliminary. Many observations are open to multiple interpretations, and many obvious questions have simply not yet been pursued. Conceptual and methodological tools from the study of psychology and religion can be combined with tools from health psychology and behavioral medicine to support the next generation of research in this area, perhaps contributing to a more definitive knowledge base.

In the meantime, those impressed by the potential contribution of this research area should make efforts to treat the findings with appropriate care and caution. If they are compelled to make clinical recommendations well beyond the justifiable implications of the available data, they should avoid the suggestion that the science of faith and health supports those recommendations. If proponents cannot resist the temptation to make a leap of faith from a limited research base to strong causal conclusions, they should at least refrain from inflicting such acrobatics on those under their care. Of course, those scholars who are skeptical or perhaps even opposed to the study of faith and health should strive for openness. Despite the protests, an impartial, perhaps even objective, review suggests that there are many valuable questions to pursue. For proponents and critics alike, this sort of advice is especially relevant at the interface of scientists' professional work and their personal convictions—be they agnostic or believers of any stripe. Such admonishments could seem like an unwise inclusion of ad hominem critiques in scholarly discourse. However, given the potentially charged nature of the discussions, it seems wise to remind ourselves of the sometimes personal nature of scientific attitudes and pursuits.

The pathway to a cumulative and convincing science of faith and health seems clear. Only through years of methodologically rigorous research will we acquire a more accurate and comprehensive view of how faith and religious practices do and do not affect health behavior and prevention efforts, psychosocial vulnerabilities, and resistance to disease, and the effects of illness on patient adjustment, and of the utility of related interventions in clinical care. Yet even methodologically sound evidence might meet with vigorous resistance. Some of the harshest critics seem to reject the endeavor outright. For them, it is essential to recall that there is no constitutional guarantee of a separation of religion and science. However, scientific standards and skepticism are no less relevant to matters of faith and health than they are in any other area of health psychology.

The recent history of health psychology and behavioral medicine may provide insight into both the stridency and merits of the current criticism of the study of faith and health and its inclusion in clinical care. Over the past few decades, many influential members of the traditional medical community resisted the emerging interest in the role of psychological factors in health. This opposition seemed to include limited access to research funding, resistance to publication of behavioral research in medical outlets, and denial of insurance coverage for effective psychological interventions for medical conditions. Despite such resistance, health psychology and behavioral medicine have made significant scientific advances and gained access to significant resources in research and health care services, to say nothing of the related public acceptance of the role of psychosocial aspects of health, illness, and medical care. These gains have been made on the generally level playing field of research methodology. The pioneers in health psychology and behavioral medicine, as well as those who have followed them, are keenly aware of the difficulty of those inroads and accomplishments. Understandably, they are often harsh critics of seemingly related developments in health research and care (e.g., "alternative medicine") that sometimes appear to adhere to a lesser scientific standard. Resistance to new and seemingly "soft science" developments in the field can be seen as an appropriate defense of the standards that were instrumental to those landmark accomplishments.

Just as clear theories and strong methods have fostered the development of a research base that has made it difficult for the remaining proponents of the traditional biomedical model to dismiss the importance of health psychology and behavioral medicine, clear theories and strong methods can ultimately help to separate the wheat from the chaff in the study of faith and health. This is especially true if the next generation of research on the topic proceeds from clearly articulated conceptual models and if the refinement and empirical integration of measures of religious and spiritual constructs proceeds with both psychometric rigor and attention to the complexity and nuance required by the nature of these activities and experiences in people's lives. In both research and practice, what might seem to some to be troubled waters are certainly navigable. The trip will be long and complex, but it might prove to be immensely productive and rewarding.

REFERENCES

Affleck, G., Zautra, A., Tennen, H., & Armeli, S. (1999). Multilevel daily process designs for consulting and clinical psychology: A guide for the perplexed. *Journal of Consulting and Clinical Psychology, 67,* 746–754.

Auerbach, S. M. (1989). Stress management and coping research in the health care setting: An overview and methodological commentary. *Journal of Consulting and Clinical Psychology, 57,* 388–395.

Baron, R. M., & Kenny, D. A. (1986). The moderator–mediator variable distinction in social psychological research: Conceptual, strategic, and statistical considerations. *Journal of Personality and Social Psychology, 51,* 1173–1182.

Chambless, D. L., & Hollon, S. D. (1998). Defining empirically supported therapies. *Journal of Consulting and Clinical Psychology, 66,* 7–18.

Clark, D. A., Cook, A., & Snow, D. (1998). Depressive symptom differences in hospitalized, medically ill, depressed psychiatric inpatients, and nonmedical controls. *Journal of Abnormal Psychology, 107,* 38–48.

Cohen, S., & Rabin, B. S. (1998). Psychologic stress, immunity, and cancer. *Journal of the National Cancer Institute, 90,* 3–4.

Cohen, S., & Rodriguez, M. (1995). Pathways linking affective disturbances and physical disorders. *Health Psychology, 14,* 374–380.

Compas, B. E., Haaga, D. A., Keefe, F. J., Leitenberg, H., & Williams, D. A. (1998). Sampling of empirically supported psychological treatments from health psychology: Smoking, chronic pain, cancer, and bulimia nervosa. *Journal of Consulting and Clinical Psychology, 66,* 89–112.

Cook, T. D., & Campbell, D. T. (1979). *Quasi-experimentation: Design and analysis issues for field settings.* Chicago: Rand McNally.

Costa, P. T., Jr., & McCrae, R. R. (1987). Neuroticism, somatic complaints, and disease: Is the bark worse than the bite? *Journal of Personality, 55,* 299–316.

Coyne, J. C., & Gotlib, I. H. (1983). The role of cognition in depression: A critical appraisal. *Psychological Bulletin, 94,* 472–505.

Coyne, J. C., & Gottlieb, B. H. (1996). The mismeasure of coping by checklist. *Journal of Personality, 64,* 959–991.

Coyne, J. C., & Smith, D. A. (1994). Couples coping with myocardial infarction: Contextual perspective on patient self-efficacy. *Journal of Family Psychology, 8,* 43–54.

Digman, J. (1990). Personality structure: Emergence of the five-factor model. *Annual Review of Psychology, 41,* 417–440.

Duffy, D., Hammerman, D., & Cohen, M. (1988). Patient–physician communication: A descriptive summary of the literature. *Patient Education and Counseling, 12,* 99–119.

Friedman, R., Subel, D., Meyers, P., Caudill, M., & Benson, H. (1995). Behavioral medicine, clinical health psychology, and cost offset. *Health Psychology, 14,* 509–518.

Funk, S. C. (1992). Hardiness: A review of theory and research. *Health Psychology, 11,* 335–346.

Gallo, L. C., & Smith, T. W. (1998). Construct validation of health-relevant personality traits: Interpersonal circumplex and five-factor model analyses of the aggression questionnaire. *International Journal of Behavioral Medicine, 5,* 129–147.

Hancock, L., Sanson-Fisher, R. W., & Redman, S. (1997). Community action for health promotion: A review of methods and outcomes 1990–1995. *American Journal of Preventive Medicine, 13,* 229–239.

Harris, A. H. S., Thoresen, C. E., McCullough, M. E., & Larson, D. B. (1999). Spiritually and religiously oriented health interventions. *Journal of Health Psychology, 4,* 413–434.

Harris, W. S., Gowda, M., Kolb, J. W., Strychacz, C. P., Vacek, J. L., Jones, P. G., Forker, A., O'Keefe, J. H., & McCallister, B. D. (1999). A randomized, controlled trial of the effects of remote, intercessory prayer on outcomes in patients admitted to the coronary care unit. *Archives of Internal Medicine, 159*(19), 2273–2278.

Holmbeck, G. N. (1997). Toward terminological, conceptual, and statistical clarity in the study of mediators and moderators: Examples from the child-clinical and pediatric psychology literatures. *Journal of Consulting and Clinical Psychology, 65,* 599–610.

Kaplan, G. A., & Camacho, T. (1983). Perceived health and mortality: A nine-year follow-up of the human population laboratory cohort. *American Journal of Epidemiology, 117,* 292–304.

Kaplan, R. M. (1984). The connection between clinical health promotion and health status: A critical overview. *American Psychologist, 39,* 755–765.

Kaplan, R. M. (2000). Two pathways to prevention. *American Psychologist, 55,* 382–396.

Kendall, P. C., Flannery-Schroeder, E., & Ford, J. (1999). Therapy outcome research methods. In P. C. Kendall, J. Butcher, & G. Holmbeck (Eds.), *Handbook of research methods in clinical psychology* (2nd ed., pp. 330–363). New York: Wiley.

Kiecolt-Glaser, J., & Glaser, R. (1995). Psychoneuroimmunology and health consequences: Data and shared mechanisms. *Psychosomatic Medicine, 57,* 269–274.

Koenig, H. G. (1997). *Is religion good for your health?: Effects of religion on mental and physical health.* Binghamton, NY: Haworth Pastoral Press.

Lazarus, R. S., & Folkman, S. (1984). *Stress, appraisal and coping.* New York: Springer.

Linden, W., Stossel, C., & Maurice, J. (1996). Psychosocial interventions for patients with coronary artery disease: A meta-analysis. *Archives of Internal Medicine, 156,* 745–752.

Lovallo, W. (1997). *Stress and health.* Thousand Oaks, CA: Sage.

Manne, S., & Zautra, A. (1989). Spouse criticism and support: Their association with coping and psychological distress among women with rheumatoid arthritis. *Journal of Personality and Social Psychology, 56,* 608–617.

McCullough, M. E., Hoyt, W. T., Larson, D. B., Koenig, H. G., & Thoresen, C. (2000). Religious involvement and mortality: A meta-analytic review. *Health Psychology, 19*(3), 211–222.

Miller, W. R. (Ed.). (1999). *Integrating spirituality into treatment: Resources for practitioners.* Washington, DC: American Psychological Association.

Norris, F. H. (1997). Frequency and structure of precautionary behavior in the domains of hazard preparedness, crime prevention, vehicular safety, and health maintenance. *Health Psychology, 16*, 566–575.

Pargament, K. I. (1997). *The psychology of religion and coping: Theory, research, practice.* New York: Guilford Press.

Peck, J., Smith, T. W., Ward, J. J., & Milano, R. (1989). Disability and depression in rheumatoid arthritis: A multi-trait, multi-method investigation. *Arthritis and Rheumatism, 32*, 1100–1106.

Rabin, B. S. (1999). *Stress, immune function, and health: The connection.* New York: Wiley-Liss.

Rhodewalt, F., & Smith, T. W. (1991). Current issues in Type A behavior, coronary proneness, and coronary heart disease. In C. R. Snyder & D. R. Forsyth (Eds.), *Handbook of social and clinical psychology* (pp. 197–220). New York: Pergamon Press.

Richards, P. S., & Bergin, A. E. (1997). *A spiritual strategy for counseling and psychotherapy.* Washington, DC: American Psychological Association.

Rozanski, A., Blumenthal, J. A., & Kaplan, J. (1999). Impact of psychological factors on the pathogenesis of cardiovascular disease and implications for therapy. *Circulation, 99*, 2192–2217.

Schneiderman, N., Weiss, S. M., & Kaufmann, P. G. (1989). *Handbook of research methods in cardiovascular behavioral medicine.* New York: Plenum.

Schulz, R., & Beach, S. (1999). Caregiving as a risk factor for mortality: The caregiver health effects study. *Journal of the American Medical Association, 282,* 2215–2219.

Schwartz, C. E., Chesney, M. A., Irvine, J., & Keefe, F. J. (1997). The control group dilemma in clinical research: Applications for psychosocial and behavioral medicine trials. *Psychosomatic Medicine, 59*, 362–371.

Shafranske, E. P. (Ed.). (1996). *Religion and the clinical practice of psychology.* Washington, DC: American Psychological Association.

Sloan, R. P., Bagiella, E., & Powell, T. (1999). Religion, spirituality, and medicine. *Lancet, 353,* 664–667.

Smith, T. W., & Gallo, L. C. (2001). Personality traits as risk factors for physical illness. In A. Baum, T. Revenson, & J. Singer (Eds.), *Handbook of health psychology* (pp. 139–172). Hillsdale, NJ: Erlbaum.

Smith, T. W., & Rhodewalt, F. (1992). Methodological challenges at the social/clinical interface. In C. R. Snyder & D. F. Forsyth (Eds.), *Handbook of social and clinical psychology* (pp. 739–756). New York: Pergamon Press.

Smith, T. W., & Ruiz, J. M. (1999). Methodological issues in adult health psychology. In P. C. Kendall, J. N. Butcher, & G. N. Holmbeck (Eds.), *Handbook of research methods in clinical psychology* (2nd ed., pp. 499–536). New York: Wiley.

Smith, T. W., & Williams, P. G. (1992). Personality and health: Advantages and limitations of the five-factor model. *Journal of Personality, 60*, 395–423.

Stone, A. A., Schwartz, J. E., Neale, J. M., Shiffman, S., Marco, C., Hickox, M., Paty, J., Porter, L., & Cruise, L. (1998). A comparison of coping assessed by ecological momentary assessment and retrospective recall. *Journal of Personality and Social Psychology, 74,* 1670–1680.

Turner, J. A., Deyo, R. A., & Loweser, J. D. (1994). The importance of placebo effects in pain treatment and research. *Journal of the American Medical Association, 271,* 1609–1614.

Waitzman, N., & Smith, K. (1998). Phantom of the area: Poverty residence and mortality in the U. S. *American Journal of Public Health, 88,* 973–976.

Waltz, J., Addis, M. E., Koerner, K., & Jacobson, N. S. (1993). Testing the integrity of a psychotherapy protocol: Assessment of adherence and competence. *Journal of Consulting and Clinical Psychology, 61,* 620–630.

Watson, D., & Pennebaker, J. W. (1989). Health complaints, stress, and distress: Exploring the central role of negative affectivity. *Psychological Review, 96,* 234–254.

Watson, D., & Tellegen, A. (1985). Toward a consensual structure of mood. *Psychological Bulletin, 98,* 219–235.

Watson, D., Weber, K., Assenheimer, J. S., Clark, L. A., Strauss, M. E., & McCormick, R. A. (1995). Testing a tripartite model: I. Evaluating the convergent and discriminant validity of anxiety and depression symptom scales. *Journal of Abnormal Psychology, 104,* 3–14.

Weinstein, N. D. (1993). Testing four competing theories of health-protective behavior. *Health Psychology, 12,* 324–333.

Weinstein, N. D., Rothman, A. J., & Sutton, S. R. (1998). Stage theories of health behavior. *Health Psychology, 17,* 211–213.

Yates, B. T. (1994). Toward the incorporation of costs, cost-effectiveness analysis, and cost-benefit analysis into clinical research. *Journal of Consulting and Clinical Psychology, 62,* 729–736.

16

◄〇►

CONCLUSIONS AND FUTURE DIRECTIONS FOR RESEARCH ON FAITH AND HEALTH

ALLEN C. SHERMAN
THOMAS G. PLANTE

Current explorations concerning health and religion span an enormously broad terrain. An expanding circle of health professionals has been drawn to this area, and the pace of research has accelerated rapidly. As the previous chapters make clear, investigations have focused on individuals from diverse walks of life with diverse health concerns. What then have we learned about the intriguing ties between health and faith? The contributors to this volume have addressed this question from a number of different vantage points, highlighting some of the promising advances associated with particular physical and mental health outcomes. In general, the quality of research is becoming more sophisticated. Clearly, however, many fundamental questions remain. Although we are becoming better acquainted with particular facets of religion or spirituality that are associated with particular dimensions of health, what these connections mean, for whom they are most important, and how we are to explain them remain matters of confusion and controversy. Given the current state of knowledge, where do we go from here? In this chapter, we summarize some of the themes from previous chapters and trace a number of salient issues that are important to address as the field moves forward. Because several previous chapters focused on methodological considerations (i.e., *how* connections between faith and health

381

might be examined more rigorously), in this chapter we underscore some of the gaps in the literature (i.e., *what* areas might be studied more productively.)

THE MANY FACES OF FAITH: MULTIDIMENSIONAL ASPECTS OF RELIGION AND SPIRITUALITY

One of the important challenges for health researchers is to cultivate a more differentiated, nuanced approach to faith. Religiousness and spirituality are not monolithic experiences; they are extraordinarily complex, dynamic, and multifaceted. Regrettably, our conceptual models and assessment tools do not always reflect this complexity—a theme highlighted by several of the contributors to this volume (e.g., Chirban, Chapter 11; Sherman & Simonton, Chapter 6; Thoresen, Harris, & Oman, Chapter 2). Investigations that arbitrarily pool together different dimensions of faith may obscure important findings. In Chapter 3, for example, McCullough summarized provocative findings from population-based studies that suggest that public religious behavior (e.g., attendance at religious services, membership in religious organizations) predicts lower mortality rates after controlling for several standard risk factors, whereas private religious practice (e.g., prayer or reading the Bible) has little predictive value. However, when the focus shifts from mortality to other health concerns, such as engaging in health-compromising behaviors (Willis, Wallston, & Johnson, Chapter 9) or coping with chronic illness (Sherman & Simonton, Chapter 7), public religiousness occupies a different role—it is no longer uniquely predictive. Charting the relationships between distinct health outcomes and different dimensions of faith remains a central task for further research. There is growing consensus among health researchers that important domains include, among others, religious or spiritual motivation; beliefs and values; commitment and identity; private practices; public involvement; personal spiritual or mystical experiences; community support and fellowship; and coping (Fetzer Institute/National Institute on Aging, 1999; Hill et al., 1998; Hood, Spilka, Hunsberger, & Gorsuch, 1996; Levin, 1996).

As investigators strive to capture some of these dimensions of faith, it would be helpful to shift the emphasis from broad, abstract indicators to more immediate, "experience-near" aspects of spirituality or religiousness. A recurrent question posed by contributors to this volume is, How does spirituality play out in everyday life? How is it expressed in emotions, cognition, behavior, and relationships, and how do these affect health? Creative approaches to assessment, such as daily monitoring, experience sampling, goal measures, and qualitative methodologies might be helpful in illuminating these experiences, complementing information from standard questionnaires. Assessment would also be enhanced by a move from "descriptive" indices, such as attendance at religious services, toward "functional" measures, such as religious coping or social support, which provide better hints about some of the myriad purposes that religion serves (Ellison & Levin, 1998).

Growing attention also has been directed to constructs that are closely linked with, though not exclusive to, spirituality and religiousness. Are there health consequences associated with forgiveness (Worthington, 1998), volunteering and altruism (Luks & Payne, 1992; Oman, Thoresen, & McMahon, 1999), empathy (Dossey, 1993), or hope (Barnum, Snyder, Rapoff, Mani, & Thompson, 1998; Snyder, Cheavens, & Michael, 1999)? Some of these concepts have been the focus of considerable study in sociology and psychology (e.g., Batson, 1998), providing a rich literature on which to draw, but their associations with health are only beginning to be scrutinized. An intriguing question is whether the health correlates of these experiences differ when they are pursued in secular as opposed to religious contexts. Forgiveness is one of the concepts that has especially captured the interest of investigators (Enright & North, 1998; McCullough, Pargament, & Thoresen, 2000; Worthington, 1998). The conceptual model outlined by Worthington, Berry, and Parrott (Chapter 5, this volume) extends the theoretical work in this area and offers a springboard for further research. Another facet of forgiveness that may be particularly compelling concerns feelings of forgiveness toward God. Difficulties forgiving God in the aftermath of tragedy or disappointment appear to be distinct from difficulties forgiving self or others, and not surprisingly, these feelings are associated with heightened distress (Exline, Yali, & Lobel, 1999; Exline, Yali & Sanderson, in press).

MULTIDIMENSIONAL ASPECTS OF HEALTH

A wide array of health outcomes might be influenced by religious or spiritual involvement. Lately, much of the attention—and much of the controversy—has focused on mortality, usually assessed in healthy community samples followed over time. Epidemiological studies also have focused on associations between religious variables and disease morbidity (e.g., incidence of cardiovascular disease, lung cancer, respiratory disease), though as discussed by Thoresen, Harris, and Oman (Chapter 2, this volume), these findings are more ambiguous. Less information is available from clinical studies that examine health outcomes among patients with established dis-

COMMENTARIES ON RESEARCH

ease or disability. Might religion play a role in how these patients fare? Among the array of clinical endpoints that are beginning to be explored are recovery following surgery (Harris et al., 1995; Pressman, Lyons, Larson, & Strain, 1990), functional disability among nursing home residents (Idler & Kasl, 1997a, 1997b), depression among elderly medical inpatients (Koenig et al., 1992), and pain among individuals with rheumatoid arthritis (Keefe et al., 2000).

Clinical research is needed to confirm preliminary findings and to explore an enormous range of other important health outcomes that have received little attention. The effects of religious or spiritual variables would be expected to vary across different diseases and different phases of pathogenesis or illness progression. Outcomes that might be relevant at different phases of illness include screening practices among nonsymptomatic individuals (e.g., Weinrich et al., 1998), health care utilization and adherence among patients confronted by a chronic condition (e.g., Harris et al., 1995), and decision making about advanced directives and end-of-life care among those who are terminally ill (e.g., Ita, 1995–1996). Within particular diseases, meaningful endpoints might include immunosuppression, infectious complications, and treatment dose reductions among cancer patients; cardiac events such as myocardial infarction or arrhythmias among individuals with cardiovascular disease; and functional status and range of motion among patients with chronic pain disorders. For the most part, this is uncharted territory.

In addition to the need for further studies regarding the trajectory of illness and recovery in selected populations, another important area for research concerns health behaviors and lifestyle (see Smith, Chapter 15, this volume). Faith may play a significant role in shaping health practices and self-care. Early studies on religion and health were driven by observations that certain denominations (e.g., Seventh Day Adventists, Mormons) had specific proscriptions governing a number of important health-risk behaviors, such as smoking, alcohol use, and diet (Jarvis & Northcott, 1987; Lyon, Klauber, Gardner, & Smart, 1976). More recent studies have moved beyond denominational affiliation to examine a broader range of religious variables that might influence health behaviors and health attitudes (Engs & Mullen, 1999; Frankel & Hewitt, 1994; Koenig, George, Meador, Blazer, & Ford, 1994; Oleckno & Blacconiere, 1991). For example, in a study of community residents followed over several decades, Strawbridge and colleagues (Strawbridge, Cohen, Shema, & Kaplan, 1997; Strawbridge, Shema, Cohen, & Kaplan, 2001) found that frequent church attenders reported better health practices (e.g., less smoking and alcohol consumption) than their less religious peers; moreover, frequent church attenders who had poor health habits initially were more likely to improve them over time. In Chapter 9,

Willis, Wallston and Johnson take this type of research a step further by crafting a more comprehensive, multidimensional approach to religious assessment. These investigators found that a constellation of religious factors, including strength of faith, God locus of control, and religious coping was associated with reduced alcohol and nicotine use among adolescents and young adults. Using similar tools, investigators might widen the net to capture other important health practices in other populations. For example, how might religion influence use of immunizations and well-baby care in a pediatric clinic, or contraceptive use and impulsive driving in a primary care practice, or nutrition and cancer screening in a geriatric setting?

Another dimension of the relationship between faith and health that warrants further study concerns adjustment to chronic illness. A growing number of studies have focused on connections between religious or spiritual involvement and quality of life among patients with particular diseases, such as HIV disease (Woods, Antoni, Ironson, & Kling, 1999), cancer (Baider et al., 1999), coronary artery disease (Falger, Sebregts, van Veen, & Franssen, 2000) and chronic pain (Keefe et al., 2000). Interesting findings concerning HIV were reviewed by Remle and Koenig (Chapter 8, this volume), and cancer was discussed by Sherman and Simonton (Chapter 7, this volume). Though results are variable, many of these studies suggest that religious individuals respond to illness with better coping or enhanced adjustment and quality of life compared with their less religious counterparts. However, health-related quality of life is a complex construct that encompasses a number of different components, including psychological well-being, social functioning, physical symptoms, and functional capacity. Psychological well-being is often further differentiated into positive affect, negative affect, and a cognitive evaluation of life satisfaction (Diener, Suh, Lucas, & Smith, 1999). Patients may function well in some of these areas and poorly in others. As yet, we know little about how religiousness or spirituality might differentially affect particular aspects of quality of life. In other words, is the pattern of relationships different for physical functioning than for psychosocial functioning, or different for life satisfaction than for distress? Moreover, to what extent might religion help maintain functioning in the face of illness or adversity (preservation of homeostasis) and to what extent might it contribute to constructive change and growth (thriving, posttraumatic growth) (Carver, 1998; Tedeschi, Park, & Calhoun, 1998)? Clearly, there is a need for investigations that examine associations between multiple dimensions of faith and multiple dimensions of quality of life across different phases of illness.

As the links between faith and health become better established, the next tier of questions begins to take on greater urgency. For which individuals, under which circumstances, are these connections most important? Are these relationships causal, and if so, what mechanisms explain them? How do they work?

FACTORS INFLUENCING THE RELATIONSHIP BETWEEN FAITH AND HEALTH: INDIVIDUAL DIFFERENCES AND CONTEXTUAL FACTORS

Spirituality and religiousness do not exist in a social or developmental vacuum. They are shaped and molded by culture, ethnicity, family, socioeconomic status, situational crises, and a host of other contextual factors. Personal characteristics such as stage of life and personality also color the relationships between faith and health. Similarly, characteristics of the illness, such as disease severity and phase of illness, may also be important. In general, religious commitment tends to be stronger among individuals from ethnic minority groups and those who are older, female, less educated, and less wealthy (Gallup, 1990; Pargament, 1997). Religious coping also appears to be stronger among individuals facing major upheaval as opposed to minor stressors (Pargament, 1997).

Nevertheless, the importance of these moderating factors varies widely across studies, so investigators need to be thoughtful about which ones should be emphasized. For example, as McCullough points out (Chapter 3, this volume), gender has emerged as an important factor in population-based studies of religion and mortality. Attendance at religious services appears to be more strongly predictive of all-cause mortality for women than for men. On the other hand, denominational affiliation is of more immediate relevance when it comes to use of medical services. Religious beliefs have little impact on whether observant Jews will accept blood transfusions, but enormous impact for Christian Scientists and Jehovah's Witnesses. When we shift our focus to coping with illness, both religious affiliation and ethnicity seem to be important. Patterns of religious coping, and their associations with distress, are different for Hispanic women with breast cancer than for non-Hispanic white patients (Culver, Alferi, Carver, Kilbourn, & Antoni, 1999); and among Hispanic women, these patterns are different for evangelical as opposed to Catholic patients (Alferi, Culver, Carver, Arena, & Antoni, 1999).

Clearly, much work has yet to be done to explore which individuals, with which cultural backgrounds and levels of risk exposure, demonstrate the strongest connections between faith and health. In particular, we know little about these relationships among followers of non-Christian theistic traditions (e.g., Muslims), adherents of polytheistic and nontheistic traditions (e.g., Hindus, Zen Buddhists), or individuals who perceive themselves as spiritual but are disaffected by organized religion.

EXPLAINING CONNECTIONS BETWEEN FAITH AND HEALTH: THE SEARCH FOR MEDIATING PATHWAYS

The bulk of evidence linking faith and health is, by necessity, descriptive and correlational (see Smith, Chapter 15, this volume). Whether these relationships are causal remains unclear. For example, does religious involvement reduce the risk of substance abuse, does substance abuse erode religiousness, or, more likely, are these connections reciprocal (Miller & Bennett, 1997)? If there are significant, causal relationships between religious or spiritual involvement and health, how can we begin to explain these connections? What mechanisms underlie them? Several conceptual schemes have been offered (Ellison & Levin, 1998; Idler, 1987; Levin, 1996; Levin & Vanderpool, 1991), but as yet evidence is limited. A comprehensive model is outlined by Thoresen and colleagues in Chapter 2 of this volume.

Among the many pathways that deserve further attention, one of the most important concerns health practices and lifestyle. Religious traditions that specifically restrict smoking, alcohol use, poor hygiene, meat consumption, sexual behavior, or violence would be expected to reduce the associated health risks among their adherents. Religious groups without specific prohibitions against these behaviors may also enhance health by generally discouraging overindulgence (Idler & Kasl, 1992). Epidemiological studies examining morbidity and mortality offer some support for these assumptions (Gardner, Sanborn, & Slattery, 1995; Jarvis & Northcott, 1987; Musick, Koenig, Larson, & Matthews, 1998; Strawbridge et al., 1997; Strawbridge et al., 2001). Conversely, as one might expect, religious traditions that limit or forbid conventional medical care confer additional health risks (Asser & Swan, 1998; Conyn-van Spaendonck, Oostvogel, van Loon, van Wijngaarden, & Kromhout, 1996; Kaunitz, Spence, Danielson, Rochat, & Grimes, 1984). On a somewhat more subtle level, traditions that regard the body as a "temple" or sacred vessel might be associated with different patterns of self-care than those that view the body with greater indifference or disdain.

Population studies with predominantly healthy individuals suggest that health practices explain some but not all of the relationship between health outcomes (e.g., mortality) and public religious involvement (Hummer, Rogers, Nam, & Ellison, 1999; Strawbridge et al., 1997; Strawbridge et al., 2000). Additional longitudinal studies that are specifically designed to test these relationships would make a valuable contribution. Of course, health behaviors and beliefs also influence outcomes for individuals who are seriously ill. How patients interpret their symptoms, seek medical care, adhere to treatment, communicate with their health providers, and take care of themselves may all be influenced by faith. Some studies have reported better treatment adherence (Harris et al., 1995) and health habits (e.g., diet, exercise, not smoking; Falger et al., 2000; Kurtz, Wyatt, & Kurtz, 1995) among religious patients relative to less religious participants. More speculatively, religiousness or spirituality might also influence disease outcomes by affecting symptom interpretation, self-advocacy for aggressive, experimental treatments, or coping through smoking and substance abuse. Few studies have examined these questions.

It seems that health practices don't tell the whole story of how faith and health are linked. Another avenue through which religiousness or spirituality might influence health involves social support. The social integration that religion provides has long been thought to promote health and well-being (Durkheim, 1897/1951). Support from a religious community might include practical assistance (e.g., transportation to medical appointments), relevant information (e.g., which doctor to see), and emotional comfort (e.g., "You are on our prayer list"), as well as affirmation of self-worth, a valued social role, and a chance to help others. The network of informal support among members of a congregation may be complemented by formal counseling from religious leaders (e.g., premarital counseling from a rabbi) or by church-based health services and outreach programs (e.g., cancer screening or weight loss services). These programs are especially prominent in minority group churches (Ellison & Levin, 1998; Erwin, Spatz, Stotts, & Hollenberg, 1999; Schorling et al., 1997). A number of studies demonstrate that stronger religious involvement is associated with larger and denser social networks and greater perceived support (Bradley, 1995; Ellison & George, 1994; Falger et al., 2000; Strawbridge et al., 1997; Strawbridge et al., 2001). Aspects of social support, in turn, have been tied to a broad range of physical and mental health outcomes (House, Landis, & Umberson, 1988; Berkman & Syme, 1979; Sarason, Sarason, & Pierce, 1990).

Thus far, however, only a few studies have directly examined ties between religiously based social support and health. Several investigations with community residents suggest that social contact accounts for part but not all of the connections between religion and health outcomes (Hummer et al., 1999; Idler & Kasl, 1992; Strawbridge et al., 1997; Strawbridge et al., 2001). Thus, although social support has been assumed to be a central mechanism linking faith and health, its mediating role remains an area of uncertainty and debate (see Thoresen et al., Chapter 2, this volume). Areas in need of further investigation include delineating which types of social support are most salient in various religious communities, examining the health correlates of negative as well as positive social exchanges within these networks, and determining whether religious social support differs in meaningful ways from secular support (Ellison & Levin, 1998).

Aside from its impact on health practices and social support, faith may also influence health by providing a foundation of existential meaning—or at least a path to guide the search (Geertz, 1966; Shafranske, Chapter 13, this volume). Religiousness or spirituality may offer a reassuring sense that life is coherent, orderly, and purposeful. Park and Folkman (1997) refer to these tacit world views or implicit beliefs about life as "global meaning." Religious or spiritual involvement may also provide an interpretive scheme for understanding particular circumstances of tragedy and suffering ("situational meaning"; Park & Folkman, 1997). Illness or adversity may be seen as part of God's plan, a "wake-up call," or a spiritual lesson rather than a random act of misfortune (Sherman & Simonton, 1999, 2001). One of us (A. S.) worked with a devout Muslim man from southern India with advanced cancer who developed severe complications in the aftermath of a bone marrow transplant. Throughout his daunting illness, he was greatly comforted by the belief that his suffering in this world would speed his way to Paradise in the next. By providing a global sense of meaning and purpose, and by coloring the way in which particular challenges are interpreted, faith may have an important impact on stress appraisal, coping, and adaptation (Park & Folkman, 1997).

Religious or spiritual involvement may also foster a sense of control (Fromm, 1950; Musick, Koenig, Larson, & Matthews, 1998). In the voluminous stress literature, perceived control has long been associated with better health practices and more favorable physiological and psychological adaptation following exposure to stressful situations, including illness (Seeman & Seeman, 1983; Wallston & Wallston, 1981). When a serious illness such as cancer, which is fraught with uncertainty, ruptures tacit assumptions about personal control, faith may restore a sense of "secondary control" (Rothbaum, Weisz, & Snyder, 1982), reducing feelings of helplessness through perceptions that "this is God's will," "God is by my side," or "this is part of the natural order of things." Studies that have focused on perceptions that God is in control (e.g., God locus of control) generally have found better health-protective behaviors (Welton, Adkins, Ingle, & Dixon, 1996; see also Willis et al., Chapter 9, this volume) and enhanced adjustment to illness (Jenkins & Pargament, 1988) among those who hold this view. Of course, the conviction that God is in control can take many different forms. Some investigators (Pargament et al., 1999; Pargament et al., 1988) have drawn interesting distinctions between a deferring approach to problem solving ("God will handle this situation; I need to turn it over to Him") versus a self-directed approach ("God gave me the resources I need to handle this on my own") or a collaborative approach ("God and I are partners and will see this through together"). Perceptions of control, and their health correlates, may differ across different religious and spiritual traditions. For example, whereas Western cultures highly value personal control and agency, Eastern cultures tend to place greater emphasis on harmonious accommodation with the community; these divergent values may have implications for health.

Faith may be translated into health through a number of other psychological channels as well. Optimism, hostility, conscientiousness, emotional expression, and neuroticism are among the cast of personality variables that are highly familiar to health researchers. Each of these might be shaped by (and in turn shape) religious or spiritual involvement. McCullough (Chapter 3, this volume) discusses a number of provocative connections among religiousness, conscientiousness, and mortality. Relative to their less meticulous peers, individuals who are highly conscientious and whose resolve is steeled by religious commitment might assume a different posture toward a broad range of health practices, such as abstinence from alcohol or adherence to complex medication regimens. Religiousness or spirituality might also promote optimism, which has been associated with better coping and adjustment over the course of serious illness (e.g., Carver et al., 1993). Moving from personality to situational variables, faith may also have an important impact on emotions (e.g., experiences of peacefulness, awe, reverence), coping (e.g., active vs. avoidant responses) and appraisal (e.g., perceiving adversity as a challenge vs. a threat), each of which might have health implications (Sherman & Simonton, Chapter 7; Remle & Koenig, Chapter 8; Plante & Sharma, Chapter 10, this volume).

Finally, it is possible that religious or spiritual involvement may influence host vulnerability to disease through its effects on neuroendocrine and immune activity (Woods et al., 1999). These effects might be mediated by some of the psychosocial variables noted above, such as social support or coping, or by other factors that remain unrecognized. As highlighted by Smith (Chapter 15, this volume), very little is known about how faith might alter physiological patterns of stress response or biological substrates of disease. Compelling demonstrations of these influences would go a long way in moving the field forward.

Recent studies of the physiological correlates of forgiveness, using laboratory simulations or imagery, demonstrate that experimental research in this area is feasible (e.g., Witvliet, Laan, & Ludwig, 2000). Intriguing findings also have emerged from correlational studies focusing on religiousness and cardiovascular activity. In a community study of healthy men, those who attached greater importance to religion and who attended services frequently demonstrated lower clinic diastolic blood pressure than their less religious peers after several standard risk factors were controlled (Larson et al., 1989). These findings were especially pronounced for smokers, who are at elevated risk for cardiovascular disease. Similarly, African American men and women who reported greater use of religious coping in their daily lives demonstrated lower ambulatory diastolic blood pressure at work, at home, and at sleep compared with those who did not rely on religious coping (Steffen, Blumenthal, Hinderliter, & Sherwood, 2000). These findings persisted after controlling for social support, stress, and depressive symptoms. Is it possible that religious or spiritual variables also affect other relevant cardiovascular indices at varying phases of pathogenesis, such as lipid levels, endothelial damage, platelet aggregation, severity of atherosclerosis, heart rate variability, or arrhythmias? Among patients with established coronary heart disease, does faith influence depression or hostility, which have been associated with heightened risk for cardiac events (Frasure-Smith, Lespérance, & Talajic, 1995; Lespérance, Frasure-Smith, Juneau, & Theroux, 2000; Davidson, 2000)? To our knowledge, this kind of programmatic research centered on specific diseases or conditions has yet to be pursued. More broadly, basic research with healthy individuals would be helpful in examining links between faith and sympathetic–adrenomedullary activity, hypothalamic–pituitary–adrenocortical activation, and immune function. Using well-established stress paradigms, the physiological responses of individuals high and low in religious involvement might be compared following exposure to acute laboratory stressors or chronic naturalistic challenges (e.g., caring for a relative with dementia). Perhaps more interestingly, investigators might examine physiological responses to ecologically relevant situations, such as opportunities for altruism, volunteering, or forgiveness.

OTHER METHODOLOGICAL
AND CONCEPTUAL CONCERNS

Earlier chapters in this volume highlighted several other important issues that merit attention as the field moves forward. Some of the research in this area has been characterized by notable methodological limitations, many of which were outlined by Sloan, Bagiella, and Powell in Chapter 14 and Smith in Chapter 15 (e.g., failure to adjust for multiple statistical tests, inadequate control for confounding factors, etc.). Studies in clinical settings often have relied on small samples, which limit the possibility of detecting significant effects. Moreover, the vast majority of clinical studies have used cross-sectional designs (i.e., measures of faith and health obtained at the same point in time), which offer no hints about temporal or causal relationships. There is a pressing need for additional longitudinal investigations in clinical populations. Designs that encompass multiple assessments over time would not only add information about how faith predicts later health outcomes but would also clarify how faith relates to changes in important explanatory variables, such as health practices or social support (Strawbridge et al., 1997).

In both clinical and epidemiological research, the role of confounding variables remains a topic of dissension (see Sloan et al., Chapter 14 and McCullough, Chapter 3, this volume). No single study can control for all extraneous influences, and which particular factors should be emphasized varies across health settings and populations. Nevertheless, investigators should be thoughtful in how they conceptualize and account for extraneous variables and how they distinguish these from mediating pathways (Levin, 1996). Statistical designs that focus on simple, bivariate associations have helped highlight areas of interest, but more sophisticated multivariate approaches (e.g., structural equation models, path analyses, growth curve models, proportional hazards modeling, etc.) are called for as investigators attempt to model the complex relationships between faith and health. Thoresen and colleagues (Chapter 2, this volume) emphasize the need for experimental and intervention research to supplement correlational studies. By the same token, qualitative studies have an important role to play in enriching our understanding of these associations.

Aside from these methodological concerns, a number of conceptual issues warrant further consideration. Under what circumstances does faith undermine or compromise health? Relatively little attention has been devoted to exploring the negative role that religion might sometimes play (e.g., Asser & Swan, 1998; Exline, Yali, & Sanderson, 2000; Exline et al., in press; Kaunitz et al., 1984; Strawbridge, Shema, Cohen, Roberts, & Kaplan, 1998; Trenholm, Trent, & Compton, 1998). The preceding chapters highlighted several examples in which faith was associated with adverse health effects. A clearer focus on these possibilities would be helpful. Pargament's influential work on religious coping represents an important step in this direction (Pargament, 1997; Pargament et al., 1998). Studies that examine changes over time would be especially useful in distinguishing transient patterns (e.g., depression or substance abuse associated with a temporary crisis of faith) from enduring ones (e.g., doctrinal prohibitions against conventional medical care).

A good deal of research concerning religion and health lacks theoretical moorings. Theory development would help guide investigators toward particular health outcomes, contextual factors, and phases of illness that may be especially important. With respect to health outcomes, some writers have complained that our focus has been too narrow. Jeffrey Levin (1996), an active researcher in this area, argues that a traditional "pathogenic" approach to research on religion and health, which emphasizes risk reduction, should be complemented by a "salutogenic" perspective, which focuses on health promotion and wellness. The factors involved in promoting health and wellness are not necessarily the same as those involved in reducing risk (e.g., Antonovsky, 1987; Benyamini, Idler, Leventhal, & Leventhal, 2000). The research of Wink and Dillon discussed in Chapter 4 of this volume, for example, found that religiosity, assessed at mid-life, predicted participants' zest for life, generativity, satisfaction with personal relationships, and community involvement several decades later. In other words, religiousness was tied to wellness and adaptation, findings that would have been missed by an exclusive focus on pathology. Levin's call for greater sensitivity to the salutary effects of faith is consistent with the growing emphasis on "positive psychology" (e.g., optimism, wisdom, creativity) that is emerging in other fields of research (Baltes & Staudinger, 2000; Seligman & Csikszentmihalyi, 2000; Simonton, 2000).

Aside from directing attention to relevant outcomes, coherent theoretical models would also highlight the situational and cultural contexts in which faith and health may be most strongly connected. For example, it is likely that some religious variables (e.g., prohibitions against alcohol use) affect health in a general way across situations, whereas others (e.g., religious coping, instrumental support from the congregation) are relevant only under circumstances of high stress. Hypotheses concerning the "buffering effects" versus "main effects" of faith have not been well defined. Not surprisingly, however, several studies suggest that the psychological benefits of religiousness are most pronounced during periods of adversity (Maton, 1989; Park, Cohen, & Herb, 1990; see also Wink & Dillon, Chapter 4, this volume).

In addition, theoretical models are needed to help delineate which religious or spiritual variables might be most relevant at which phases of illness. The dimensions of faith that are important for risk exposure or disease onset may be very different from those associated with disease progression. For example, a religious woman who avoids multiple sexual partners as an expression of religious devotion may thereby reduce her risk of contracting human papillomavirus infection, which is associated with cervical dysplasia and, over the course of many years, cervical cancer. Once she has developed cervical cancer, however, it is unlikely that her religiously motivated sexual abstinence would have much impact on whether the tumor subsequently metastasizes to other areas of her body. And if her religious community is one that promotes intense shame about cancer and harbors mistrust of physicians, she might experience a poorer outcome than a nonreligious peer with similar disease.

The need for theory-building or model development has begun to be taken up by a number of intrepid writers, including Worthington and colleagues (Chapter 5) and Thoresen and associates (Chapter 2) in this volume. Moreover, the psychology of religion literature contains several theoretical models that have spawned social science research for decades and that merit consideration by health researchers (e.g., models of intrinsic and quest orientations; Allport & Ross, 1967; Batson & Schoenrade, 1991). This legacy is often ignored or poorly understood by health professionals. And of course there are a number of well-established models in health research that might readily incorporate religious and spiritual variables, perhaps enriching these frameworks and providing a useful guide for further research. For example, these variables might be encompassed within broader models of health behavior (Rosenstack, 1974; Salovey, Rothman, & Rodin, 1998), psychoneuroimmunology (Goodkin, Antoni, Sevin, & Fox, 1993; Andersen, Kiecolt-Glaser, & Glaser, 1994) or stress, coping, and self-regulation (Carver & Scheier, 1998; Lazarus & Folkman, 1984), or within more discreet models of posttraumatic growth (Tedeschi et al., 1998), benefit finding (Tennen & Affleck, 1999), or resilience and thriving (Carver, 1998; O'Leary & Ickovics, 1995).

CLINICAL IMPLICATIONS

Thus far our discussion has focused on research—how can we better understand the complex ties between faith and health? A final set of questions concerns clinical applications. How should findings be translated from the laboratory to the clinic? There is growing recognition among health professionals that religiousness and spirituality are important areas to understand and assess. As noted in previous chapters in this book, the ethical guidelines promoted by the American Psychological Association (1992) and by several other professional organizations (e.g., American Psychiatric Association Committee on Religion and Psychiatry, 1990) require sensitivity to religious and cultural diversity. Chirban (Chapter 11, this volume) discussed helpful guidelines for assessment of religious concerns in the psychotherapy setting, and Sherman and Simonton (Chapter 6) reviewed formal measures of religiousness, some of which might be used as screening tools to facilitate discussion in medical settings.

Beyond sensitive assessment and respectful accommodation, however, the role of clinicians becomes more complicated and controversial (e.g., Sloan et al., 2000). Should therapists make use of spiritual interventions with their religious clients, or should this be handled by referral to religiously affiliated counselors or clergy? Is it appropriate for physicians or other medical providers to issue religious recommendations? What are the preferences and opinions of patients and clinicians?

Whether and how spirituality and religiousness should be integrated into treatment is the subject of a rapidly expanding literature (e.g., Kelly, 1995; Miller, 1999; Richards & Bergin, 2000; Shafranske, 1996). Nevertheless, the boundary conditions concerning which types of interventions might be appropriately implemented by which professionals for which patients remain to be consensually defined. Introducing personal prayer within an individual psychotherapy session clearly is not quite the same as offering smoking cessation classes in a local church to reach underserved populations, though superficially both might be labeled "religious interventions." Moreover, the appropriate role for psychotherapists would be expected to differ from that of medical staff, who typically function within different professional boundaries. Clients who are highly religious or who seek help with spiritual conflicts should elicit a therapeutic stance different from one used with those who are less religious or whose presenting concerns are distal from their spiritual views. And those who are seriously ill may have different spiritual needs than patients who are more healthy.

The contributors to this volume have presented a broad spectrum of views about spiritually oriented interventions. In Chapter 14, Sloan, Bagiella, and Powell raised a number of ethical objections with respect to medical providers becoming involved in religious matters, including the potential for coercion and abuse of authority; additional caveats about issuing clinical recommendations based on current research were presented by Smith in Chapter 15. A different perspective was outlined in Chapter 12 by Tan and Dong, who discussed how a range of spiritual interventions might be incorporated within clinical practice, by mental health clinicians as well as by medical staff. In Chapter 13, Shafranske examined attitudes toward religion and use of religious interventions among clinicians working in rehabilitation settings, in which spiritual concerns are often very poignant. Shafranske's findings add to a growing number of surveys conducted with health professionals from different disciplines (e.g., Ellis, Vinson, & Ewigman, 1999; Koenig, Bearon, & Dayringer, 1989; Kristeller, Zumbrun, & Schilling, 1999). Most clinicians seem to feel that patients' spiritual concerns are important, that professional education in this area is woefully inadequate, and that clergy are a central but underutilized resource. There is less consensus about whether and how clinicians from different disciplines working in various settings should address spiritual issues. Most of the contributors to this volume highlighted the need to insure that clinical services are grounded in informed consent, are culturally sensitive and respectful of personal preferences, and are targeted toward relevant treatment goals. Clearly, there is no room for proselytizing or exploiting the power of the clinician's role. They also echoed the need for additional training in this area— a change that is beginning to emerge in medical school curricula but has yet to materialize in psychology training programs.

CONCLUSION

The interface between religion, spirituality, and health is an extraordinarily rich area for scientific investigation. For many, a concern with the sacred or transcendent goes to the heart of what it means to be human. Health professionals are beginning to appreciate the possibility that spiritual commitment may have relevance beyond the pew and the pulpit. The chapters in this volume have examined some of the ways in which attempts to live a spiritual or religious life may have implications for mental and physical health. Exploring the meaning, magnitude, and mechanisms of these connections is the major challenge that lies ahead. This endeavor is apt to tax the creative talents of health researchers for some time to come. If the contributions to this volume provide any indication, however, the quest should be an exciting and provocative one.

REFERENCES

Alferi, S. M., Culver, J. L., Carver, C. S., Arena, P. L., & Antoni, M. H. (1999). Religiosity, religious coping, and distress: A prospective study of Catholic and Evangelical women in treatment for early-stage breast cancer. *Journal of Health Psychology, 4,* 343–356.

Allport, G. W., & Ross, J. M. (1967). Personal religious orientation and prejudice. *Journal of Personality and Social Psychology, 5,* 432–443.

American Psychiatric Association Committee on Religion and Psychiatry. (1990). Guidelines regarding the possible conflict between psychiatrists' religious commitment and psychiatric practice. *American Journal of Psychiatry, 197,* 542.

American Psychological Association. (1992). Ethical principles of psychologists and code of conduct. *American Psychologist, 47,* 1597–1611.

Andersen, B. L., Kiecolt-Glaser, J. K., & Glaser, R. (1994). A biobehavioral model of cancer stress and disease course. *American Psychologist, 49,* 389–404.

Antonovsky, A. (1987). *Unraveling the mystery of health: How people manage stress and stay well.* San Francisco: Jossey-Bass.

Asser, S. M., & Swan, R. (1998). Child fatalities from religion-motivated medical neglect. *Pediatrics, 101*(4, Part 1), 625–629.

Baider, L., Russak, S. M., Perry, S., Kash, K., Gronert, M., Fox, B., Holland, J., & Kaplan-Denour, A. (1999). The role of religious and spiritual beliefs in coping with malignant melanoma: An Israeli sample. *Psycho-Oncology, 8,* 27–35.

Baltes, P. B., & Staudinger, U. M. (2000). Wisdom: A metaheuristic (pragmatic) to orchestrate mind and virtue toward excellence. *American Psychologist, 55,* 122–136.

Barnum, D. D., Snyder, C. R., Rapoff, M. A., Mani, M. M., & Thompson, R. (1998). Hope and social support in the psychological adjustment of pediatric burn survivors and matched controls. *Children's Health Care, 27,* 15–30.

Batson, C. D. (1998). Altruism and prosocial behavior. In D. T. Gilbert, S. T. Fiske, & G. Lindzey (Eds.), *The handbook of social psychology* (4th ed., vol. 2, pp. 282–316). New York: McGraw-Hill.

Batson, C. D., & Schoenrade, P. (1991). Measuring religion as quest: 1. Validity concerns. *Journal for the Scientific Study of Religion, 30,* 416–429.

Benyamini, Y., Idler, E. L., Leventhal H., & Leventhal, E. A. (2000). Positive affect and function as influences on self-assessments of health: Expanding our view beyond illness and disability. *Journal of Gerontology, 55B,* P107–P116.

Berkman, L. F., & Syme, S. L. (1979). Social networks, host resistance, and mortality: A nine year follow-up of Alameda County residents. *American Journal of Epidemiology, 109,* 186–204.

Bradley, D. E. (1995). Religious involvement and social resources: Evidence from the data set "Americans' Changing Lives. " *Journal for the Scientific Study of Religion, 34,*259–267.

Carver, C. S. (1998). Resilience and thriving: Issues, models, and linkages. *Journal of Social Issues, 54*(2), 245–266.

Carver, C. S., Pozo, C., Harris, S. D., Noriega, V., Scheier, M. F., Robinson, D. S., Ketcham, A. S., Moffat, F. L., Jr., & Clark, K. C. (1993). How coping mediates the effect of optimism on distress: A study of women with early stage breast cancer. *Journal of Personality and Social Psychology, 65,* 375–390.

Carver, C. S., & Scheier, M. F. (1998). *On the self-regulation of behavior.* New York: Cambridge University Press.

Conyn-van Spaendonck, M. A., Oostvogel, P. M., van Loon, A. M., van Wijngaarden, J. K., & Kromhout, D. (1996). Circulation of the poliovirus during the poliomyelitis outbreak in the Netherlands in 1992–1993. *American Journal of Epidemiology, 143,* 929–935.

Culver, J. L., Alferi, S. M., Carver, C. S., Kilbourn, K. M., & Antoni, M. H. (1999). Ethnic differences in coping strategies among early-stage breast cancer patients [Abstract]. *Annals of Behavioral Medicine, 21*(Suppl.), S230.

Davidson, K. W. (2000, March). *Dose-response relations between hostility reductions and cardiac-related hospitalizations.* Paper presented at the annual meeting of the American Psychosomatic Society, Savannah, GA.

Diener, E., Suh, E. M., Lucas, R. E., & Smith, H. L. (1999). Subjective well-being: Three decades of progress. *Psychological Bulletin, 125,* 276–302.

Dossey, L. (1993). Love and healing. In *Healing words: The power of prayer and the practice of medicine* (pp. 109–117). San Francisco: Harper.

Durkheim, E. (1951). *Suicide: A study in sociology* (J. A. Spaulding & G. Simpson, Trans.). New York: Free Press. (Original work published 1897)

Ellis, M. R., Vinson, D. C., & Ewigman, B. (1999). Addressing spiritual concerns of patients: Family physicians' attitudes and practices. *Journal of Family Practice, 48,* 105–109.

Ellison, C. G., & George, L. K. (1994). Religious involvement, social ties, and social support in a Southeastern community. *Journal for the Scientific Study of Religion, 33,* 46–61.

Ellison, C. G., & Levin, J. S. (1998). The religion–health connection: Evidence, theory, and future directions. *Health Education and Behavior, 25,* 700–720.

Engs, R., & Mullen, K. (1999). The effect of religion and religiosity on drug use among a selected sample of postsecondary students in Scotland. *Addiction Research, 7,* 149–170.

Enright, R. D., & North, J. (Eds.). (1998). *Exploring forgiveness.* Madison, WI: University of Wisconsin Press.

Erwin, D. O., Spatz, T. S., Stotts, R. C., & Hollenberg, J. A. (1999). Increasing mammography practice by African American women. *Cancer Practice, 7,* 78–85.

Exline, J. J., Yali, A. M., & Lobel, M. (1999). When God disappoints: Difficulty forgiving God and its role in negative emotion. *Journal of Health Psychology, 4,* 365–379.

Exline, J. J., Yali, A. M., & Sanderson, W. C. (2000). Guilt, discord, and alienation: The role of the religious strain in depression and suicidality. *Journal of Clinical Psychology, 56*(12), 1481–1496.

Exline, J. J., Yali, A. M., & Sanderson, W. C. (in press). Comfort and strain in religious life: Associations with mental health. *Journal of Clinical Psychology.*

Falger, P. R. J., Sebregts, E. H. W. J., van Veen, G., & Franssen, A. (2000, April). *Religiosity, life quality and lifestyles after a coronary event: 1-year follow-up.* Paper presented at the annual meeting of the Society of Behavioral Medicine, Nashville, TN.

Fetzer Institute/National Institute on Aging. (1999). *Multidimensional measurement of religiousness/spirituality for use in health research.* Kalamazoo, MI: John E. Fetzer Institute.

Frankel, B. G., & Hewitt, W. E. (1994). Religion and well-being among Canadian university students: The role of faith groups on campus. *Journal for the Scientific Study of Religion, 33,* 62–73.

Frasure-Smith, N., Lespérance, F., & Talajic, M. (1995). The impact of negative emotions on prognosis following myocardial infarction: Is it more than depression? *Health Psychology, 14,* 388–398.

Fromm, E. (1950). *Psychoanalysis and religion.* New Haven: Yale University Press.

Gardner, J. W., Sanborn, J. S., & Slattery, M. L. (1995). Behavioral factors explaining the low risk for cervical cancer in Utah Mormon women. *Epidemiology, 6,* 187–189.

Gallup, G., Jr. (1990). *Religion in America: 1990.* Princeton, NJ: Princeton Religious Research Center.

Geertz, C. (1966). Religion as a cultural system. In M. Banton (Ed.), *Anthropological approaches to the study of religion* (pp. 1–46). London: Tavistock.

Goodkin, K., Antoni, M. H., Sevin, B., & Fox, B. H. (1993). A partially testable, predictive model of psychosocial factors in the etiology of cervical cancer: II. Bioimmunological, psychoimmunological and socioimmunological aspects, critique and prospective integration. *Psycho-Oncology, 2,* 99–121.

Harris, R. C., Dew, M. A., Lee, A., Amaya, M., Buches, L., Reetz, D., & Coleman, G. (1995). The role of religion in heart-transplant recipients' long-term health and well-being. *Journal of Religion and Health, 34,* 17–31.

Hill, P. C., & Hood, R. W., Jr. (Eds.). (1999). *Measures of religiosity.* Birmingham, AL: Religious Education Press.

Hill, P. C., Pargament, K. I., Swyers, J. P., Gorsuch, R. L., McCullough, M. E., Hood, R. W., & Baumeister, R. F. (1998). Definitions of religion and spirituality. In D. B. Larson, J. P. Swyers, & M. E. McCullough (Eds.), *Scientific research on spirituality and health: A consensus report* (pp. 14–30). Rockville, MD: National Institute for Healthcare Research.

Hood, R. W., Jr., Spilka, B., Hunsberger, B., & Gorsuch, R. (1996). *The psychology of religion: An empirical approach* (2nd ed). New York: Guilford Press.

House, J. S., Landis, K. R., & Umberson, P. (1988). Social relationships and health. *Science, 241*(4865), 540–545.

Hummer, R. A., Rogers, R. G., Nam, C. B., & Ellison, C. G. (1999). Religious involvement and U. S. adult mortality. *Demography, 36,* 272–285.

Idler, E. (1987). Religious involvement and the health of the elderly: Some hypotheses and an initial test. *Social Forces, 66,* 226–238.

Idler, E., & Kasl, S. (1992). Religion, disability, depression, and the timing of death. *American Journal of Sociology, 97,* 1052–1079.

Idler, E., & Kasl, S. (1997a). Religion among disabled elderly persons: I. Cross-sectional patterns in health practices, social activities, and well-being. *Journals of Gerontology Series B—Psychological Sciences and Social Sciences, 52B,* S294–S305.

Idler, E. L., & Kasl, S. V. (1997b). Religion among disabled and non-disabled elderly persons: II. Attendance at religious services as a predictor of the course of disability. *Journals of Gerontology Series B—Psychological Sciences and Social Sciences, 52B,* S306–S316.

Ita, D. J. (1995–1996). Testing of a causal model: Acceptance of death in hospice patients. *Omega, 32,* 81–92.

Jarvis, G. K., & Northcott, H. C. (1987). Religion and differences in morbidity and mortality. *Social Science and Medicine, 25,* 813–824.

Jenkins, R. A., & Pargament, K. I. (1988). Cognitive appraisals in cancer patients. *Social Science and Medicine, 26,* 625–633.

Kaunitz, A. M., Spence, C., Danielson, T. S., Rochat, R. W., & Grimes, D. A. (1984). Perinatal and maternal mortality in a religious group avoiding obstetric care. *American Journal of Obstetrics and Gynecology, 150,* 826–831.

Keefe, F. J., Affleck, G., Lefebvre, J., Underwood, L., Caldwell, D. S., Drew, J., Gibson, J., & Pargament, K. (2000, March). *Coping with arthritis pain: The role of daily spiritual experiences and religious and spiritual coping.* Paper presented at the annual meeting of the American Psychosomatic Society, Savannah, GA.

Kelly, E. W., Jr. (1995). *Spirituality and religion in counseling and psychotherapy: Diversity in theory and practice.* Alexandria, VA: American Counseling Association.

Koenig, H. G., Bearon, L. B., & Dayringer, R. (1989). Physician perspectives on the role of religion in the physician–older patient relationship. *Journal of Family Practice, 28,*441– 448.

Koenig, H. G., Cohen, H. J., Blazer, D. G., Pieper, C., Meador, K. G., Shelp, F., Goli, V., & DiPasquale, B. (1992). Religious coping and depression among elderly, hospitalized medically ill men. *American Journal of Psychiatry, 149,* 1693–1700.

Koenig, H. G., George, L. K., Meador, K. G., Blazer, D. G., & Ford, S. M. (1994). Religious practices and alcoholism in a Southern adult population. *Hospital and Community Psychiatry, 45,* 225–231.

Kristeller, J. L., Zumbrun, C. S., & Shilling, R. F. (1999). "I would if I could": How oncologists and oncology nurses address spiritual distress in cancer patients. *Psycho-Oncology, 8,* 451–458.

Kurtz, M. E., Wyatt, G., & Kurtz, J. C. (1995). Psychological and sexual well-being, philosophical/spiritual views, and health habits of long-term cancer survivors. *Health Care for Women International, 16,* 253–262.

Larson, D. B., Koenig, H. G., Kaplan, B. H., Greenberg, R. S., Logue, E., & Tyroler, H. A. (1989). The impact of religion on men's blood pressure. *Journal of Religion and Health, 28,* 265–278.

Lazarus, R., & Folkman, S. (1984). Coping and adaptation. In W. D. Gentry (Ed.), *The handbook of behavioral medicine* (pp. 282–325). New York: Guilford Press.

Lespérance, F., Frasure-Smith, N., Juneau, M., & Theroux, P. (2000). Depression and 1-year prognosis in unstable angina. *Archives of Internal Medicine, 160*(9), 1354–1460.

Levin, J. S. (1996). How religion influences morbidity and mortality and health: Reflections on natural history, salutogenesis, and host resistance. *Social Science and Medicine, 43,* 849–864.

Levin, J. S., & Vanderpool, H. Y. (1991). Religious factors in physical health and the prevention of illness. *Prevention in Human Services, 9,* 41–64.

Luks, A., & Payne, P. (1992). *The healing power of doing good: The health and spiritual benefits of helping others.* New York: Fawcett Columbine.

Lyon, J. L., Klauber, M. R., Gardner, J. W., & Smart, C. R. (1976). Cancer incidence in Mormons and non-Mormons in Utah, 1966–1970. *New England Journal of Medicine, 294,* 129–133.

Maton, K. (1989). The stress-buffering role of spiritual support: Cross-sectional and prospective investigations. *Journal for the Scientific Study of Religion, 28*(3), 310–323.

McCullough, M. E., Pargament, K. I., & Thoresen, C. E. (Eds.). (2000). *Forgiveness: Theory, research, and practice.* New York: Guilford Press.

Miller, W. R. (Ed.). (1999). *Integrating spirituality into treatment: Resources for practitioners.* Washington, DC: American Psychological Association.

Miller, W. R., & Bennett, M. E. (1997). Addictions: Alcohol/drug problems. In D. Larson, J. P. Swyers, & M. E. McCullough (Eds.), *Scientific research on spirituality and health: A consensus report* (pp. 68–82). Rockville, MD: National Institute for Healthcare Research.

Musick, M. A., Koenig, H. G., Larson, D. B., & Matthews, D. (1998). Religion and spiritual beliefs. In J. Holland (Ed.), *Psycho-oncology* (pp. 780–789). New York: Oxford University Press.

O'Leary, V. E., & Ickovics, J. R. (1995). Resilience and thriving in response to challenge: An opportunity for a paradigm shift in women's health. *Women's Health: Research on Gender, Behavior, and Policy, 1,* 121–142.

Oleckno, W. A., & Blacconiere, M. J. (1991). Relationship of religiosity to wellness and other health-related behaviors and outcomes. *Psychological Reports, 68,* 819–826.

Oman, D., Thoresen, C. E., & McMahon, K. (1999). Volunteerism and mortality. *Journal of Health Psychology, 4,* 301–316.

Pargament, K. I. (1997). *The psychology of religion and coping: Theory, research, practice.* New York: Guilford Press.

Pargament, K. I., Cole, B., VandeCreek, L., Belavich, T., Brant, C., & Perez, L. (1999). The vigil: Religion and the search for control in the hospital waiting room. *Journal of Health Psychology, 4,* 327–341.

Pargament, K. I., Kennell, J., Hathaway, W., Grevengoed, N., Newman, J., & Jones, W. (1988). Religion and the problem-solving process: Three styles of coping. *Journal for the Scientific Study of Religion, 27,* 90–104.

Pargament, K. I., Zinnbauer, B. J., Scott, A. B., Butter, E. M., Zerowin, J., & Stanik, P. (1998). Red flags and religious coping: Identifying some religious warning signs among people in crisis. *Journal of Clinical Psychology, 54,* 77–89.

Park, C., Cohen, L. H., & Herb, L. (1990). Intrinsic religiousness and religious coping as life stress moderators for Catholics versus Protestants. *Journal of Personality and Social Psychology, 59,* 562–574.

Park, C. L., & Folkman, S. (1997). Meaning in the context of stress and coping. *Review of General Psychology, 1,* 115–144.

Pressman, P., Lyons, J. S., Larson, D. B., & Strain, J. J. (1990). Religious belief, depression, and ambulation status in elderly women with broken hips. *American Journal of Psychiatry, 147,* 758–760.

Richards, P. S., & Bergin, A. E. (2000). *Handbook of psychotherapy and religious diversity.* Washington, DC: American Psychological Association.

Rosenstock, I. M. (1974). Historical origins of the health belief model. *Health Education Monographs, 2,* 328–335.

Rothbaum, R., Weisz, J. R., & Snyder, S. S. (1982). Changing the world and changing the self: A two-process model of perceived control. *Journal of Personality and Social Psychology, 42,* 5–37.

Salovey, P., Rothman, A. J., & Rodin, J. (1998). Health behavior. In D. T. Gilbert, S. T. Fiske, & G. Lindzey (Eds.), *The handbook of social psychology* (4th ed., vol. 2, pp. 633–683). New York: McGraw-Hill.

Sarason, B. R., Sarason, I. G., & Pierce, G. R. (Eds.). (1990). *Social support: An interactional view.* New York: Wiley.

Schorling, J. B., Roach, J., Siegel, M., Baturka, N., Hunt, D. E., Guterbock, T. M., & Stewart, H. L. (1997). A trial of church-based smoking cessation interventions for rural African Americans. *Preventative Medicine, 26,* 92–101.

Seeman, M., & Seeman, T. E. (1983). Health behavior and personal autonomy: A longitudinal study of control in illness. *Journal of Health and Social Behavior, 24,* 144–160.

Seligman, M. E. P., & Csikszentmihalyi, M. (2000). Positive psychology: An introduction. *American Psychologist, 55,* 5–14.

Shafranske, E. P. (Ed.). (1996). *Religion and the clinical practice of psychology.* Washington, DC: American Psychological Association.

Sherman, A. C., & Simonton, S. (1999). Family therapy for cancer patients: Clinical issues and interventions. *Family Journal, 7,* 38–49.

Sherman, A. C., & Simonton, S. (2001). Coping with cancer in the family. *Family Journal, 9,* 193–200.

Simonton, D. K. (2000). Creativity: Cognitive, personal, developmental, and social aspects. *American Psychologist, 55,* 151–158.

Sloan, R. P., Bagiella, E., VandeCreek, L., Hover, M., Casalone, C., Hirsch, T. J., Hasan, Y., Kreger, R., & Poulos, P. (2000). Should physicians prescribe religious activities? [sounding board]. *New England Journal of Medicine, 342*(25), 1913–1916.

Snyder, C. R., Cheavens, J., & Michael, S. T. (1999). Hoping. In C. R. Snyder (Ed.), *Coping: The psychology of what works* (pp. 205–227). New York: Oxford University Press.

Steffen, P., Blumenthal, J., Hinderliter, A., & Sherwood, A. (2000, March). *Religious coping, ethnicity, and ambulatory blood pressure.* Paper presented at the annual meeting of the American Psychosomatic Society, Savannah, GA.

Strawbridge, W. J., Cohen, R. D., Shema, S. J., & Kaplan, G. A. (1997). Frequent attendance at religious services and mortality over 28 years. *American Journal of Public Health, 87,* 957–961.

Strawbridge, W. J., Shema, S. J., Cohen, R. D., & Kaplan, G. A. (2001). Religious attendance increases survival by improving and maintaining good health behaviors, mental health, and social relationships. *Annals of Behavioral Medicine,* 23(1), 68–74.

Strawbridge, W. J., Shema, S. J., Cohen, R. D., Roberts, R. E., & Kaplan, G. A. (1998). Religiosity buffers effects of some stressors on depression but exacerbates others. *Journals of Gerontology Series B—Psychological Sciences and Social Sciences,* 53(3), 5118–5126.

Tedeschi, R. G., Park, C. L., & Calhoun, L. G. (1998). *Posttraumatic growth: Positive changes in the aftermath of crisis.* Mahwah, NJ: Erlbaum.

Tennen, H., & Affleck, G. (1999). Finding benefits in adversity. In C. R. Snyder (Ed.), *Coping: The psychology of what works* (pp. 205–227). New York: Oxford University Press.

Trenholm, P., Trent, J., & Compton, W. C. (1998). Negative religious conflict as a predictor of panic disorder. *Journal of Clinical Psychology, 54,* 59–65.

Wallston, K. A., & Wallston, B. S. (1981). Health locus of control scales. In H. M. Lefcourt (Ed.), *Research with the locus of control concept* (Vol. 1, pp. 189–243). New York: Academic Press.

Weinrich, S., Holdford, D., Boyd, M., Creanga, D., Cover, K., Johnson, A., Frank-Stromborg, M., & Weinrich, M. (1998). Prostate cancer education in African American churches. *Public Health Nursing, 15,* 188–195.

Welton, G. L., Adkins, A. G., Ingle, S. L. & Dixon, W. A. (1996). God control: The fourth dimension. *Journal of Psychology and Theology, 24,* 13–25.

Witvliet, C., Laan, K. V., & Ludwig, T. E. (2000, April). *To forgive or not to forgive: Effects on heart rate, blood pressure, skin conductance, and facial EMG.* Paper presented at the annual meeting of the Society of Behavioral Medicine, Nashville, TN.

Woods, T. E., Antoni, M. H., Ironson, G. H., & Kling, D. W. (1999). Religiosity is associated with affective and immune status in symptomatic HIV-infected gay men. *Journal of Psychosomatic Research, 46,* 165–176.

Worthington, E. L., Jr. (Ed.). (1998). *Dimensions of forgiveness: Psychological research and theoretical perspectives.* Philadelphia: Templeton Foundation Press.

INDEX

Church membership, Gallup data, 18
Churches
    and cancer screening, 184, 185
    and health services, 388
    and social support, 388
    and substance abuse prevention, 233
Clinical intervention (religion/spirituality-
    based) (see also Psychotherapy)
    approaches to, 297–305
    cognitive therapy, 34, 37
    cost effectiveness, 361, 362
    ethical concerns, 306, 347–350, 374,
        394, 395, 396
    ethical guidelines/recommendations, 277–
        282, 296, 297, 315–317, 332
    evaluation of, 360–362, 372, 373
    guidelines, 296, 297
    HIV/AIDS patients, 207, 208
    substance use/abuse, 249–251
    young adults, 232–234
Clinical trials, 345
Coercion, danger of, 348 (see Clinical
    interventions; Ethical issues and
    guidelines)
Cognitive-behavioral therapy and
    religiousness, 34, 37
Community involvement and religiousness,
    97–101
Community of caring, 305
Community-based religious interventions,
    303–305
Conceptual models, 40–42, 67–69, 358,
    359–360, 364, 365, 367, 368–369,
    370, 377, 382–383, 392–394
    forgiveness, 107–138
    religiousness and health, 40–42, 392–394
    religiousness and spirituality, 5–8, 22–24,
        168–169, 292–293
Confounding variables, 21, 341–345, 366,
    367, 392
Confucian principles, 294
Conscientiousness
    and health behavior, 367, 390
    and religiousness–mortality association,
        65, 66
    and unforgiveness, 111, 112, 119, 120, 127
    health link, 127
Conscientiousness-based virtues, 119–120
    (see Warmth-based virtues)
Construct validity, 358
Control (see Health locus of control;
    Perceived control of health)

COPE Inventory, 148, 176, 218, 222
Coping Responses Inventory, 148
Coping behaviors (see also Religious coping)
    and alcohol/tobacco use, young adults,
        220–231
    and disability, 312–315
    assessment, 218, 371
    emotion- and problem-focused, 218, 219
    interview assessment, 274
Coronary heart disease (see Heart disease)
Cortisol hypersecretion, 117
Cost effectiveness, interventions, 361, 362
Countertransference regarding religious
    issues, 281
Creative activities and religiousness in older
    adults, 97–101
Cross-lag panel analysis, 30, 31
Cross-sectional research on religiousness/
    spirituality and health, 38, 43, 76,
    82–87, 172, 178, 185, 220–229,
    244, 363, 392
Cultural factors
    and assessment of religiousness/
        spirituality, 276, 277
    and forgiveness, 123
    and religious clinical interventions, 255,
        294, 316
    Asian Americans, religious beliefs of,
        294, 295
    religiousness and anxiety, 248
    religiousness and depression, 244, 245
    religiousness and health, 386–387
    religiousness and HIV, 209
    religiousness and schizophrenia, 252, 253

Daily experience sampling, 44, 371, 382
    (see also Momentary ecological
    assessment)
Dealing with Illness Inventory—Revised, 148
Death anxiety, 247, 248
Defensiveness, and unforgiveness, 116, 117
Delusions, 252
Demon possession, 252
Denial
    alcohol use risk factor, 230
    and unforgiveness, 116, 117
Depression, 243–246
    and religious coping among HIV patients,
        245
    and religiousness, 33, 36, 37, 243, 246
    and religiousness among caregivers, 245
    and religiousness in elderly, 245, 246